'This deeply informative book addresses the single issue of wellbeing within the complex environment of the city. In doing so, it reveals, one elegant chapter at a time, how human lives are impacted by systems of urban systems: including mobility, infrastructure, the built and natural environment, industry and culture. In calling for better data and better tools to understand the interdependencies that influence wellbeing, the authors quite correctly place the importance of caring for the way we live in cities alongside the urgency of the climate emergency.'

—*Tim Stonor, Space Syntax*

'The chapters gathered for *Designing Future Cities* provide important insights into how an individual's health and wellbeing are shaped by a diverse array of issues ranging from urban density, transport and walkability, to access to nature, culture and food.'

—*Laura Vaughan, Bartlett School of Architecture, University College London, UK*

'Wellbeing is perhaps the most important hidden issue of our time. It features neither in the business models that guide city investments, nor adequately in sustainability and resilience debates, yet it largely determines our quality of life. This book helps rebalance the discourse on 21st Century city development and should be required reading for urban professionals.'

—*Professor Chris Rogers, University of Birmingham, UK*

DESIGNING FUTURE CITIES FOR WELLBEING

Designing Future Cities for Wellbeing draws on original research that brings together dimensions of cities we know have a bearing on our health and wellbeing – including transportation, housing, energy, and foodways – and illustrates the role of design in delivering cities in the future that can enhance our health and wellbeing. It aims to demonstrate that cities are a complex interplay of these various dimensions that both shape and are shaped by existing and emerging city structures, governance, design, and planning. Explaining how to consider these interconnecting dimensions in the way in which professionals and citizens think about and design the city for future generations' health and wellbeing, therefore, is key. The chapters draw on UK case and research examples and make comparison to international cities and examples.

This book will be of great interest to researchers and students in planning, public policy, public health, and design.

Christopher T. Boyko is a 50th Anniversary Lecturer in Design at Lancaster University. He explores critical connections between urban design and behaviour, informing both design practice and policy. He has undertaken research on the relationship between wellbeing, sharing, and neighbourhoods for the *Liveable Cities* project; urban density and decision-making processes on *Urban Futures*; and urban design decision-making process and sustainability for *VivaCity2020*. He is currently working on the *Remembering Resistance* project, focussing on activism and public space.

Rachel Cooper OBE is Distinguished Professor of Design Management and Policy at Lancaster University. She was a Lead Expert for the UK Government Foresight programme on the Future of Cities, and the Academy of Medical Sciences addressing 'the health of the public 2040'. She is now on the Expert Steering Group for the UK Partnership for Prevention Research and a UK representative on the ICSU Scientific Committee for Health and Wellbeing in the Changing Urban Environment.

Nick Dunn is Professor of Urban Design and Executive Director of Imagination, the design research lab at Lancaster University, UK. He is Senior Fellow at the Institute for Social Futures, exploring new ways to envision and analyse the futures of people, places, and planet. He has authored numerous books, journal articles, and commissioned reports. Nick's expertise on cities, design, futures, and health has led to curated exhibitions and keynotes around the world.

DESIGNING FUTURE CITIES FOR WELLBEING

Edited by
Christopher T. Boyko, Rachel Cooper and Nick Dunn

Routledge
Taylor & Francis Group
NEW YORK AND LONDON

First published 2021
by Routledge
52 Vanderbilt Avenue, New York, NY 10017

and by Routledge
2 Park Square, Milton Park, Abingdon, Oxon, OX14 4RN

Routledge is an imprint of the Taylor & Francis Group, an informa business

Library of Congress Cataloging-in-Publication Data
Names: Boyko, Christopher, editor. | Cooper, Rachel, 1953– editor. | Dunn, Nick, 1974– editor.
Title: Designing future cities for wellbeing / edited by Christopher T. Boyko, Rachel Cooper and Nick Dunn.
Description: New York : Routledge, 2020. | Includes bibliographical references and index.
Identifiers: LCCN 2020016173 (print) | LCCN 2020016174 (ebook) | ISBN 9781138600775 (hardback) | ISBN 9781138600782 (paperback) | ISBN 9780429470684 (ebook)
Subjects: LCSH: City planning—Environmental aspects. | Cities and towns—Technological innovations. | Political planning. | Public health.
Classification: LCC HT166 .D38677 2020 (print) | LCC HT166 (ebook) | DDC 307.1/216—dc23
LC record available at https://lccn.loc.gov/2020016173
LC ebook record available at https://lccn.loc.gov/2020016174

ISBN: 978-1-138-60077-5 (hbk)
ISBN: 978-0-429-47068-4 (ebk)

Typeset in Bembo
by codeMantra

CONTENTS

FIGURES

TABLES

PREFACE

The purpose of this book is to examine the different dimensions of cities that we know have an impact on our health and well-being. In doing this, the book aims to demonstrate the significant role of design in delivering cities in the future that can enhance our health and well-being. An important aspect of this collection is its emphasis toward actively and consciously improving well-being and quality of life so that future generations may flourish. This is in contrast to many existing approaches to designing cities that simply seek to cope with demand. It is useful to know that this book was written before the global crisis around the coronavirus pandemic. At the time of writing, the impacts of Covid-19 are still being felt in manifold ways and with varying degrees of severity in different contexts, including many cities. From the current position, there appear to be some emergent themes that will form part of the way cities respond to this viral outbreak and its consequences, which further highlight the relationship between the design of cities and health and well-being. One immediate action is likely to concern digital infrastructures and the ability of cities to have access to open and transparent health data of their citizens to support strategies, such as tracking and tracing the movement of viruses. It is also increasingly apparent that the value of active mobility, with its multiple benefits and reduction in pressure on public transportation systems, will cause many cities to reconsider the role and provision of infrastructures and space for cycling and walking. Concerns regarding density and its correlation to the spread of infections have not been borne out in all urban contexts, and given the many advantages of cities, it will be interesting to see how they reconfigure themselves to provide safe and healthy places while retaining their vibrancy and appeal. Reconsidering density and the design of living space will play a key role as shifts in working arrangements change and their flexibility increases, including the repurposing of some traditional workplaces, such as office blocks. In relation to this latter issue, it is possible that cities, which are currently considered to be second- or third-tier cities, may prosper much more favourably because they may have better green and blue infrastructure provision, more affordable housing, and, crucially, the political will and urban space through which to develop effectively. Prior to the global pandemic, a number of cities were already considering the implementation of self-sufficient neighbourhoods where leisure and work are purposefully located within proximity to homes. Given the radical changes to work patterns and places where work can be done for many people due to the lockdown measures introduced during the pandemic, it is highly likely that these types of initiatives will increase in number as we re-evaluate our relationships with work within a wider context that puts greater emphasis on our health and well-being through the life course. The contributions collected in this book point toward a better, collective future that will promote health and well-being in cities, in some cases through radical step-changes and alternatives to existing pathways. One fundamental outcome of the global pandemic has been the new level of attention and reflection given to how we live, what we value and why. It is in the pursuit of enabling as many people as possible to "do well, feel good, do good and feel well" that this book has been written.

Nick Dunn

CONTRIBUTORS

AbuBakr S. Bahaj leads the 55-strong Energy and Climate Change Division and the Sustainable Energy Research Group at the University of Southampton, where he holds a Personal Chair in Sustainable Energy. Professor Bahaj has pioneered sustainable energy research and established the energy theme within the University. Professor Bahaj's work has resulted in over 300 articles, published in international refereed journals and conferences. He is a Fellow of the Institution of Civil Engineers, Institution of Engineering Technologies and the Royal Academy of Arts. He is also the Chief Scientific Advisor to Southampton City Council, believed to be the first such appointment in the UK. In 2014, Professor Bahaj was named by the UK's Science Council as one of the UK's 100 leading practising scientists.

Luke Blunden is a Researcher in the Sustainable Energy Research Group (SERG energy.soton.ac.uk) within Engineering and Physical Sciences at the University of Southampton. Research interests include marine renewable energy generation, energy for development, the energy performance of buildings in the context of user behaviour and evaluating potential for energy efficiency retrofit measures on the scale of cities. Since joining SERG, Blunden has worked on the simulation of tidal power effects on coastal seas; tagged fish in Sweden; designed and constructed solar power plants in East Africa and Saudi Arabia and carried out household energy and environment monitoring studies in the UK and China.

Leonidas Bourikas is Lecturer in Future Living at ImaginationLancaster, Lancaster University. Leo undertakes interdisciplinary research related to environmental design, energy and the built environment. The work has a people-based focus and includes user behaviour in the home and at work, alongside wider neighbourhood and city scale analysis. His research interests are in the interactions of urban living and digital technology with occupants' behaviours and data interpretations, and how these socio-spatial interactions could enable sustainable future living with a focus on health and societal wellbeing. Leo is currently a researcher in the radical Beyond Imagination project that looks at the creation of a healthier, more prosperous and sustainable world through cutting-edge design research (www.lancaster.ac.uk/lica/research/imaginationlancaster). Email: l.bourikas@lancaster.ac.uk | Twitter: @lbourik | Publications: goo.gl/Z2xNxm.

Christopher T. Boyko is a 50th Anniversary Lecturer in Design at Lancaster University. He explores critical connections between urban design and behaviour, informing both design practice and policy. He has undertaken research on the relationship between wellbeing, sharing and neighbourhoods for the *Liveable Cities* project; urban density and decision-making processes on *Urban Futures* and urban design decision-making process and sustainability for *VivaCity2020*. He is currently working on the *Remembering Resistance* project, focussing on activism and public space.

Milena Büchs is Associate Professor in Sustainability, Economics and Low Carbon Transition at the University of Leeds. Büchs' research focusses on sustainable welfare, especially on the inequality of carbon emissions and fairness of carbon reduction, as well as wellbeing implications of the zero-carbon transition. She is currently PI of the EU-funded Marie Skłodowska-Curie Fellowship project 'ShaRe – The potential of Sharing Resources for mitigating carbon emissions and other environmental impacts', and is Co-I on the UKRI-funded Centre for Research on Energy Demand Reduction (www.creds.ac.uk). One of her recent papers has won the Elsevier Atlas award: Büchs, M., & Koch, M. (2019). Challenges for the degrowth transition: The debate about wellbeing. *Futures, 105,* 155–165, https://doi.org/10.1016/j.futures.2018.09.002.

Stephen Clune is a sustainable designer, researcher and educator with over 10 years' experience. This includes working as a Senior Lecturer and researcher in sustainable design at ImaginationLancaster at Lancaster University, UK. Prior to this, Stephen was a Research Fellow at the Centre for Design, RMIT, University in Melbourne. Stephen's core interest focusses on how design – and design thinking – can assist in the move towards a sustainable society, with a particular interest in design as a facilitator of change. Stephen is committed to assisting organisations and communities to enhance their sustainability, drawing on a diverse range of tools from social practice theory, behavioural change, life cycle analysis and design thinking.

Ricardo Codinhoto is an Associate Professor in Architecture and Design in the Built Environment at the University of Bath, where he has worked for the last five years. His research and scholarship are internationally recognised.

His focus is on integrated design and design theories, particularly on the built environment's impact on people, processes and services. His publications span: built environment design and behaviour, health and wellbeing, co-design and mediated intelligence, evidence-based design, integrated design management, stakeholder requirements and engagement, systematic design methods, parametrical design and building information modelling. He is a member of various national and international professional and academic groups. He has been a keynote speaker, competition panel member and researcher in numerous countries including Australia, Brazil, Colombia, Finland, Japan, Italy and Portugal.

Cary Cooper CBE is the 50th Anniversary Professor of Organizational Psychology and Health at ALLIANCE Manchester Business School of the University of Manchester, President of the Chartered Institute of Personnel and Development (HR professional body), Immediate Past President of the British Academy of Management, President of the Institute of Welfare and Founding Chair of the National Forum of Health and Wellbeing at Work (an employer body comprised of 38 major/global employers). He is the author/editor of over 170 books and over 400 scholarly articles on organisational psychology and HR topics.

Rachel Cooper OBE is Distinguished Professor of Design Management and Policy at Lancaster University. She was a Lead Expert for the UK Government Foresight programme on the Future of Cities, and the Academy of Medical Sciences addressing 'the health of the public 2040'. She is now on the Expert Steering Group for the UK Partnership for Prevention Research and a UK representative on the ICSU Scientific Committee for Health and Wellbeing in the Changing Urban Environment.

Claire Coulton is a Project Manager and Coordinator in ImaginationLancaster, Lancaster University. Over the last seven years, she has worked in a number of different roles, primarily supporting, conducting and managing research, including in the Engineering and Physical Sciences (EPSRC)-funded *Liveable Cities* and *PETRAS* projects. Many of the projects she has worked on have centred on future cities, urban design, wellbeing and the Internet of Things. Claire is also the editor of the ImaginationLancaster Little Book series.

Antony Darby is a Reader in Structural Engineering at the University of Bath, where he has worked for the last 20 years. He received his Doctorate from the University of Cambridge followed by a Post-doctoral position at the University of Oxford before taking up his current position. In between, he has also worked for petrochemical contractor, M.W. Kellogg, and satellite designers, Matra-Marconi Space. His research interests cover a breadth of subjects from use of composites in concrete construction to human factors in building design. His most recent research involves the development of a facility, known as VSimulator, designed to replicate sway motion, environmental conditions and physical surroundings in tall buildings to assess impact on human comfort, wellbeing and productivity.

Matthew Dennis is a Lecturer in Geography in the School of Environment, Education and Development at the University of Manchester. His research background is in social-ecological systems with a focus on highly managed landscapes. His work looks at the spatial considerations that inform our understanding of nature conservation, human health and wellbeing, and (social-)ecological resilience. A key element of this work involves the application of geo-statistical techniques to developing appropriate and accurate characterisations of the natural environment, effective environmental monitoring, and the modelling and evaluation of social-ecological outcomes.

Nick Dunn is Professor of Urban Design and Executive Director of Imagination, the design research lab at Lancaster University, UK. He is Senior Fellow at the Institute for Social Futures, exploring new ways to envision and analyse the futures of people, places and planet. He has authored numerous books, journal articles and commissioned reports. Nick's expertise on cities, design, futures and health has led to curated exhibitions and keynotes around the world.

James D. Hale has been active in the field of sustainable development for over 20 years. Following a master's degree in ecology, he worked as an environmental/spatial planner within local government, and then spent the next 10 years as an academic researcher. He collaborated broadly to better understand the interdependencies between ecological habitats, built infrastructure and human activities. He is a firm believer in the systems-approach to research and practice, particularly the integration of social and ecological perspectives. James now works as a sustainability consultant, helping organisations to address some particularly challenging areas in this field, such as identifying complex dependencies, unintended consequences, tensions between sustainable development goals, and future-proofing strategies for sustainable development projects.

Mark Hammond is a Senior Lecturer at Manchester School of Architecture – a joint institute between the University of Manchester and Manchester Metropolitan University. His research investigates the links between urban ageing and various facets of urban development, including collaborative housing and neighbourhood regeneration. Since 2018, he has split his time between MSA and the Greater Manchester Combined Authority, where he develops research-engaged policy and strategies as part of the GM Ageing Hub.

Ian Hesketh is the Wellbeing Lead at the UK College of Policing and the Senior Responsible Owner (SRO) for the National Police Wellbeing Service in the UK. Ian also supports the National Forum for Health and Wellbeing at Manchester University Alliance Business School. He is an Honorary Researcher at Lancaster

University Management School and a Visiting Fellow at the Open University Business School. He holds a PhD in Management and Social Psychology and an MBA from Lancaster University. His research interests are centred on Wellbeing, Resilience and Transformation in the context of working life, and most notably he introduced the concept and phenomena of *Leaveism* to explain human behaviours associated with workplace workload and stress.

Patrick James is a physicist and Professor of Energy and Buildings specialising in micro-generation and large-scale energy-based field trials. His work sits at the interface of technology and people in both the residential and office environments. He has published over 170 articles in proceedings / key journals, is a Chartered Engineer and is a Fellow of the Chartered Institute of Building Service Engineers (FCIBSE).

Philip James is Professor of Ecology and leads the Ecosystem and Environment Research Centre in the School of Science, Engineering and Environment at the University of Salford. His research interests include urban ecology, sustainable development, green infrastructure and social-ecological systems. Philip is a member of the Natural Capital Board for Greater Manchester and recently co-delivered DEFRA's Urban Pioneer project in Greater Manchester. His particular concern was to ensure that the values associated with private gardens was fully appreciated. Philip's current activities are focussed on the role of green infrastructure in climate change mitigation as part of the IGNITION project. Philp has authored or co-authored three books on urban ecology/biology.

Helene Joffe is a social-health psychologist at University College London. Having worked on how the public engages with a range or risks including climate change, earthquakes and emerging infectious diseases, Helene's current research examines how to maximise wellbeing in urban environments and how to change earthquake and fire-related behaviour and build resilience in seismic parts of the world. It has been supported by the Economic and Social Research Council (ESRC), EPSRC, Faraday Institute and Rail Safety & Standards Board. She is the co-Leader of UCL's Human Wellbeing Grand Challenge and co-founder of EPICENTRE (Earthquake and People Interaction Centre). Among her 100+ publications, she has written *Risk and 'the Other'* (Cambridge University Press) and edited *Living with Perils in 21st century* (Springer). She has pioneered a research method – the 'Grid Elaboration Method' – published in 2014 in an American Psychological Association journal.

Andrew Laing, PhD, is a consultant and teacher focussed on the nature of work, workplaces, technology and cities. Since 2007, he has been a visiting lecturer at Princeton University, in urban theory and architecture. He headed workplace strategy and design at Bridgewater Associates, 2016–2018. Until 2016, he was a global leader for workplace strategy services at AECOM (formerly DEGW).

He joined DEGW in London in 1989, working on research and consulting services worldwide. He founded the North American DEGW practice in 1998. He received a doctorate in Urban Studies and Planning from MIT in 1988; he studied architecture and planning at University College London. He co-authored *The Responsible Workplace* (1994) and *New Environments for Working* (1998) with Frank Duffy and has published many articles.

Margaret Watson qualified as a pharmacist in 1987, and worked in secondary care and public health. In 1998, she received her PhD and has spent over 25 years as a health services researcher. Her main research interests include the synthesis and translation of evidence into practice, particularly concerning medicines use and pharmaceutical care. In 2018, she started Watson Research and Training Ltd, providing consultancy on research and research training, as well as coaching and mentoring. In July 2019, she was invited to join the Strathclyde Institute of Pharmacy and Biomedical Sciences as a Global Talent Attraction Platform Professor. She divides her time between her university and consultancy roles. In 2019, she was made a Fellow of the Royal Pharmaceutical Society (UK).

Christopher Phillipson is Professor of Sociology and Social Gerontology at the University of Manchester, UK. He has a number of research interests relating to age-friendly cities, work and retirement, and critical gerontology. His most recent book is *Precarity and Ageing: Understanding Risk and Insecurity in Later Life* (edited with Amanda Grenier and Rick Settersten, Policy Press, 2020).

Serena Pollastri is a Lecturer in Design and Urban Futures at ImaginationLancaster in the UK. Through a mix of critical visual design practice and research she develops processes and artefacts for articulating pluralistic, polyphonic and multispecies pasts, presents and futures. Serena has previously worked in China as a Lecturer at the Lancaster University/Beijing Jiaotong University double degree programme in Media Art and Design, and before that as a senior designer and researcher at Tektao Urban Design Lab and Tongji University. Here she was mostly involved in the DesignHarvests project, investigating ways of fostering urban-rural connections through acupuncture design actions with food, crafts and IT.

Andy C. Pratt is Professor of Cultural Economy at City, University of London. He specialises in the analysis of the cultural industries globally. This research has three strands. The first focusses on the social and economic dynamics of clustering and knowledge exchange. The second strand concerns the definition and measurement of employment in the cultural, or creative, industries. The third concerns cultural governance and policy making at the national, regional and urban scales. His current research concerns trans-local cultural production chains and is funded by EU Horizon 2020; see https://cicerone-project.eu.

Katerina Psarikidou is Lecturer at the Science Policy Research Unit (SPRU) at Sussex University. Her research revolves around the study of the sustainability and innovation potential of alternative agro-food networks and low-carbon mobility systems. She has been researcher and investigator for a series of EC, EPSRC, Higher Education Funding Council For England (HEFCE)-funded interdisciplinary and cooperative research programmes (e.g. PAGANINI, FAAN, Liveable Cities, AgriFood Resilience). Her research has been published in journals and edited books of international impact (e.g. *Sustainability: Science, Practice and Policy, Local Environment, Sustainability, Ephemera*, etc.). She is co-editor of the book *Cycling Societies: Emerging Innovations, Inequalities and Governance* (with Routledge). She is author of the monograph *Reclaiming the Knowledge Economy: the case of Alternative Agro-Food Networks* (with Palgrave MacMillan).

Nicholas Smith is a social-environmental psychologist with research interests in the perception and communication of risk issues. He is particularly interested in public awareness, understanding and communication of climate change and his research is mixed methodological. He received a BA in Environmental Management in 2004 from the University of Leeds and an MSc in Psychological Research Methods from UCL in 2005. He completed his PhD at UCL in 2010 exploring social representations of climate change. Since finishing his PhD, he worked as a post-doctoral research associate with the Yale Program on Climate Change Communication and subsequently at UCL as a research fellow on the Liveable Cities project. He became a Lecturer in the department of psychology at the University of Westminster in 2014.

Nick Tyler is the Chadwick Professor of Civil Engineering at UCL. His work fuses music, engineering and design and is inspired by lives in many parts of the world. He is actively involved in helping people in London, Beirut, Japan and several cities in Latin America to create sustainable and equitable environments where they can freely interact with each other (what he calls 'Sociality'), sometimes challenging the urban status quo of planning, design and politics.

Konstantinos Tzoulas is a Senior Lecturer in Environmental Management at Manchester Metropolitan University. His research interests include urban ecology, sustainable development, green infrastructure planning and public health. Konstantinos' current research evaluates the social and economic benefits of peri-urban sphagnum farming. Recently he worked on evaluating the wellbeing benefits of urban parks for people with early stage dementia. He has also worked on co-developing a pubic action plan for enhancing the ecological and wellbeing benefits of private gardens. In the past, Konstantinos worked with local authorities on urban regeneration policy, and he currently leads the biodiversity policy for Manchester Metropolitan University.

Marcella Ucci is an Associate Professor in Environmental and Healthy Buildings at the UCL Institute for Environmental Design and Engineering, within the Bartlett Faculty of the Built Environment. Her research focusses on the interactions/tensions between sustainable building design/operation and occupant comfort, health and wellbeing. Her expertise includes building performance monitoring and modelling, evaluation of indoor air quality (especially in relation to moisture and dampness in buildings), active design and operational aspects of buildings – particularly occupant behaviour. She has led the development and launch of a new Master's Degree, 'Health, Wellbeing and Sustainable Buildings', is on the Editorial Board of 'Architectural Science Review' and 'Indoor and Built Environment' (previously Deputy Editor) and is Secretary of the UK Indoor Environments Group (previously Chair: 2012–2017).

Stefan White is joint Head of the Manchester School of Architecture. He is an architect researching and practising the architecture and urbanism of social and environmental sustainability. He is director of the PHASE Place-Health research and delivery group at the Manchester School of Architecture – working collaboratively to understand and create healthier places with the UK Government, Regional Health and Care providers, City Councils, Registered Housing Providers and Local Communities.

Yue Wu (吴越or Phil), BSc, MSc, PhD, is a researcher in Sustainable Energy at the University of Southampton. His research focusses on the deployment of renewable energy systems in urban areas and its impact on a wide range of social and environmental aspects such as fuel poverty, thermal comfort and energy usage behaviour. His research has contributed to a number of real-life applications. In 2019, he was awarded an Enterprise Fellowship by the Royal Academy of Engineering, UK, for his development of Solar City.

Victoria Zeeb is a psychologist interested in the study of wellbeing, mental health and existential meaning. She received a PhD in Psychology from UCL for her work on social connection in cities and its impact on wellbeing. She is currently a Trainee Counselling Psychologist at City University where she is continuing to pursue her research interests while also training as a practitioner, working one-on-one with people experiencing mental health difficulties.

1

INTRODUCTION

Christopher T. Boyko

Wellbeing in cities is vital for our collective future. Amid major sociodemographic, cultural, political, technological, environmental and economic upheaval, shift and change, the planet continues to urbanise and people are moving into urban areas, whether by choice or by force. Further, as the processes of urbanisation continue to affect greater areas of the planet, their impact in terms of climate change and other environmental issues is being felt by many who live in non-urban areas. Clearly, the challenges facing cities to ensure healthy populations are significant and appear intractable. To cope with this influx of people, cities are expanding horizontally and vertically, with new housing, roads, sewers and other vital infrastructure being designed, planned and built every day. However, coping is not enough these days: the current design, development and planning tools we use are proving incapable of capturing the messiness, the dynamic nature and the (im)possibilities of places and people (see Albrechts & Balducci, 2013; Albrechts, 2017).

Moreover, as our cities swell, citizens are becoming even more unhealthy. Levels of obesity, diabetes and malnutrition in cities are becoming worse (Feng et al., 2010; Pouliou & Elliott, 2010). The prevalence of private vehicles on our roads suggests we are not walking or cycling as much for commuting and leisure, and sitting in traffic amidst poor air quality (da Schio et al., 2019; Glazener & Khreis, 2019; Nieuwenhuijsen & Khreis, 2019; Stevenson & Gleeson, 2019). In an era of 'digital convenience', incidences of loneliness and isolation are on the increase (Knowles & Hanson, 2018; Nowland et al., 2018). And for those of us in employment, our work-life balance is on a knife-edge, with increases in both Leaveism (Hesketh & Cooper, 2010) and Presenteeism (Johns, 2010). Again, we are coping, but only just.

To counter this, we need to be designing our cities for more than just coping. Some smaller parts of cities, like neighbourhoods or developments, may be designed, planned and built, so that their inhabitants feel safe(r) and they experience a greater sense of privacy, or that the area embodies the principles of environmental sustainability. However, not many places, from building to city scale, start from a position of actively and consciously improving the wellbeing, health and/or quality of life of their citizens through design. In the UK, the National Health Service (NHS) began an initiative in 2014 to create several Healthy New Towns (NHS, 2014, 2015). These places are attempting to adopt 'place-shaping' urban design and housing to promote health and wellbeing while improving the delivery of health and social care. Internationally, the World Health Organization (WHO) has established two programmes that seek to improve health in cities. The first, WHO Healthy Cities, originated in 1978 and was inspired by the WHO European Health for All strategy and the Health21 targets. It aims to put health and public health on the political and social radar of cities around the world, highlighting the need for equity, interdisciplinary and intersectoral collaboration and action, participatory governance and solidarity (WHO, 2018). The second, WHO's Age-Friendly Cities and Communities, formalised in 2006, endeavours to create age-friendly environments that progressively improve the match between people, their needs and the environments in which they live, work and recreate (Buffel et al., 2018). Such cities and communities can foster healthy and active ageing, ageing safely in-place and achieving positive contributions to the community while concomitantly retaining autonomy and dignity, and freedom from poverty (GNAFCC, 2017).

All three of these schemes have 'health' and 'healthy' at their core, yet are doing slightly different things. The first one embraces a 'starting from scratch' mentality and essentially is exploring how to save the nationally funded NHS money by thinking preventively. The latter two prioritise mending what we have in our cities to ensure that public health and ageing, respectively, are not overlooked in policy. But is 'health' and 'healthy' different from 'wellbeing'? Is there an advantage to 'starting from scratch' versus a 'mending' approach when designing cities for wellbeing? And if we are getting better at designing cities with health/healthy in mind, can we also design cities of the future for wellbeing? In order to answer these questions, we will first look into the concept of wellbeing and discuss its relevance to this book.

What Is Wellbeing?

As with most concepts being defined by academics, finding an accepted definition of wellbeing is difficult. In part, this is because there are so many ways of achieving wellbeing, and how one defines it will very much depend on what is valued or viewed as important (Kahneman, 2011; Dodge et al., 2012). The concept of wellbeing also has had a long and rich history, beginning with scholars in Ancient Greece and finding homes in the fields of economics, geography, health, neuroscience, philosophy, psychology, social sciences, sociology and policymaking (van Hoorn, 2007), meaning that many different ideas from many different people have been interwoven into our understanding(s) (Stoll, 2014).

Traditionally, notions of wellbeing were divided into two camps: hedonia and eudaimonia. Hedonia primarily concerns the experience of pleasure and enjoyment. Aristippus first explained it as the physical pursuit of pleasure, with Epicurus suggesting that hedonism was attained through the intellectual enlightenment of one's environment and the absence of pain (later took up by Bentham and others as they explored the balance between pleasure and pain). More recently, positive psychologists and behavioural economists have referred to hedonia as the presence of positive emotions/affect, the absence of negative emotions/affect and satisfaction (Thompson & Marks, 2008). Such a focus implies that the individual or a subjective approach to evaluating life events is the best way to measure hedonia (Diener et al., 1999).

Alternatively, eudaimonia refers to the attainment of wellbeing through worthwhile undertakings and the pursuit of what Aristotle called a virtuous, 'good life' (Henderson & Knight, 2012). Instead of a focus on achieving individual needs or desires – not all of which will result in wellbeing if fulfilled – eudaimonia emphasises personal growth and self-actualisation (Ryan & Deci, 2001). This may be accomplished through particular acts of kindness, honesty and justice (Henderson & Knight, 2012), which Waterman (1993) suggests are rooted in human nature. In terms of measuring eudaimonia, then, scholars believe that a more objective approach is needed, one that involves people being holistically engaged and challenged to attain positive psychological functioning through characteristics including autonomy, environmental mastery, personal growth, positive relationships, purpose in life and self-acceptance (Ryff, 1995).

In recent years, more integrated approaches have been developed in recognition of the multi-dimensionality of wellbeing (e.g. Diener, 2009; Michaelson et al., 2009; Stiglitz et al., 2009). One of the most prominent is 'flourishing', which concerns the experience of life going well, and of feeling good and functioning effectively (Huppert & So, 2013). Flourishing pertains not just to the absence of disorder, but includes both hedonic and eudaimonic components. It also involves maintaining a high level of mental wellbeing (Ryff & Singer 1998; Keyes, 2002; Huppert & So, 2009a, b, 2013). Seligman's (2011) PERMA model offers one way to understand wellbeing via flourishing. Through five building blocks for a flourishing life – positive emotion, engagement, relationships, meaning and accomplishment – Seligman affirms that wellbeing is not just one, single concept, but is multi-dimensional in scale and should be measured both subjectively and objectively.

Given what we know about wellbeing from the above section, and taking inspiration from Huppert and So's (2013) definition of flourishing, the following description feels appropriate for this book: *wellbeing is about doing well, feeling good, doing good and feeling well* (White, 2010)[1] (see Figure 1.1).

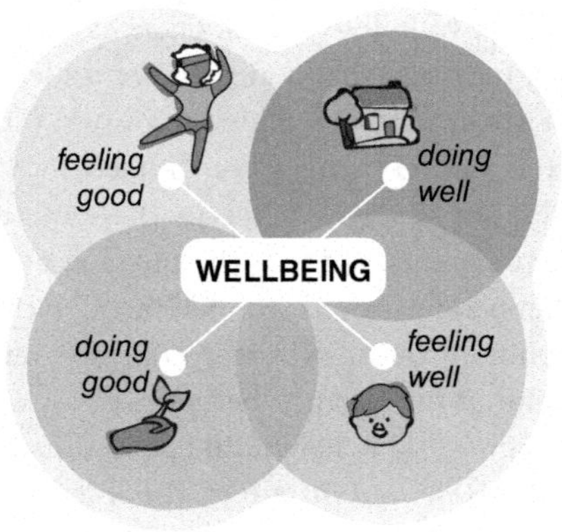

FIGURE 1.1 A conceptualisation of White's (2010) definition of wellbeing.
Source: Serena Pollastri.

'Doing well' refers to a certain, material standard of living and/or economic prosperity. 'Feeling good' involves personal, subjective perceptions of levels of satisfaction. 'Doing good' relates to a more collective, shared understanding of how the world is and should be. 'Feeling well' stresses the significance of health to wellbeing. Thus, White's (2010) definition includes both subjective and objective dimensions alongside personal and collective notions of wellbeing. It also incorporates the idea of effective functioning via a link to health. Finally, this description demonstrates that wellbeing is not static; rather, it is a dynamic concept that allows people to assess and compare how they are doing, both at present and in the past. But what about *future* wellbeing? How can we assess our wellbeing at a later point in life? And can cities be designed with our future wellbeing in mind?

How Does Wellbeing Feature in the Design of Future Cities?

Visions for future cities have existed for hundreds of years, driven by a strong desire for change in the urban environment and in transforming our links with urban space (Mansfield, 1990; Easton, 2002). Through radical grand plans, like Frank Lloyd Wright's Broadacre City, to slightly smaller – and still radical! – ideas, such as Jack Lynn and Ivor Smith's Park Hill estate in Sheffield, visions of cities have challenged the status quo, sought to raise or resolve problems facing societies and have acted as critical sounding boards for the evaluation of city form. However, while most visualisations are successful at suggesting how and where people will live, work and move around, they rarely are converted into concrete plans. As Dunn et al. (2014) state: 'Even in those projects where the design was subsequently constructed in reality the subtleties and *joie de vivre* are lost' (p. 13, emphasis author).

On the whole, visions that are created for cities of the future tend to be quite binary in their outlook: either dystopian or utopian. With the former, places are uncomfortably divided into haves and have nots. A small minority of people often possess all of the resources and power (should a complete breakdown of governance not already exist), leaving the majority to live in squalor and fear. With the latter, there is a presumption that everyone is benefiting from living in a 'perfect' world of sustainability and benevolence. Nonetheless, this may not be true, as someone always seems to be left out of nirvana.

In unpacking these visions, the wellbeing of the people within dystopian or utopian futures may seem obvious: a minority of people with the power are happy in dystopian futures and everyone is happy in utopian futures. However, this might not be the case, and wellbeing may be a far more subtle thing to assess. For example, some residents living in 'have-not' areas, such as slums, may perceive a high level of community spirit that contradicts what outsiders would believe such areas to possess (Busby, 2017) (see also the NBC television show, *The Good Place*, for a great example of people experiencing illbeing in a place of wellbeing). Thus, understanding the subtleties of wellbeing is key if future cities are to be designed to support people in urban areas and make them flourish. Using wellbeing as a lens, we can critique and interrogate what we currently know about cities and apply this knowledge in the design of future visions for cities.

What to Expect from the Rest of the Book

This book contains a wealth of information across 15 chapters, each of which provides insight into a multitude of significant topics and issues, spanning transport, healthcare, home, neighbourhoods, work, culture, technology, energy, nature and the human lifespan. All of these undoubtedly impact – and will continue to impact – the design of cities and the health and wellbeing of the people who live in them.

In Chapter 2, Helene Joffe, Nicholas Smith and Victoria Zeeb investigate aspirations that people have for themselves and for cities of the future. Adopting a naturalistic, mixed methods approach to their research, the authors explore city-dwellers' aspirations in the UK's two largest cities: London and Birmingham. Across the 96 city-dwellers they interviewed and surveyed in both cities, the theme of social connection emerged repeatedly.

Chapter 3 sees Katerina Psarikidou exploring the notion of mobilities and its connection to wellbeing in cities. Using sociologist John Urry's (2007) conceptualisation of mobilities and applying it to her research, Psarikidou asks the important question: how can our current mobility patterns in cities be more sustainable without sacrificing what many of us see as the 'good life'?

Continuing with the theme of movement in Chapter 4, Nick Tyler explores how our current transport systems might evolve in the future to enable human wellbeing in cities. He believes that understanding people and how they function, and how the city assists these functions, is paramount to developing transport systems that reach their full potential in terms of wellbeing. To do this, Tyler examines transport for a future city from three different perspectives: the person, the city and the implications of these perspectives on the design of transport systems.

The focus of Chapter 5 is on nature more generally and its association with health and wellbeing in cities. In their writing, Philip James, Konstantinos Tzoulas and Matthew Dennis posit that some twenty-first-century illnesses affecting urbanites create low-level, chronic inflammation, which are a direct consequence of the environments we inhabit. They believe that a reframing of nature in our urban environments via both policy and practice is what is needed to counter the onset of these illnesses.

In Chapter 6, we turn our attention to household energy and its relationship with health, wellbeing, income and access to greenspace. A team from the University of Southampton (UK), involving AbuBakr' Bahaj, Luke Blunden, Leonidas Bourikas, Milena Büchs, Patrick James and Yue Wu, conducted a multi-disciplinary, in-depth study, looking at the above relationship in an area of Southampton where people were likely to own two or more cars. The authors share their work and conclude with a discussion about the complexity of reducing energy use in cities while also improving people's wellbeing.

Chapter 7 brings to light a fundamental issue relating to cities, both at present and in the future: food. In particular, Stephen Clune and Serena Pollastri explore the relationship between food and wellbeing in cities, and target the role that design can play in thinking about food and wellbeing in the future. Their chapter discusses the concept of 'food-related illbeing' in cities and how this concept can be used to frame the challenges in which designers engage when redesigning food systems for wellbeing.

In Chapter 8, Marcella Ucci looks at the significant impact of housing on children and their health and wellbeing. Through a review of the latest and established evidence, Ucci reveals three housing dimensions that play a key role in children's health and wellbeing: physical hazards, fit to needs and security and stability. The author then considers the design and research implications for housing for children at both building and urban scales in cities of the future.

Shifting to the other end of the lifespan, Chapter 9 introduces us to the concept of precarity within the context of the World Health Organization's Age-Friendly Cities and Communities programme. Via the Manchester Age-Friendly Neighbourhoods project, Mark Hammond, Stefan White and Christopher Philipson examine how co-creating local plans and small-scale interventions between older people and other organisations within neighbourhoods can facilitate long-term interdependence and reduce some uncertainty about their future. The authors believe that co-creation can help to combat precarity and associated issues, such as spatial exclusion and social isolation, thus improving the wellbeing of older people in their neighbourhoods.

Within Chapter 10, the authors concentrate on health and social care provision within cities. Ricardo Codinhoto, Christopher Boyko, Antony Darby and Margaret Watson explore how global transitions in disease, demography and urbanisation are changing the way we think about health and wellbeing. Focussing on the importance of the physical environment, the authors suggest that a holistic and integrated view of health and wellbeing is needed to counter our current, fragmented care system, and that architecture and urban design should be facilitating this integration by designing in health and care prevention wherever possible.

Taking a closer look at the physical environment, Chapter 11 investigates the following question: do high-density, high-deprivation neighbourhoods hinder wellbeing among its residents and discourage walkability through its design? Christopher Boyko, Rachel Cooper, Claire Coulton and James Hale explore the relationships between density and wellbeing, deprivation and wellbeing, and walkability and health in a quantitative study across three UK cities. The authors share their significant findings and contemplate what these mean for practice and policy in terms of designing future cities with wellbeing in mind.

Offering a different perspective to the overall themes of the book, Chapter 12 emphasises the co-development of culture and cities, and the challenges and opportunities presented by both in relation to wellbeing. To do this, Andy Pratt unpacks the dramatic changes in culture over time in the UK as well as the complexities of cities. Through his analysis, Pratt shows how components of those changes and complexities possess their own dynamics that can mesh together to generate space for culture and positively impact wellbeing.

For Chapter 14, we visit the smart city concept and consider the relationship between technology and wellbeing in the city. Through a series of provocations, Andrew Laing argues that current discourses on the smart city emphasise utility and efficiency, which restrict users and citizens from fully participating in the making of their collective wellbeing in cities. To counter this, Laing suggests alternative views of the future smart city, including the creation of a 'new civics' that would enable more democratic forms of governance.

Chapter 13 examines the changing nature of working life and the changing demographics of workers, positing how both affect wellbeing in cities. Ian Hesketh and Cary Cooper explore current and future issues, comprising work-life balance, the increase of service and knowledge-based economies and the rise of portfolio workers, and connect them to notions of wellbeing and work. The authors end by reflecting on potential opportunities for design to improve wellbeing and employment in cities of the future, including discussion of biophilic design.

The final chapter sees Rachel Cooper and Nick Dunn take stock of what was written in the previous chapters and attempt to synthesise some of the key arguments, ideas, concerns and challenges. The authors then will offer guidance and recommendations about what cities of the future can do to design for wellbeing.

In bringing together these various perspectives of how we design future cities for wellbeing, this book aims to share key insights and present new concepts to enable collective life to flourish. Understanding how and why these interconnecting dimensions both shape and are shaped by existing and emerging cities enables us to think about, and design for, future generations' health and wellbeing. This is of critical importance. As we travel further through the twenty-first century, the challenges that face us are complex and interrelated. Ensuring that we have the necessary approaches to best apply our creativity, diversity and innovation will help safeguard populations, both in cities and beyond, and those that follow in the future.

Note

1 The author acknowledges that many other definitions exist that capture the essence of wellbeing, some of which will be explored and analysed in this book (see, e.g. Andrew & Whitney, 1976; Dodge et al., 2012; Steuer & Marks, 2008).

References

Albrechts, L. (2017). Some ontological and epistemological challenges. In L. Albrechts, A. Balducci, & J. Hillier (Eds.), *Situated practices of strategic planning: An international perspective* (pp. 1–12). Abingdon: Routledge.

Albrechts, L., & Balducci, A. (2013). Practicing strategic planning: In search for critical features to explain the strategic character of plans. *disP - The Planning Review, 49* (3), 16–27.

Andrews, F. M., & Whitney, S. B. (1976). *Social indicators of wellbeing: Americans' perceptions of life quality.* New York: Plenum Press.

Buffel, T., Handler, S., & Phillipson, C. (2018). *Age-friendly cities and communities: A global perspective.* Bristol: Policy Press.

Busby, S. (2017). Finding a concrete utopia in the dystopia of a 'sub-city'. *Research in Drama Education: The Journal of Applied Theatre and Performance, 22* (1), 92–103.

da Schio, N., Boussauw, K., & Sansen, J. (2019). Accessibility versus air pollution: A geography of externalities in the Brussels agglomeration. *Cities, 84*, 178–189.

Diener, E. (Ed.). (2009). Subjective wellbeing. In *The science of wellbeing: The collected work of Ed Diener* (pp. 11–58). New York: Springer.

Diener, E., Suh, E. M., Lucas, R. E., & Smith, H. L. (1999). Subjective wellbeing: Three decades of progress. *Psychological Bulletin, 125* (2), 276–302.

Dodge, R., Daly, A. P., Huyton, J., & Sanders, L. D. (2012). The challenge of defining wellbeing. *International Journal of Wellbeing, 2* (3), 222–235.

Dunn, N., Cureton, P., & Pollastri, S. (2014). A visual history of the future. *Future of cities: working paper.* London: Foresight, Government Office for Science.

Easton, R. (2002). *Ideal cities: Utopianism and the (un)built environment.* London: Thames and Hudson.

Feng, J., Glass, T. A., Curriero, F. C., Stewart, W. F., Schwartz, B. S. (2010). The built environment and obesity: A systematic review of the epidemiological evidence. *Health & Place, 16* (2), 175–190.

Glazener, A., & Khreis, H. (2019). Transforming our cities: Best practices towards clean air and active pollution. *Current Environmental Health Reports*, 1–16. https://doi.org/10.1007/s40572-019-0228-1

GNAFCC. (2017). Membership in the global network of age-friendly cities and communities. Available from http://www.who.int/ageing/age-friendly-environments/GNAFCC-membership-en.pdf?ua=1

Henderson, L. W., & Knight, T. (2012). Integrating the hedonic and eudaimonic perspectives to more comprehensively understand wellbeing and pathways to wellbeing. *International Journal of Wellbeing, 2* (3), 196–221.

Hesketh, I., & Cooper, C. (2014). Leaveism at work. *Occupational Medicine, 64* (3), 146–147.

Huppert, F. A., Abbott, R. A., Ploubidis, G. B., Richards, M., & Kuh, D. (2009). Parental practices predict psychological wellbeing in midlife: Life-course associations among women in the 1946 British birth cohort. *Psychological Medicine, 40* (9), 1507–1518.

Huppert, F. A., Marks, N., Clark, A., Siegrist, J., Stutzer, A., Vittersø, J., & Wahrendorf, M. (2009). Measuring wellbeing across Europe: Description of the ESS wellbeing module and preliminary findings. *Social Indicators Research, 91* (3), 301–315.

Huppert, F. A., & So, T. T. C. (2013). Flourishing across Europe: Application of a new conceptual framework for defining wellbeing. *Social Indicators Research, 110* (3), 837–861.

Johns, G. (2010). Presenteeism in the workplace: A review and research agenda. *Journal of Organizational Behavior, 31*, 519–542.

Kahneman, D. (2011). *Thinking, fast and slow.* Toronto: Doubleday Canada.

Keyes, C. L. M., (2002). The mental health continuum: From languishing to flourishing in life. *Journal of Health and Behaviour Research, 43*, 207–222.

Knowles, B., & Hanson, V. L. (2018). The wisdom of older technology (non)users. *Communications of the ACM, 61* (3), 72–77.

Mansfield, H. (1990). *Cosmopolis: Yesterday's cities of the future.* New Brunswick, NJ: Center for Urban Policy Research.

Michaelson, J., Abdallah, S., Steuer, N., Thompson, S., & Marks, N. (2009). *National accounts of wellbeing: Bringing real wealth onto the balance sheet.* London: New Economics Foundation.

NHS. (2014). *Five year forward view.* London: NHS.

NHS. (2015). *The forward view into action: Registering interest to join the healthy new towns programme.* London: NHS.

Nieuwenhuijsen, M., & Khreis, H. (Eds.). (2019). Urban and transport planning, environment and health. In *Integrating human health into urban and transport planning* (pp. 3–16). Cham: Springer.

Nowland, R., Necka, E. A., & Cacioppo, J. T. (2018). Loneliness and social Internet use: Pathways to reconnection in a digital world? *Perspectives on Psychological Science, 13* (1), 70–87.

Pouliou, T., & Elliott, S. J. (2010). Individual and socio-environmental determinants of overweight and obesity in Urban Canada. *Health & Place, 16* (2), 389–398.

Ryan, R. M., & Deci, E. L. (2001). On happiness and human potentials: A review of research on hedonic and eudaimonic wellbeing. *Annual Review of Psychology, 52*, 141–66.

Ryff, C. D. (1995). Wellbeing in adult life. *Current Directions in Psychological Science, 4* (4), 99–104.

Ryff, C. D., & Singer, B. (1998). Middle age and wellbeing. In H. S. Friedman (Ed.), *Encyclopedia of mental health* (2nd ed., pp. 707–719). New York: Academic Press.

Seligman, M. (2011). *Flourish: A visionary new understanding of happiness and well-being.* New York: Free Press.

Steuer, N., & Marks, N. (2008). *Local wellbeing: Can we measure it?* London: Young Foundation.

Stevenson, M., & Gleeson, B. (2019). Complex urban systems: Compact cities, transport and health. In M. Nieuwenhuijsen and H. Khreis (Eds.), *Integrating human health into urban and transport planning* (pp. 271–286). Cham: Springer.

Stiglitz, J., Sen, A., & Fitoussi, J. P. (2009). Report by the commission on the measurement of economic performance and social progress. Available from http://files.harmonywithnatureun.org/uploads/upload112.pdf

Stoll, L. (2014). A short history of wellbeing research. In D. McDaid & C. L. Cooper (Eds.), *The Economics of Wellbeing* (pp. 1–19). Oxford: Wiley Blackwell.

Thompson, S., & Marks, N. (2008). *Measuring wellbeing in policy: Issues and applications.* London: New Economics Foundation.

Urry, J. (2007). *Mobilities.* Cambridge: Polity.

Van Hoorn, A. (2007, 2–3 April). A short introduction to subjective wellbeing: Its measurement, correlates and policy uses. Paper presented at *Is happiness measureable and what do those measures mean for policy?*, Rome, Italy.

Waterman, A. S. (1993). Two conceptions of happiness Contrasts of personal expressiveness (eudaimonia) and hedonic enjoyment. *Journal of Personality and Social Psychology, 64* (4), 678–691.

White, S. C. (2010). Analysing wellbeing: A framework for development practice. *Development in Practice, 20* (2), 158–172.

WHO. (2018). What is a healthy city? Available from http://www.euro.who.int/en/health-topics/environment-and-health/urban-health/who-european-healthy-cities-network/what-is-a-healthy-city

2

WHAT DO CITY DWELLERS WANT FOR THEMSELVES AND THEIR CITIES? IMPLICATIONS FOR PLANNING LIVEABLE CITIES

Helene Joffe, Nicholas Smith and Victoria Zeeb

Introduction

Set against a backdrop of cities continuing to grow in size and number, how can they accommodate the aspirations and wellbeing of those who dwell in them? What are city dwellers' priorities for their own futures and what do they want from future cities? Understanding the human dimension of city living is central for planning future cities to deliver wellbeing for their inhabitants.

This chapter explores the aspirations of city dwellers living in the UK's two largest cities, London and Birmingham. We explore these city dwellers' aspirations both for themselves and for the cities of the future. We thereby assess city dwellers' priorities *and* what they see as facilitating their sense of wellbeing. Before exploring what people feel gives them wellbeing, we review theoretical writings and empirical evidence concerning wellbeing and the city. By combining existing knowledge with our study of subjective wellbeing, we can inform the design of human-centred cities that enhance wellbeing.

Wellbeing and the City

Personal wellbeing is a happy, healthy and prosperous condition that includes a sense of life satisfaction and lack of anxiety. Specific factors that improve personal wellbeing, at an individual level, are fivefold: connecting with other people, being active, taking notice (embodied in 'mindfulness'), ongoing learning and giving of oneself (Aked et al., 2009; Ruggeri et al., 2016) In particular, robust evidence demonstrates that connecting with others is crucial for wellbeing (Hold-Lunstad et al., 2015; Leung et al., 2011), and that relatedness is a key human need (Ryan et al., 2008). This relatedness refers to not only the need to feel connected to others in one's social environment, but to experience a sense of belonging and to care for, and be cared for, by others (Deci & Ryan, 2002). Cross-cultural studies demonstrate a positive link between such relatedness and wellbeing (Chirkov, 2009; Deci et al., 2001; Schmuck et al., 2000); building and maintaining connections with significant others form a key buffer against mental ill-health (Jenkins et al., 2008; Morrow, 2001). Such connections are two-fold: 'strong ties' are relationships to people to whom one has long-term attachments that are emotionally intimate. Family, romantic partners and friends tend to fall into this category. The second type of social tie is the 'weak tie', characterised by being more limited in frequency, intimacy and emotional intensity than the strong tie. Acquaintances and strangers can fall into this latter category. Simply aspiring to relatedness, rather than aspiring to goals that are guided by extrinsic values, such as money or fame, is positively linked to wellbeing (Kasser & Ryan, 2001).

The city provides a complex context within which interpersonal connection takes place. A long-standing theoretical debate examines the effects of city life on people. Key social theorists have argued that city life is characterised by social conventions that hamper social interactions. Since city dwellers are deemed to be overwhelmed by the sheer number of people encountered, they protect themselves from the stimulus overload by displaying a blasé and unfriendly attitude (Milgram, 1974; Simmel, 1903). This allows them to successfully navigate public space without feeling threatened (Proshansky, 1978; Proshansky et al., 1983). However, it can lead to a profoundly alienating and insular experience (Durkheim, 1951; Marx, 1978).

By way of contrast, other theorists argue that casual contact between dwellers in public spaces can produce a vivacious atmosphere, a sense of joy and 'collective effervescence' (Jacobs, 1961; Jovchelovitch & Priego-Hernandez, 2013; Simmel & Hughes, 1949). Effervescent social contact takes place on the streets as well as in 'third places' (Oldenburg & Brissett, 1982): places separate from the usual social environments of home and work. Third places vary by culture, and include spaces such as French cafés, German beer gardens and English pubs (Oldenburg, 1999). They provide the space for important experiences and relationships to develop and foster a sense of wellbeing because people congregate in them primarily to enjoy each other's company. People do so directly, by starting conversations, or indirectly, by enjoying being in the presence of others.

Set against these more theoretical writings, there is developing empirical evidence that casts light on both the negative and positive sides of city living. On the one hand, the built environment can foster social connectedness and trust by creating meeting places, local shops and street networks (Balducci & Cheeci, 2009; Joffe & Smith, 2016; Wood et al., 2008). 'Active sidewalks', where people socialise outside of both home and work contexts, can nurture this sense of social connectedness and trust between city residents (Gehl, 2013; Jacobs, 1961). In addition, people gain a sense of wellbeing from having convenient public transport and accessible cultural and leisure facilities (Leyden et al., 2011).[1]

The 'walkability' of a city is also important (Frank et al., 2006; Saelens et al., 2003), with research identifying that those who live in walkable and mixed-use neighbourhoods are more likely to know and trust their neighbours; they are, also, more socially and politically engaged with the community than those living in car-dependent suburbs (Leyden, 2003). Furthermore, there are tangible physical and mental health benefits when 'walkable' spaces are green (Bell et al., 2008; Ellaway et al., 2005; Thompson et al., 2012).

Despite the links between city design and subjective wellbeing, high-density living is associated with increased levels of obesity (Arambepola et al., 2008), respiratory problems linked with urban pollutants (Environmental Audit Committee, 2014) and high crime rates (Corrado et al., 2013; Howley et al., 2009). In addition to the physical implications, living in densely populated urban areas is related to mental illness (Oher et al., 2014), which Lederbogen et al. (2011) link to city dwellers' over-responsiveness to stress. Furthermore, connections have been found between urban living and schizophrenia (Krabbendam & Van Os, 2005; Peen et al., 2010), and population density in highly urbanised environments is strongly related to the onset of first episode psychosis (Oher et al., 2014).

Beyond the debate and empirical evidence concerning whether city living is alienating or invigorating, cities are shaped by societal trends. Late modernity has led to more flexibility in the construction of the life course (Giddens, 1991). Individuals are less confined to specific types of relationships. This is most noticeable in the construction and deconstruction of family, partnership and household formation. Just as the roles of these social relationships change, so too do the roles played by non-kin relations, such as friends and community (Allan, 2008). Set against this backdrop, we explored what people from Britain's largest cities wanted for their own futures and for cities of the future. We did so by way of a free association method, so that we were able to enter people's own perspectives without imposing pre-conceived views on them.

Methods

A mixed-methods approach was used to investigate personal aspirations and aspirations for cities of the future for London and Birmingham city dwellers. Detailed methodological information is provided in Joffe and Smith (2016). In brief, a recruitment agency was used to recruit 96 city dwellers, split evenly across both cities (and sampled to be representative of age, gender, ethnicity, socio-economic status and all areas of the city). The Grid Elaboration Method (Joffe & Elsey, 2014) was used to elicit city dweller free associations concerning their aspirations for their own futures and for future cities. Participants were then asked to elaborate their own free associations in an in-depth interview, and the data were analysed using thematic analysis (Joffe, 2012). Survey data were also collected from each of the participants and analysed using SPSS, though the focus below is on the interview-based data.

In the results presented below, people's personal aspirations are presented first, followed by their aspirations for cities of the future. The social connection theme forms the focus of the personal aspiration results, due to its prevalence in the data. Reference to social connectedness is also present in many aspects of people's aspirations for cities of the future.

Results: What Do People Want for Their Own Lives?

City dweller's personal aspirations fell into two broad categories: tangible and intangible. Thematic analysis revealed that the most prevalent tangible aspirations were for job/career (58%), money (56%) and travel (53%). The most prevalent intangible aspirations were for social connection (81%), happiness/contentment (51%) and security (34%). The aspiration for social connection was the most prevalent theme in the interview data. It was, therefore, chosen as the focus of the analysis presented in this chapter, with reference to the other aspirations.

Aspiration for Social Connection

City dwellers aspired to connect with both strong ties – family/partners (67%) and friends (25%) as well as weak ties – people in their local area (13%), people they encounter in the city (non-local) (18%), people in working life (13%) and people outside of the city (13%). It is the aspirations for weak ties that we will explore in this chapter since many facets of this kind of connection are particular to city living. Furthermore, the bulk of existing evidence linking social connectedness with wellbeing focusses on strong ties and so this focus on weak ties works towards increasing understanding of the role played by weak ties in the city. The data were examined for demographic differences along gender, age, socioeconomic status and city of residence lines. Evident differences are reported.

Aspiration for Social Connection with Weak Ties in Local Area

A substantial portion of the sample talked of the importance of weak ties in describing their aspirations. Weak ties included neighbours and others in one's local area. Weak ties were associated with enjoyment, wanting to share with others and having impact beyond the family unit. They also enabled escape from everyday stress and improvement of quality of life. Saying 'hello' to people on the street or in a shop, and stopping for a quick chat was seen as making everyday activities more enjoyable. This 'neighbourly' attitude was anchored to a representation of neighbourliness found in smaller towns or villages:

> ...when we go up to the local shop they know us by name ... I always read the headlines and they always ask me, just jokingly, oh what's in the

> headlines today, do you want a report back? And it's just because they know us, it's neighbourly, it's really neighbourly, it's like a... the feeling of a small little village or town but ... in the middle of the city.
>
> *[Female, 36–54, higher SES, BME, Birmingham]*

Beyond enjoyment, the aspiration for social connection with local people was linked to helping and acknowledging one another: 'It's a matter of knocking on your neighbour's door and saying I'm just going to the shop, do you need anything, it takes 2 minutes' [Male, 36–54, lower SES, White, Birmingham].

The majority of dwellers who wanted to connect with others in their local area spoke of wanting to be part of a community. City dwellers with this aspiration used the words 'community', 'local area' and 'neighbourhood' interchangeably. Being part of a community was equated with having a support system. There was a particular interest in supporting others in the community, either financially or by volunteering time. An aspiration for social solidarity was also present in the data. In particular, this aspiration was related to working together to have an impact:

> [It] takes, I would say, a community effort to change a lot of things that needs [sic] to be changed. You know, so you, as a father, individual, a man, you're doing your best within your home, you know, within your little area but if you did want changes, serious changes within politics, government, community, it's then going to take a big effort so I guess to live in a good community is important.
>
> *[Male, 36–54, lower SES, BME, Birmingham]*

The aspiration for local community was linked to a sense of nostalgia. A common comparison was made between neighbourhood connection nowadays and that of yesteryear. There was a consensus that people who do not know many of their neighbours in the present would have known them 20–30 years ago. This view was equally distributed among all age groups. Knowing and trusting those around one was associated with a purported feeling of safety that prevailed in the past and allowed children to play happily on the street, and people to leave their front doors open or unlocked without worry. Finally, in both the London and the Birmingham data, there was a sense that society had become more selfish, and that people did not 'pull together like they used to':

> I mean I guess maybe 20 years... even maybe 30 years... ago, people, you know, neighbours used to interact quite freely, your neighbours were your friends, things like that. In this day and age, you know, if it doesn't concern me then I'm not really that bothered. I mean we see people that are being beaten up on the street, mugged and we turn a blind eye like we didn't see it. ... I feel like society, we're so egocentric.
>
> *[Male, 18–35, higher SES, BME, London]*

Aspiration for Social Connection with Weak Ties in the City (Non-local)

City dwellers also wished to engage with others in the city outside of their local area. One avenue for connection was via group activities and clubs in the city at large. This aspiration was only present in the London data. Londoners aspired to join group activities, such as cycling, dog walking or running with other like-minded city dwellers. Here, conceptions of connecting with weak ties were closely related to achieving a particular goal, such as health:

> I've spent years before in the past joining a gym and it's just solitary. I mean what I do now is outdoors, it's boot camps and running but it's with a group, you know, with people and realizing that that's what I've needed … more of a social element.
>
> *[Female, 36–54, higher SES, BME, London]*

This 'social element' increased both the enjoyment of the activity and the motivation to persist. Like the aspiration to connect with people locally, the aspiration to connect with non-local weak ties was found mostly within the 36–54-year-olds.

Beyond the wish to engage directly with others through activities, there was a strong desire for small-scale interactions with people in public spaces (shops; third places, such as pubs, parks and streets) that were pleasant and enjoyable. City dwellers aspired to connect with these weak ties by adopting a positive demeanour towards them. In Birmingham, this demeanour was further defined by the desire to be friendly, kind and show concern for others. In London there was a slightly stronger emphasis on being respectful and polite, rather than friendly:

> If you've lived on the Earth, you've lived in this world, you've interacted with maybe millions of people on a daily basis consciously or subconsciously, purposely or, you know, by accident, and you want to feel like you've made a mark somehow in a strange kind of way, whether, you know, it's just opening a door for someone or just being polite.
>
> *[Male, 18–35, higher SES, BME, London]*

Dwellers spoke of the visceral feelings of enjoyment that come from low intensity and positive connection: 'my nature is just to say hello to people because if people, if somebody says hello to me that I don't know, it kind of gives me a nice, just a nice feeling' [Male, 36–54, higher SES, BME, Birmingham].

Finally, this desire for face-to-face connection with others in the city also extended to the way in which dwellers wanted services to be provided in the city:

> I'd rather walk up to someone in a ticket office and say excuse me, how do you get there, than being on a machine … it's a shame because we

> are humans and it's nice to see a face if you're talking to someone, but everything seems to be going away from that and talking to screens.
>
> *[Male, 36–54, lower SES, White, London]*

This aspiration for face-to-face connection highlights the way in which connection with others is seen by the city dwellers as part of humans' inherently social nature.

Aspiration for Social Connection with Weak Ties in Working Life

Social connection with weak ties was also sought in working life where it was primarily related to two goals: achieving something positive by having an impact on others and the world around one, and enjoying oneself.

The vast majority of those who aspired to social connection at work did so to have an impact on others. This was associated with an aspiration to create positive change. Some young people, for example, aspired to being teachers in order to help children achieve their potential. This was seen to give meaning and purpose to their lives, which was linked to a sense of achievement, as well as success:

> The aspiration is to be successful in the future with what I'm doing for others.
>
> *[Female, 36–54, higher SES, BME, Birmingham]*

Having a positive impact on other people's lives was described as inherently rewarding.

Social connection at work was also associated, by a small number of people, with enjoying one's work. Interacting with others was seen as pleasurable and active, as opposed to being 'static', sitting behind a computer and not speaking to anyone:

> There's times when people come to you and talk to you and trust you with stuff and it's just nice to always talk. Rather than, be … on a computer all day you don't speak to no-one and it's just, I just love interacting with people.
>
> *[Male, 18–35, higher SES, White British, Birmingham]*

Aspiration for Social Connection with Weak Ties Outside of the City

Finally, city dwellers also aspired to connect with weak ties outside of the city. This type of social connection linked to the aspiration for travel. Connecting with people while travelling was seen as part of an authentic experience that allowed for learning about different ways of living:

> By travelling you meet people as well, you can have good, you know, relationships with people abroad in which you can exchange... you can say, 'You know what? Come and spend some time with me over here and see how we live in England'.
>
> *[Male, 36–54, lower SES, BME, Birmingham]*

Aspiration for Disconnection

A tiny proportion (3%) of city dwellers expressed an aspiration to disconnect from others and to be alone. This aspiration was associated with two qualities. The first was seeing other people, either at work or at home, as a source of stress and ill-being.

> Well, I mean it is just time for yourself, for me really just to walk in the park with the dogs, you know, and have some time to yourself. I don't have to answer to anybody, I haven't got to please anybody.
>
> *[Female, 55–67, higher SES, White British, Birmingham]*

The second aspect of the aspiration for disconnection was that some city dwellers who had experienced 'quite a bit of solitude' had become accustomed to the sense of freedom and peace that it provided. This was very different to the dominant description of social disconnection in the data, which presented being alone or disconnected from others as lonely, boring or embarrassing.

Results: What Do People Want from Cities of the Future?

Having discussed people's aspirations for their own lives, and focussed on their aspirations for city-based, 'weak tie' connections, we turn to examining what people wanted for cities of the future. The most expressed aspiration is for desirable facilities and services: social, cultural, retail and municipal (79%), with transport attracting a lot of specific attention (60%). In addition, nature is highly prized (68%), as is a sense of community (66%) and safety (53%).

Aspirational Facilities and Services

People want future cities to contain a range of services and facilities, such as restaurants, cafés, pubs and clubs. These are associated with high levels of personal wellbeing, providing good opportunities to socialise. Dwellers, particularly those of a higher socio-economic status in the two cities, talked of the 'buzz' and 'vibe' generated in these lively and exciting places. Such facilities were also seen to be needed to counteract the pressures created by city living. These social spaces were sometimes seen as an escape, which was particularly important for female dwellers, who had a greater tendency than the male dwellers to find the city to be too busy and noisy:

> I think if you're going to be in a city, which is quite busy and quite stressful sometimes, it's nice to be social and go out with your friends... just to go and meet someone in a bar or see friends between work... cities have a lot to offer, I think, with restaurants and bars and cinemas and clubs and things, that you don't really get anywhere else.
>
> *[Female, 18–35, higher SES, White British, London]*

A rich culture and heritage were also revealed as hallmarks of a desirable British city, particularly for the white, as opposed to the British minority ethnic, respondents. London dwellers, in particular, were impressed by the cultural facilities that their own city had to offer, even if they had not yet visited them:

> ...there's so many things in London that I haven't even done or that I hear about that I want to go and see. I haven't even had a chance to go to the Science Museum, which is shocking considering I did science but there's just so much to do. And I just think it's great that it's got so much history.
>
> *[Female, 18–35, higher SES, White British, London]*

In addition, cities were places where people expected to find a wide range of shopping facilities. This was particularly salient for female dwellers. The appeal of 'local' shopping facilities was widely mentioned, in part for their convenience. Alongside enjoyment of local shopping facilities, a minority of dwellers reflected on the demise of the local, British high street since it had been filled with chain shops. There was a preference for independent shops. Chain shops and larger supermarkets were seen as eroding the enjoyment associated with the social experience of shopping, such as chatting to a familiar owner. This evoked feelings of ill-being and sadness.

Several dwellers specifically identified the vulnerability of the young and the old and the need for governments to provide sufficient services to look after these populations. Local community centres were heralded as the glue that held a community together and kept young people from 'roaming the streets'. Several spoke of their demise due to lack of funding.

Transport was a key service that people discussed. Accessible and efficient transport was highly valued. Many dwellers spoke of their enjoyment of being able to move around their city easily by public transport. Where cycling was mentioned, it tended to be connected to a healthy lifestyle, rather than to reducing carbon emissions within a city.

By way of contrast to more positive references regarding transport, for most, transport evoked feelings of anger and frustration. Several Londoners talked about the tension created by 'cramped' conditions and being 'shoved' and 'pushed' by 'robotic' commuters on peak rush hour services. The car was often seen as the less stressful and more efficient option, both within London and Birmingham. However, transport, both public and private, was also seen as a source of pollution and dirt, which evoked strong disgust.

Aspiration for Nature

Green and blue space was a salient feature of the city aspirations. In the majority of such associations, nature was experienced as contributing to wellbeing. Green and blue spaces were seen as places of health and exercise, relaxation, escape and planetary wellbeing.

> Yeah, it just kind of smells … fresh and it's kind of relaxing and tranquil. That's why I like to go there like on my breaks … let everything kind of just go behind me, work, whatever, and just kind of have a moment for myself and then get back to the hustle and bustle after.
>
> *[Female, 18–35, higher SES, BME British, London]*

There was less emphasis on socialising in nature than in the built environment. Tranquillity could be gained by solitude in such places. Yet despite strong idealisation of what such spaces could provide, people, particularly women, worried about their vulnerability to attack in such open spaces.

Aspiration for a Sense of Community and Safety

Not surprisingly given their personal aspirations for social connectedness, the desire for a strong sense of community in cities of the future was expressed by approximately two-thirds of dwellers. Friendliness was seen as a defining characteristic, particularly for Birmingham dwellers and for younger dwellers across the two cities. The importance of friendly communities co-existed with the desire to live in close-knit, warm communities:

> Well, since we've moved here, this bit of the street where we are, they're just, like, very friendly. Everybody talks to each other and I just think it's lovely.
>
> *[Female, 18–35, higher SES, White British, Birmingham]*

Having good neighbours aided a sense of community and many highlighted the important functions neighbours provide, including increased feelings of safety:

> I couldn't imagine living somewhere where I didn't know my neighbours … that's alien to me, I can't imagine living next door to somebody and not actually knowing their first name, or being able to knock in an emergency if something was needed.
>
> *[Female, 36–54, lower SES, White British, London]*

A sense of happiness was also regularly associated with being involved in community activities. High levels of involvement in the community were associated with a strong community spirit and a sense of belonging. Several city dwellers spoke of community events and the sense of intimacy they created including the Royal Wedding, the Queen's Diamond Jubilee and the London Olympics:

> ...I quite liked it in London when the Olympics were going on and when there was a royal wedding, so like big things that involve the whole city ... everyone just seemed... a bit happier. ... everyone sort of came together even though you don't know anyone it was quite nice.
>
> *[Female, 18–35, lower SES, White British, London]*

A sense of community was seen by the majority of dwellers as a highly important attribute of a future liveable city. Major regret was expressed concerning its erosion. In particular, many lamented the loss of what life was like in cities when they were younger. Communities were places where people knew their neighbours and looked out for one another: local children played outside on the streets in a carefree way. This symbolised how socially connected the neighbourhood was. Children of the present, by contrast, were represented as isolating themselves in their rooms surfing the Internet and playing 'X box'. Moreover, certain groups, or gangs of children, were symbolised as threatening and dangerous. Many also felt that contemporary communities were defined by a general lack of mutual respect, often exacerbated by increasingly hectic and technologised lifestyles. The sense was that nobody invested time in maintaining neighbourly relationships.

City dwellers from both cities also aspired to live in safe cities. Several dwellers spoke about their desire to live in safe neighbourhoods and not to be scared of leaving their houses. As such, a fear of crime was a salient contributor to ill-being. Reflecting on the past, many saw the communities and cities in which they currently lived as more dangerous:

> I'd like to think that the city we lived in was secure. I'd be much happier feeling that me and my family are living in a secure place where the crime rate isn't so high, where there wasn't a drug problem... which my kids don't see because, you know, our kids don't play out on the street. I was allowed to when I was a kid but things were different then.... People did leave their door open and times have changed so much.
>
> *[Male, 36–54, lower SES, White, Birmingham]*

An awareness of crime was also linked to the desire for stronger law enforcement. Enforcement was seen to have 'no teeth' nowadays, thereby increasing crime. A more visible police service was seen as a solution. The desire for a safer neighbourhood was symbolised by the 'the local bobby' who knows everybody by name and identifies local hotspots of trouble, walking the street.

Dwellers also spoke of derogated and stigmatised 'others' who many regarded as responsible for these increases in crime. 'Gangs', 'hoodies' and 'youths' were seen as key perpetrators and symbolised as threatening and dangerous. Several dwellers linked these derogated societal groups to the negative aspects of living in a multicultural society:

> You go in the town at night and there's young gangs of different ethnic communities mooching around and they get together... the wrong thing's said, you know, fists are flying. There's gunshot wounds every week in Birmingham, it's not good.
>
> *[Male, 55–67, lower SES, White British, Birmingham]*

Discussion

This study shows that social connection is highly prized in the city. Using a naturalistic, novel method, the chapter highlights that social connection is the most prevalent aspiration when people talk about their aspirations for their futures and highly salient in their aspirations for cities of the future. From the range of what could have been mentioned, not only does social connection prevail, it includes both strong and weak ties. Weak ties give people far more opportunities for connection and, therefore, wellbeing than had been explored previously. City dwellers are motivated by a desire to matter to others and to enjoy life. Corroborating the mattering literature and extending it to weak ties, people want to enter the awareness of others, be relied upon by them and feel important to them (Rosenberg & McCullough, 1981). In particular, the salience bestowed on small-scale, face-to-face, pleasant interactions on the streets and in third places demonstrates that city dwellers desire to live in cities that foster the opportunity for interactions that are friendly and polite.

This challenges the classical conception of cities as full of disinterested and blasé strangers, indifferent to the people they encounter (Simmel, 1903). The extent to which participants want to matter to weak ties provides a new perspective for the mattering literature, which has so far focussed on strong ties. People highly value the transformation of instrumental/informational exchange into social interaction. Our work, reported here and elsewhere (Joffe & Smith, 2016), indicates that the 'smart' agenda, which promotes efficiency, is unlikely to bolster this sense of mattering and consequent wellbeing.

Beyond mattering, the desire for social connection is most commonly motivated by enjoyment. Even when talking about services in cities, face-to-face connection is not aspired to because it is seen as more efficient, but because it is regarded as more pleasant and enjoyable. Providing evidence for the suppositions of Jacobs (1961) and Simmel and Huges (1949), the aspirations evident in this study point to a conception of the city as a place of potential 'collective effervescence' – a place in which joy can be felt by the sheer presence of others. Having observed the centrality of this desire and corroborating the findings of Cattell et al. (2008), there is a need to create urban spaces in which people feel they can linger and connect with others in ways that are exciting and joyful.

While visceral pleasure is gained from connectedness in both cities, the sense given is that Londoners value politeness and aspire, for their weak ties, to connect with people in the city at large, whereas Birmingham dwellers aspire to friendliness and focus on connecting with people in their local area. The relative sizes of the two cities, with London approaching a mega-city size and Birmingham considerably smaller, may underpin these differences. The role played by politeness in softening the stresses of mega-city living may provide a fruitful area of study. The ways in which politeness or other such qualities may be valued cross-culturally would provide another fertile area for future study.

Finally, city dweller aspirations for social connection are shaped by a strong sense of nostalgia. Participants' aspirations for social connection in the future hark back to an imagined, ideal past. This manifests itself in their longing for a time when community was close-knit and people knew their neighbours. These longings are associated with feelings of trust and safety. Contemporary cities are represented as having generated youthful gangs and shopping centres filled with dreary chain shops. The character of the city is threatened by these symbols of an anxiety-generating, broken community. While one could argue that nostalgia is out of kilter with the highly mobile communities and variegated family units found in contemporary society (Sweeney, 2010; Urry, 2000), city planners could draw on this longing. They could design so that face-to-face, communal elements that recreated imagined ways of old were reintroduced.

In juxtaposition to the massive research attention given to the 'smart' city, with its implications of technological fixes for city dweller concerns, interpersonal interaction is key for British, large-city dwellers' sense of the liveability of their cities; people want to see the bobby walking on the street, they want to interact with friendly people in shops, fetes and pubs, they crave a sense of community.

Beyond the emphasis on social connection, a connection to nature was emphasised. Green space was viewed highly positively by the majority of those who mentioned it. For city dwellers, public green spaces provide one of the few avenues for direct contact with nature (Fuller et al., 2007). Furthermore, the way in which buildings and cities are designed also has a significant impact on the wellbeing of city residents. Cities that contained beautiful buildings, both modern and historical, but designed in a way that was sensitive to the particular city's cultural heritage, were highly valued. There was far less focus on the creativity, ingenuity and technological know-how reflected in many new buildings. Again, the 'smart' agenda was not at the fore of most people's visions.

The appeal of efficient transport systems was also a central design feature for the aspirational city and was related to both a desire for improved accessibility and lower urban pollution levels. In particular, images of a dirty and polluted city were prevalent and reviled. This echoes findings from other studies that identify a strong loathing of pollution (O'Neill & Nicholson-Cole, 2009; O'Neill et al., 2013).

Conclusion: What Is the Relationship between City-Dweller Aspirations and Their Wellbeing?

Aspirations for cities of the future are synonymous with what people feel will make them happy in a city (Goldberg et al., 2012). A key quality that the majority of city dwellers wished for was a strong sense of social connectedness and community. Empirical evidence regarding the causes of personal wellbeing aligns with this wish: feeling connected to, and involved with, one's community is an important predictor of wellbeing and overall happiness (Leyden et al., 2011).

The design and aesthetics of cities have a major impact on the personal wellbeing of their residents in part because of the social interactions that design fosters. Communal spaces facilitate the interactions that are central to wellbeing. Social ties nurture a deep sense of belonging and rootedness (Cattell et al., 2008). This speaks to a broader conceptualisation of cities as places where 'collective effervescence' (Jacobs, 1961) can be fostered. While the piazza symbolises this in hotter countries, in colder countries such as the UK, internal piazzas might take on this role. The 'collective joy' fostered in the ritualistic coming together of strangers who share a sense of collective identity (Ehrenreich, 2007; Novelli et al., 2013) can foster wellbeing in city dwellers.

Note

1 High-density urban environments can also increase the sharing of resources (e.g. public transportation), financial investment in better quality amenities and greater productivity and employment opportunities (see Boyko & Cooper, 2011, for a full review).

References

Aked, J., Marks, N., Cordon, C., & Thompson, S. (2009). *Five ways to wellbeing.* London: New Economics Foundation.

Allan, G. (2008). Flexibility, friendship, and family. *Personal Relationships, 15*(1), p1–16.

Arambepola, C., Allender, S., Ekanayake, R., & Fernando, D. (2008). Urban living and obesity: is it independent of its population and lifestyle characteristics? *Tropical Medicine & International Health, 13*(4), p448–457.

Balducci, A., & Checchi, D. (2009). Happiness and quality of city life: the Case of Milan, the Richest Italian City. *International Planning Studies, 14*(1), p25–64.

Bell, J. F., Wilson, J. S., & Liu, G. C. (2008). Neighborhood greenness and 2-year changes in body mass index of children and youth. *American Journal of Preventive Medicine, 35*(6), p547–553.

Cattell, V., Dines, N., Gesler, W., & Curtis, S. (2008). Mingling, observing, and lingering: everyday public spaces and their implications for wellbeing and social relations. *Health & Place, 14,* p522–561.

Chirkov, V. I. (2009). A cross-cultural analysis of autonomy in education: a self-determination theory perspective. *Theory and Research in Education,* 7(2), p253–262.

Corrado, G., Corrado, L., & Santoro, E. (2013). On the individual and social determinants of neighbourhood satisfaction and attachment. *Regional Studies, 47*(4), p544–562.

Deci, E. L., & Ryan, R. (2002). Overview of self-determination theory: an organismic dialectical perspective. In E. L. Deci & R. M. Ryan (Eds.), *Handbook of self-determination research* (p3–33). Rochester, NY: The University of Rochester Press.

Deci, E. L., Ryan, R. M., Gagné, M., Leone, D. R., Usunov, J., & Kornazheva, B. P. (2001). Need satisfaction, motivation, and wellbeing in the work organizations of a former eastern bloc country: a cross-cultural study of self-determination. *Personality and Social Psychology Bulletin, 27*(8), p930–942.

Durkheim, E. (1951). *Suicide: a study in sociology.* Glencoe, IL: The Free Press.

Ehrenreich, B. (2007). *Dancing in the streets: a history of collective joy.* New York: Metropolitan Books.

Ellaway, A., Macintyre, S., & Bonnefoy, X. (2005). Graffiti, greenery, and obesity in adults: secondary analysis of European cross sectional survey. *BMJ, 331*(7517), p611–612.

Environmental Audit Committee. (2014). *Action on air quality.* London: House of Commons.

Frank, L. D., Sallis, J. F., Conway, T. L., Chapman, J. E., Saelens, B. E., & Bachman, W. (2006). Many pathways from land use to health: associations between neighborhood walkability and active transportation, body mass index, and air quality. *Journal of the American Planning Association, 72*(1), p75–87.

Fuller, R. A., Irvine, K. N., Devine-Wright, P., Warren, P. H., & Gaston, K. J. (2007). Psychological benefits of greenspace increase with biodiversity. *Biology Letters, 3*(4), 390–394.

Gehl, J. (2013). *Cities for people.* Washington, DC: Island Press.

Giddens, A. (1991). *Modernity and self-identity: self and society in the late modern age.* Stanford, CA: Stanford University Press.

Goldberg, A., Leyden, K. M., & Scotto, T. J. (2012). Untangling what makes cities liveable: happiness in five cities. *Proceedings of the Institution of Civil Engineers-Urban Design and Planning, 165*(3), p127–136.

Holt-Lunstad, J., Smith, T. B., Baker, M., Harris, T., & Stephenson, D. (2015). Loneliness and social isolation as risk factors for mortality: a meta-analytic review. *Perspectives on Psychological Science, 10*(2), p227–237. doi: 10.1177/1745691614568352

Howley, P., Scott, M., & Redmond, D. (2009). Sustainability versus liveability: an investigation of neighbourhood satisfaction. *Journal of Environmental Planning and Management, 52*(6), p847–864.

Jacobs, J. (1961). *The death and life of great American cities.* New York: Random House.

Jenkins, R., Meltzer, H., Jones, P., Brugha, T., Bebbington, P., Farrell, M., & Crepaz-Keay, D. (2008). *Foresight mental capital and wellbeing project. Mental health: future challenges.* The Government Office for Science.

Joffe, H. (2012). Thematic analysis. In D. Harper & A. R. Thompson (Eds.), *Qualitative research methods in mental health and psychotherapy: a guide for students and practitioners* (p209–223). Chichester: John Wiley & Sons, Ltd.

Joffe, H., & Elsey, J. W. (2014). Free association in psychology and the grid elaboration method. *Review of General Psychology, 18*(3), p173–185.

Joffe, H., & Smith, N. (2016). City dweller aspirations for cities of the future: how do environmental and personal wellbeing feature? *Cities, 59*, p102–112.

Jovchelovitch, S., & Priego-Hernandez, J. (2013). *Underground Sociabilities: identity, culture and resistance in Rio de Janeiro's favelas.* Brasilia: UNESCO.

Kasser, T., & Ryan, R. M. (2001). Be careful what you wish for: optimal functioning and the relative attainment of intrinsic and extrinsic goals. In P. Schmuck & K. Sheldon (Eds.), *Life goals and wellbeing: towards a positive psychology of human striving* (p116–131). Gottingen: Hogrefe.

Krabbendam, L., & Van Os, J. (2005). Schizophrenia and urbanicity: a major environmental influence—conditional on genetic risk. *Schizophrenia Bulletin, 31*(4), p795–799.
Lederbogen, F., Kirsch, P., Haddad, L., Streit, F., Tost, H., Schuch, P., … Deuschle, M. (2011). City living and urban upbringing affect neural social stress processing in humans. *Nature, 474*(7352), p498–501.
Leung, A., Kier, C., Fung, T., Fung, L., & Sproule, R. (2011). Searching for happiness: the importance of social capital. *Journal of Happiness Studies, 12*(3), p443–462.
Leyden, K. M. (2003). Social capital and the built environment: the importance of walkable neighborhoods. *American Journal of Public Health, 93*(9), p1546–1551.
Leyden, K. M., Goldberg, A., & Michelbach, P. (2011). Understanding the pursuit of happiness in ten major cities. *Urban Affairs Review, 47*(6), p861–888.
Marx, K. (1978). Alienation and social classes. In R. C. Tucker (Ed.), *The Marx-Engels reader* (2nd ed., p133–135). New York: W. W. Norton.
Milgram, S. (1974). The experience of living in cities. *Crowding and Behavior, 167*, p41.
Morrow, V. (2001). *Networks and neighbourhoods: children's and young people's perspectives.* London: NHS Health Development Agency.
Novelli, D., Drury, J., Reicher, S., & Stott, C. (2013). Crowdedness mediates the effect of social identification on positive emotion in a crowd: a survey of two crowd events. *PLOS One, 8*(11), e78983.
O'Neill, S., & Nicholson-Cole, S. (2009). "Fear won't do it" promoting positive engagement with climate change through visual and iconic representations. *Science Communication, 30*(3), p355–379.
O'Neill, S. J., Boykoff, M., Niemeyer, S., & Day, S. A. (2013). On the use of imagery for climate change engagement. *Global Environmental Change, 23*(2), p413–421.
Oher, F., Demjaha, A., Jackson, D., Morgan, C., Dazzan, P., Morgan, K., … Bentall, R. (2014). The effect of the environment on symptom dimensions in the first episode of psychosis: a multilevel study. *Psychological Medicine, 44*(11), p2419–2430.
Oldenburg, R. (1999). *The great good place: cafés, coffee shops, bookstores, bars, hair salons, and other hangouts at the heart of a community* (3rd ed.). New York: Marlowe & Company.
Oldenburg, R., & Brissett, D. (1982). The third place. *Qualitative Sociology, 5*(4), p265–284.
Peen, J., Schoevers, R. A., Beekman, A. T., & Dekker, J. (2010). The current status of urban-rural differences in psychiatric disorders. *Acta Psychiatrica Scandinavica, 121*(2), p84–93.
Proshansky, H. M. (1978). The city and self-identity. *Environment and Behavior, 10*(2), p147–169. doi: 10.1177/0013916578102002
Proshansky, H. M., Fabian, A. K., & Kaminoff, R. T. (1983). Place identity: physical world socialization of the self. *Journal of Environmental Psychology, 3*, p57–83.
Rosenberg, M., & McCullough, B. C. (1981). Mattering: inferred significance and mental health among adolescents. *Research in Community & Mental Health, 2*, p163–182.
Ruggeri, K., Garcia-Garzon, E., Maguire, Á., & Huppert, F. A. (2016). Inequalities in well-being: Insights from a comprehensive well-being measure. *ESRC Policy Report.* Available from https://neweconomics.org/uploads/files/7831bc5dbdb172539e_64m6brzrn.pdf
Ryan, R. M., Huta, V., & Deci, E. L. (2008). Living well: a self-determination theory perspective on eudaimonia. *Journal of Happiness Studies, 9*(1), p139–170.
Saelens, B. E., Sallis, J. F., & Frank, L. D. (2003). Environmental correlates of walking and cycling: findings from the transportation, urban design, and planning literatures. *Annals of Behavioral Medicine, 25*(2), p80–91.
Schmuck, P., Kasser, T., & Ryan, R. M. (2000). Intrinsic and extrinsic goals: their structure and relationship to wellbeing in German and US college students. *Social Indicators Research, 50*(2), p225–241.

Simmel, G. (1903). The metropolis and mental life. In K. H. Wolff (Ed.), *The Sociology of Georg Simmel* (p409–426). Glencoe, IL: The Free Press.

Simmel, G., & Hughes, E. (1949). The sociology of sociability. *American Journal of Sociology, 55*(3), p254–261.

Sweeney, M. M. (2010). Remarriage and stepfamilies: strategic sites for family scholarship in the 21st century. *Journal of Marriage and Family, 72*(3), p667–684.

Thompson, C. W., Roe, J., Aspinall, P., Mitchell, R., Clow, A., & Miller, D. (2012). More green space is linked to less stress in deprived communities: evidence from salivary cortisol patterns. *Landscape and Urban Planning, 105*(3), p221–229.

Urry, J. (2000). *Sociology beyond societies.* London: Sage.

Wood, L., Shannon, T., Bulsara, M., Pikora, T., McCormack, G., & Giles-Corti, B. (2008). The anatomy of the safe and social suburb: an exploratory study of the built environment, social capital and residents' perceptions of safety. *Health & Place, 14*(1), p15–31.

3

MOBILITIES FOR WELLBEING

Hedonism or Eudaimonism?

Katerina Psarikidou

Introduction

Contemporary lives are very much dependent on movement. People, things, information and ideas are on a constant move. In his *Mobilities* book, John Urry (2007) said, 'it sometimes seems as if all the world is on the move' (p. 3). So, can you imagine if the world stopped moving? What would be the implications of such a prospect for people and societies? This chapter aims to unpack the diverse and complex interconnections between Mobilities[1] and wellbeing in cities. More specifically, it aims to contribute to emerging debates on the ways we can transform mobility systems in cities without compromising people's current levels and experiences of wellbeing and quality of life in cities.

There is no doubt: there is an increasing number of people living in cities. The more people live in cities, the more cities are transformed into places of constant movement. And, the more cities are transformed into places of constant movement, the more they become key to people's experiences of wellbeing and quality of life (Amin & Thirft, 2002; Sheller & Urry, 2006). They can host, facilitate as well as impede our movement and contribute to the production of both mobilities and immobilities that are key to our experiences of a 'good life' in cities (O'Neil, 2006; Urry, 2007). However, the more cities become places of constant movement, the greater the need for fuelling movements, the more energy is depleted and the more carbon emissions are produced (Sims et al., 2014). Addressing this double-sided effect of movement is a great societal challenge: how can we transform our current mobility patterns towards a more sustainable direction without compromising our experiences of the 'good life' in cities? This chapter aims to address this question. However, by doing so, it also raises the questions: what do we mean by 'good life'? And, how does this link to the idea of mobilities (and immobilities) in cities?

There are increasing number of studies that underline the interlinkages between mobilities and wellbeing (Nordbakke & Schwanen, 2014; Ziegler & Schwanen, 2011). However, as will be discussed in this chapter, most of them are based on a narrow, mostly quantitative approach to wellbeing and mobilities, mainly reduced to analyses of travel satisfaction. This chapter opens up to a more multifaceted analysis that considers both hedonic/individual and eudaimonic/social approaches to wellbeing (Christie & Nash, 1998; Nussbaum, 2000; O'Neil, 2006; Sayer, 2004) in order to explore Mobilities for wellbeing in cities. It starts by providing a critical overview of the different conceptualisations of wellbeing and their use in existing research on mobility and transport. It then focusses on our research for the Liveable Cities programme in order to offer an analysis that helps us understand mobility practices not only as a means towards wellbeing through the accomplishment of other social practices of wellbeing, but also as a practice of wellbeing itself. Through such analysis, I discuss the more blurred and complex intersections between hedonic and eudaimonic, individual and social wellbeing, and suggest that only if we develop a more holistic approach to wellbeing will we be able to re-design mobility systems in ways that can contribute to the pursuit and delivery of wellbeing in cities.

Mobilities and Wellbeing: A Critical Overview

Wellbeing: A Contested Concept

No doubt, wellbeing is a contested concept. It is a broad term that has been gaining prominence in government policy and academic circles (e.g. Marks & Thompson, 2008; Reid & Hunter, 2011; Waldron, 2010). However, its meaning can vary. As Galloway et al. (2006) put it, 'what is considered "the good life" varies between individuals, and between societies and cultures' (p. 28).

The historical roots of wellbeing can be found in the philosophical debate concerning what the 'good life' means, linked also to ideas of a 'good society'. A distinction between hedonic and eudaimonic approaches to wellbeing has been key in this debate.

On the one hand, following a utilitarian logic to wellbeing, hedonic approaches underline the significance of happiness or pleasure as the key criterion for a person's wellbeing through the satisfaction of their own preferences and desires (Diener, 2009). Contemporary 'consumer societies' are a manifestation of such a logic in which wellbeing is expected to be pursued through increased personal wealth and material consumption (O'Neil, 2006). In this context, an individualistic logic becomes prominent: wellbeing is narrowly perceived as the property of an individual that can be pursued only through personal life satisfaction (Bauman, 2000). However, a calculative rationality also prevails (Weber, 1978), in which wellbeing turns into a measurable unit reduced to indicators, including money, income and commodities.

Such calculative logic is also evident in the distinction between 'objective' and 'subjective' wellbeing (Phillips, 2006; Rapley, 2003; Ringen, 1995). According to Hird (2003), objective dimensions of wellbeing are the quantifiable material and social attributes (e.g. income, education and health status), whereas the subjective dimensions of wellbeing are based on people's personal evaluations of their lives, their thoughts and feelings about their quality of life. The first are widely used among policy makers and professionals interested in social welfare and health, whereas the second is principally developed by psychologists and economists to evaluate individual life satisfaction and happiness (Dolan et al., 2006; Reid & Hunter, 2011). Despite their differences, both dimensions share a quantitative understanding of wellbeing, usually translated into a number of indicators that are set and defined *a priori* by 'experts' in the field (Nordbakke & Schwanen, 2014).

Aristotle's concept of 'eudaimonia' provides the grounds for an alternative conceptualisation of 'wellbeing' beyond individual happiness and personal satisfaction. In this context, wellbeing is achieved through a purposeful public engagement, contributing to the building of a 'good society' (Bruni & Porta, 2005; O'Neill, 1993). Although it can still focus on the individual as an agent of public participation, as opposed to the hedonic framework, it is more than a property of an individual; wellbeing is both conceptualised and achieved within the context of the society. As Bruni and Porta (2005) put it, it is a 'relational' concept through which human flourishing arises as people function and interact within society – for example, through participation in civil life and friendships. This eudaimonic framework also offers a different, more qualitative and bottom-up understanding of wellbeing: a wellbeing that is not reduced to a number of indicators but is based on people's descriptive narratives and perceptions and experiences of a 'good life'. This 'good life' is perceived beyond an individualistic, consumerist logic, by situating an individual's human flourishing in 'the social': their active participation, engagement and contribution to society.

Wellbeing in Mobility Research

There is no doubt that mobility is an integral element for the accomplishment of a lot of everyday practices that contribute to wellbeing and quality of life, in terms of both fulfilling basic human needs, and other, more pleasure-seeking experiences of everyday life (Cass et al., 2005; Shove et al., 2012). For example, as part of our everyday lives, most of us need to 'move' in order to get to work or do our shopping, to go to the cinema, meet friends, participate in other leisure activities. Such direct connections between mobility and wellbeing are also acknowledged in the existing academic literature, both in transport studies (Duarte et al., 2010; Ettema et al., 2010) and in Mobilities research[2] (Freudendal-Pedersen, 2009; Urry, 2007; Ziegler & Schawanen, 2011).

Existing studies on mobility and wellbeing adopt a narrow approach to mobility, primarily associating it with transport. As a result, an instrumental approach to mobility becomes prevalent: mobility appears to mainly refer to movement from A to B in physical space for the accomplishment of an activity or activities at the end destination. There is also a narrow focus on the type of activities accomplished. Much attention has been paid to everyday activities in the city (e.g. shopping, meeting others, etc.), whereas research has relatively ignored the study of other activities that involve travelling elsewhere (e.g. visiting friends/family; going on holiday). Finally, a strong focus is also given to certain socio-demographic groups, with prioritisation given to the study of mobility among the elderly. Despite its limited focus, such research can provide interesting insights for understanding the interconnections between Mobilities and wellbeing and for researching the impact of mobility on the wellbeing of a wider and more diverse spectrum of the population living in cities.

Current studies point our attention to specific dimensions that are important in understanding the role of mobility in the accomplishment of a 'good life' in cities. In many cases, especially among transport studies, a quantitative approach to studying mobility and wellbeing prevails. For example, existing research has found a statistical association between indicators of out-of-home activities, trip-making, availability of transport and unfulfilled transport needs, on the one hand, and measures of wellbeing, on the other (e.g. Banister & Bowling, 2004; Cvitkovich & Wister, 2001; Mollenkopf et al., 2005; Spinney et al., 2009). Such quantitative studies are not, of course, unrelated to the above-discussed calculative understanding of 'wellbeing' as a set of indicators for 'subjective' or 'objective' wellbeing. Within this context, travel satisfaction – also conceptualised as 'customer satisfaction' (see Ettema et al., 2010) – appears as a key unit of measurement. Such discourses on 'satisfaction' also reinforce a hedonic understanding of wellbeing that primarily adopts an individualistic, pleasure-seeking and consumption-centred approach to mobility. However, they also seem to prioritise a focus on certain transport modes (e.g. public transport, the car), while paying less attention to other transport modes (e.g. cycling, walking) or other mobility patterns (e.g. Information and Communication Technologies).

So, how about moving towards a more 'eudaimonic' approach to wellbeing for the study of mobility? How about developing a more qualitative and bottom-up understanding of the correlations between wellbeing and mobility in cities? John Urry's Mobilities paradigm is key for developing a more qualitative and holistic approach to the study of mobility, not only by realising the wellbeing aspects of mobility, but also for reinforcing a more 'social' understanding of wellbeing for the study of mobility in cities by attending to the social relations that can be afforded between people and places that are physically distant. Of course, here, the concept of immobility is also important, highlighting the centrality of questions of access and inclusion in the study of Mobilities for wellbeing. In order to understand the interconnections of mobility and wellbeing, we also need to pay more attention to non-movement, as well as explore the interconnections between movement and non-movement – for example, the ways a person's movement can also impede the movement of others.

Existing studies on mobility and wellbeing have also attempted to develop a more qualitative understanding of such interconnections. Such studies primarily focus on movement in physical space in order to explore its role in fulfilling basic human needs, as well as meeting others or visiting places (e.g. Metz, 2000; Psarikidou, 2018). Due to a primary concern with mobility for the elderly, in many cases, immobility has also explored in the context of the physical affordances of a person to move and the subsequent implications on the elderly's every day out-of-home movement. Within this context, a narrow focus on 'the car' as an indicator of wellbeing also prevails. Driving cessation has been variously discussed as an important event with significant wellbeing implications for the elderly, in terms of both fulfilling basic needs and meeting others (Adler & Rottunda 2006; Marottoli et al., 1997; Ragland et al., 2005). In the context, perceptions of wellbeing have been associated with feelings of independence, self-confidence and autonomy, as well as sense of community-belonging, socialisation and social inclusion (e.g. Allen, 2008; Davey, 2007; Mollenkopf et al., 2011; Psarikidou, 2020; Smith et al., 2002).

This chapter is inspired by the above theoretical and empirical frameworks in order to develop a more multifaceted analysis of Mobilities and wellbeing in cities, based on both hedonic and eudaimonic approaches to wellbeing (Christie, 1998; O'Neill, 2006). It specifically focusses on research conducted for the EPSRC Liveable Cities programme in the city of Birmingham, one of the largest and most car-dependent cities in the UK.

Mobilities for Wellbeing in our Research

Birmingham as a 'Liveable City'? Nowadays, an increasing number of cities aspire to be 'liveable cities'. Every year different cities compete to be *the most* liveable city. Every year they develop their own criteria and indices of liveability to be met by themselves and others. As a result, every year not only do we come across different lists of liveable cities, but also different definitions of liveable cities, as well as different indicators under which cities can be considered as 'liveable' (e.g. The Economist, 2017). Of course, this trend is not unrelated to the above-discussed narrow, calculative approach to wellbeing, which also reinforces a reductionist approach to the definition of 'liveable cities' (please see also Section 'Wellbeing: a contested concept').

Although the aim of this chapter is not to provide an overview of different definitions of 'liveable cities', it is worth identifying if there are any common frameworks of thought in the definition of 'liveability' in cities. However, according to some official research and policy web resources, 'liveable cities' are described as 'places that people want to live', 'places that promote healthy and happy people and community wellbeing', 'healthy cities promoting health, wellbeing and equity', and 'good life in a healthy city' (see the Conversation, 2018; Davern et al., 2018). From the above, we understand that 'good life' and 'wellbeing' become key words in defining 'liveability'. And, considering the contested nature of the concept of 'wellbeing' itself, an ambiguity with regard to the concept of 'liveable cities' becomes inevitable. However, what we also understand is the centrality of 'mobility' in the materialisation of the above visions of a 'liveable city' (Davern et al., 2018; see also www.sharedmobilityprinciples.org).

Birmingham is an interesting city for researching wellbeing and mobility in cities. With the largest population in the UK outside London, Birmingham is the sixth most deprived local authority in the UK, with 40% of the population living in the 10% most deprived areas in the country and 44.3% of the population being economically inactive (Birmingham City Council, 2013a). At the same time, Birmingham is a very car-centric and car-dependent city.[3] Its historic, economic dependence on car manufacturing not only contributed significantly to the wider, socio-spatial organisation of the city around the car (Cherry, 1994), it also carries important wellbeing implications for the local population. On the one hand, it provided a source of income and employment for the local population. On the other hand, in more recent times, its decline signalled a rise of unemployment and economic deprivation across the city. Such correlations between wellbeing and mobility are also obvious in different local policy and transport documents. Again, the car is the dominant mobility pattern with an impact on local people's wellbeing. It appears as a key indicator of liveability that not only provided a source of employment in the past, but is also the key mode for accessing employment in the present. Car ownership is also an indicator for measuring deprivation in cities, with 36% of households in the city not owning a car or van (Centro, 2011). Despite a reported increase of car ownership in Birmingham, fuel and transport poverty – also due to rising prices of oil and public transport fares – remain important indicators of inequalities and immobilities – both physical and social – across the city (Birmingham City Council, 2013b).

A correlation between deprivation and car ownership was also prevalent in our research. The car was the dominant mode of transport in areas of low deprivation, despite the local residents' environmental concerns and low-carbon aspirations. On the contrary, public transport (especially the bus) was reported as the key mode of transport for residents of high-deprivation areas, despite their personal aspirations to own and drive a car. Thus, for both resident groups, the car was a symbol of 'good life'. It appeared as a signifier of 'distinction' and social status (Bourdieu, 1984) that was not unrelated to modern 'consumer culture' and its dominant, hedonic understanding of 'wellbeing' (Bauman, 2000). Here, social stigma (Goffman, 1963) of different transport modes is also important for understanding as well as explaining people's aspirations for, or disassociations from, certain modes of transport. For example, in our research, the higher car insurance fees in high-deprivation areas were due to the stigmatisation of such areas as areas of higher criminality. And, such stigmatising assumptions were key for turning 'the car' into a symbol of social status and an object for aspiration among residents of high-deprivation areas. However, in low-deprivation areas, the social stigma of 'dirt' and 'unsafety' attributed to public transport were important factors for high car use rates in such areas. Recent, local public transport authorities' plans reiterate such ideas of social stigma of the existing public transport. In order to encourage wider public transport use, they plan to introduce the new luxurious 'platinum bus' across Birmingham, equipped with high-quality seating and special services for combatting crime (e.g. lighting and CCTV cameras) (see National Express West Midlands, 2015).

Thus, our research in Birmingham has helped us understand that changing people's mobility patterns towards a more low-carbon direction without compromising current levels of wellbeing is a much more complex challenge. In the case of car-centric Birmingham, it is not only about how we can get people out of the car, without affecting their current levels of wellbeing, it is also about how we can change their current perceptions and aspirations of wellbeing that are currently associated with certain modes of transport. Or else, putting it more broadly, it was about identifying ways to move from a hedonic, consumerist and pleasure-seeking framework of wellbeing to a more eudaimonic approach to wellbeing and mobility in cities.

Mobility and Wellbeing in Birmingham

For the Liveable Cities project, we organised a series of focus groups in wards with contrasting levels of deprivation. As discussed above, in our research, deprivation appeared not only as an interesting indicator for 'wellbeing', but also as an interesting socio-demographic characteristic shaping people's perceptions of 'good life' in their cities. We believed that a comparative analysis between high- and low-deprivation areas would help us better understand the connection between deprivation and wellbeing, but also further investigate the role of mobility in shaping such perceptions of wellbeing. In other words, we believed that this distinction would be important for understanding how people's perceptions of a 'good life' are affected by the mobility options that are accessible by them and the areas in which they live.

Drawing on different conceptualisations of wellbeing, we were interested in developing a more qualitative, bottom-up understanding of wellbeing that would be based on people's descriptive narratives and perceptions of 'good life'. We thus asked people to give us an overview of different practices that contribute to their 'good life' in cities. We specifically asked people from wards with different levels of deprivation what they do and they like doing. By doing so, we were interested in encompassing a broad utilitarian approach to wellbeing, perceived both as fulfilment of basic needs and as satisfaction of personal preferences and desires (see Metz, 2000). Research participants provided us with a long list of practices that are linked to their experiences and perceptions of 'good life'. We call such practices as 'practices of wellbeing' which can be divided into three categories:

- Everyday practices linked to their basic livelihood and health needs (e.g. work, doing the school run, going to school/other classes; shopping; walking; visiting doctors);

- Everyday/common leisure practices conduced frequently in the city (e.g. going out for coffee, volunteering, attending local community groups, visiting the library, attending sports/dance or other activities, going to cinema or concerts, drumming, jogging, cycling);
- More unusual practices linked to their experiences of good life, also going beyond the boundaries of the city (e.g. visiting family in other cities, travelling elsewhere for bird-watching, photography, butterfly-watching, going on holiday).

As becomes prevalent in this list, there is a convergence between hedonic and eudaimonic traditions in what makes a 'good life'. Research participants described practices that focus on the individual's personal satisfaction as a key criterion for pursuing a 'good life' (e.g. shopping, bird-watching, jogging). However, the majority of practices reveal a more 'social' and 'relational' approach through which wellbeing is achieved in the context of 'being with' others (e.g. visiting family, going out, meeting friends, etc.). Such 'practices of wellbeing' can again be clustered into two different categories depending on their contribution to the wellbeing of an individual or the society. For example, some research participants reported their active engagement and meetingness with others as a means towards their individual, personal wellbeing (e.g. going on holiday). However, for some others, the very same practices could go beyond an individualistic focus, constituting practices of political acts and purposeful engagement in society as a whole (e.g. volunteering, attending community groups and social activities) (see Hetherington, 1998; Szerszynski, 2005).

The role of mobilities was also key in understanding people's perceptions and experiences of wellbeing in cities. Drawing on current studies on mobility and wellbeing, we were also interested in finding out more about how people travel in order to accomplish their 'practices of wellbeing'. In this context, an instrumental approach to mobility prevailed through which mobility was mainly considered as 'a means' to a 'good life' that was usually accomplished through undertaking another practice at the end destination. Of course, as described above, such practices could vary in terms of their relation to wellbeing. Some of them could have an individual focus, while others a societal focus; some of them would follow a more hedonic approach, while others, a more eudaimonic approach to wellbeing (e.g. work, shopping, volunteering, meeting friends).

However, in our research, mobility seemed to go beyond an instrumental role for wellbeing. In many cases, research participants described the intrinsic value of mobility as a 'practice of wellbeing' itself. For example, mobility practices, such as walking and cycling, have been considered as practices with a direct implication on people's wellbeing. Research participants have specifically described the aesthetic and personal health benefits of both walking and cycling. In this context, motility was also discussed as a significant contributor to people's experiences of wellbeing. For example, people discussed how being physically able or affording to move could change their overall experiences of wellbeing.

Also, despite their primary, instrumental role, some mobility practices could also be perceived as 'practices of wellbeing'. The example of 'going on holiday' is indicative towards such a direction. On the one hand, participants described travelling to the airport only as a means for getting closer to their holidays. On the other hand, some other participants described their journey as also part of their holidays, and thus as significant part of their experience and perception of wellbeing (see Figures 3.1 and 3.2).

The comparison of these two journeys allows us to make some interesting observations about the interconnections of mobility, wellbeing and deprivation.

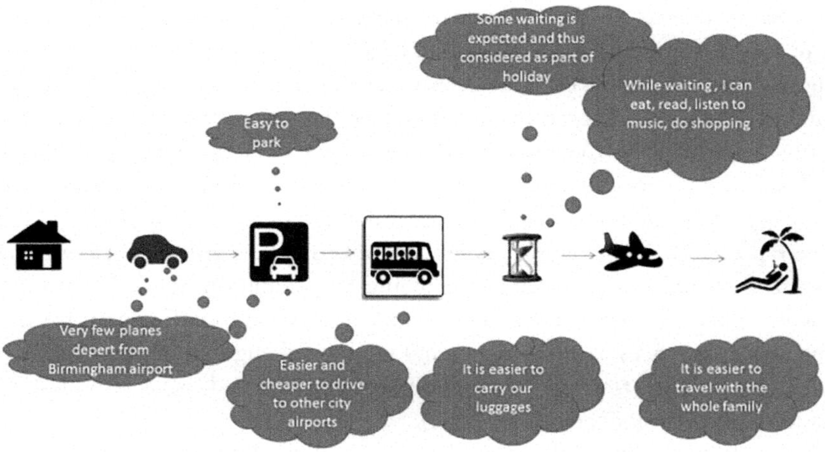

FIGURE 3.1 Travelling to the airport by car.
Source: Author.

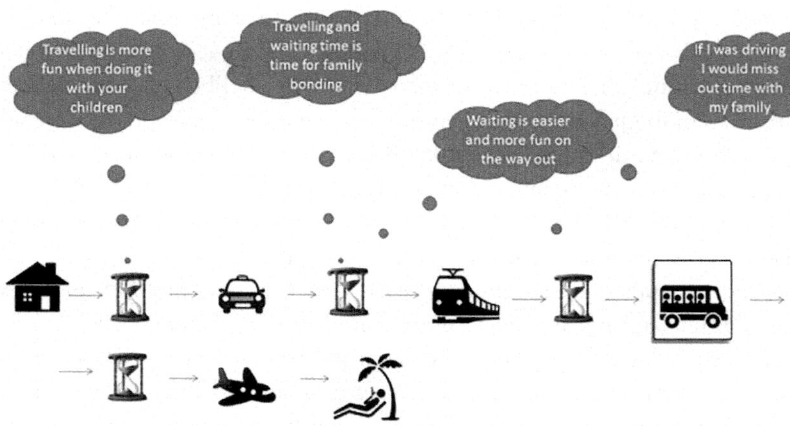

FIGURE 3.2 Travelling to the airport by train.
Source: Author.

First, a car/public transport divide still prevails. This confirms the above discussion about the car being the dominant transport mode in low-deprivation areas, as opposed to public transport being commonly used in high-deprivation areas. However, both participants gave positive expressions of wellbeing in relation to their mobility patterns. In the case of the car, convenience and speed were discussed as key contributors to participant's wellbeing, whereas fun family time during travelling was discussed by the second participant as a significant contributor to their wellbeing that would also compensate for the possible longer duration and slower speed of their journey. Thus, we understand that a possibility to change people's mobility patterns is possible if people change their approaches to different mobility practices and identify the ways they can contribute to their experience of 'good life' in cities. Thus, based on this example, a shift from the car to public transport can be possible if people value their alternative differently and appreciate the ways it can contribute to their wellbeing. However, we understand that, in order for such a shift to take place, we also need to change dominant perceptions of 'good life', and move from a hedonic to a more eudaimonic approach to wellbeing. Looking again at the above example, driving the car is described as an individualistic practice, also linked to the research participant's personal satisfaction at the end destination. However, a more 'social' approach to wellbeing becomes obvious in the description of the train journey. The research participant not only described the train journey as part of their wider experience of wellbeing, but also described it as an experience of wellbeing that can only be materialised socially, that is, while being with others.

A more social approach to wellbeing is also essential for overcoming immobilities in cities. Our research helped us understand that movement does relate not only to our movement, but also to the movement of others around us. This was very evident in the examples of the 'school run', where walking the kids to school or walking the dog were also important parts that shape the way our movement relates to the wellbeing of others around us, but also the way we move can have an impact on the way that others move. It revealed that our movement can facilitate, change, reduce or impede the movement of others; and, the movement of others can also have a significant impact on the way we move or not move. Such observations encourage us to move beyond an individualist approach to movement. However, they also encourage us to move beyond an individualist approach to wellbeing, too. They help us understand that our movement is not only about our wellbeing, but also the wellbeing of others around us. Furthermore, other people's movement or need to move is not only about those people's wellbeing, but also about the wellbeing of others around them. Thus, once more, it has helped us realise the significance of 'the social' in understanding both mobility and wellbeing in cities, that is, in order for people to choose the ways they move, they also need to think of their movement in the wider context of society and consider the implications of their movement on the movement and the wellbeing of themselves and others.

Conclusions: Hedonism or Eudaimonism?

This chapter attempted to unpack the diverse and complex interconnections between Mobilities and wellbeing in cities. More specifically, it focussed on contributing to emerging debates over how we can transform mobility systems in cities without compromising people's experiences of wellbeing in cities. However, the chapter also pointed out that, in order to do so, we first need to better understand what we mean by 'wellbeing', and how this links to the idea of 'mobilities' in cities. It has argued that a narrow, calculative, individualistic and consumerist logic to wellbeing prevails, and that this is also manifested in dominant instrumental approaches to the role of 'mobilities' in the pursuit of a 'good life'. Moreover, this chapter has opened up to a more multifaceted, qualitative analysis of wellbeing and mobilities in cities, based on both hedonic/individual and eudaimonic/social approaches to wellbeing (Christie, 1998; O'Neil, 2006). It has drawn on research in the city of Birmingham, one of the most car-dependent cities in the UK, with some of the highest rates of deprivation and unemployment in the country.

Our research revealed that there is a multiple and complex convergence between hedonic and eudaimonic traditions that shape people's perceptions of wellbeing, and thus their mobility patterns in cities. First, it has helped us to understand that mobility practices are not only means towards other 'practices of wellbeing' (e.g. work, meeting friends, bird-watching), but also 'practices of wellbeing', themselves (e.g. walking, cycling). Second, it raised the significance of 'motility' as an enabler of wellbeing, that is, the significance of knowing that you are 'able to move', even when you are not 'on the move'. Furthermore, it has pointed our attention to a more holistic understanding of 'wellbeing' within the context of mobilities in cities. Thus, we realised that, although research participants' descriptive narratives revealed an individualistic approach to 'wellbeing', most of these practices are, at the same time, 'social', that is accomplished through, or while, being with others. And, although some of these 'social' 'practices of wellbeing' are accomplished within the context of an individualistic logic to wellbeing (e.g. for personal satisfaction), some others meet the principles of a more eudaimonic approach to wellbeing (e.g. for human flourishing through purposeful engagement and contribution to society).

Thus, our analysis has helped us realise that a more holistic approach to wellbeing is necessary for re-designing mobility systems in cities without compromising people's current levels of wellbeing. It has also pointed our attention to the significance of the relatively ignored social dimension of wellbeing for designing mobility systems. In other words, it has helped us realise that we need to develop a more qualitative approach to wellbeing that can be based on people's descriptive narratives of wellbeing and thus go beyond a series of indicators measuring 'liveability' in cities. Such qualitative understandings of wellbeing are also important for reframing our questions and challenges in ways that would meet people's needs and achieve sustainable mobilities for liveable cities. In order to develop mobilities for wellbeing in the cities, we should be asking, 'How we can change people's mobility patterns without affecting their levels of wellbeing?'

However, we should also be asking: 'how we can change people's perceptions and aspirations of wellbeing that are currently associated with certain mobility patterns?', and 'how can we make people realise the wellbeing potential of other mobility practices in their lives in cities?' Of course, for such a change to take place, a shift from a purely hedonic to a more eudaimonic approach to wellbeing is pivotal: an approach that underlines the significance of 'the social' and 'the relational' in understanding and experiencing both mobility and wellbeing, and thus researching and designing 'sustainable mobilities for liveable cities'.

Notes

1 By *Mobilities,* I hereby refer to the concept introduced by John Urry to describe a wider set of movements of people, objects, information and ideas (Urry, 2007).
2 Transport Studies refer to an interdisciplinary field that focusses solely on transport for the study of mobility. Mobilities research refers to the interdisciplinary research area pioneered by the Sociologist, John Urry, referring to the wider set of corporeal, physical, imaginative, communicative and virtual movements that we need to consider for the study mobility (see Urry, 2007).
3 According to recent statistics, car use amounts to 42.2% of daily journeys, followed by bus with 29.2%, rail 27%, metro and cycling less than 2% (Centro, 2011).

References

Adler, G., & Rottunda, G. (2006). Older Adults' Perspectives on Driving Cessation. *Journal of Aging Studies*, 20 (3), p227–235.

Allen, J. (2008). Older People and Wellbeing. Institute for Public Policy Research, London. Retrieved 20 June 2018. Available online at https://www.ippr.org/files/images/media/files/publication/2011/05/older_people_and_wellbeing_1651.pdf

Amin, A., & Thrift, N. (2002). *Cities: Reimagining the Urban*. Cambridge: Polity Press.

Banister, D., & Bowling, A. (2004). Quality of Life for the Elderly: The Transport Dimension. *Transport Policy,* 11, p105–115.

Bauman, Z. (2000). *Liquid Modernity*. Cambridge: Polity Press.

Birmingham City Council. (2013a). *Birmingham Carbon Plan Analysis: An Illustrative Look at Future Emissions in Birmingham*. Available online at www.birmingham.gov.uk. Accessed on 25 August 2013.

Birmingham City Council. (2013b). *Changing Gear. Transforming Urban Movement Through Cycling and Walking in Birmingham*. A Report from Overview and Scrutiny. Available online at http://www.pushbikes.org.uk/dnl/changinggear.pdf. Accessed on 15 September 2013.

Bourdieu, P. (1984). *Distinction: A Social Critique of the Judgement of Taste*. Trl. by Richard Nic. London: Harvard College, Routledge and Kegan Paul.

Bruni, L., & Porta, P. L. (Eds.). (2005). *Economics and Happiness, Framing the Analysis*. Oxford: Oxford University Press.

Cass, N., Shove, E., & Urry, J. (2005). Social Exclusion, Mobility and Access. *Sociological Review*, 53(3), p539–555.

Centro. (2011). *Annual Statistical Report 2011*. Available online at http://www.centro.org.uk/. Accessed on 20 August 2013.

Cherry, G. E. (1994). *Birmingham: A Study in Geography, History, and Planning*. Belhaven World Cities Series. Chichester: Wiley.

Christie, I. & Nash, E. (1998). *The Good Life*. London: DEMOS Publishing Creative Commons.

Cvitkovich, Y., & Wister, A. (2001). The Importance of Transportation and Prioritization of Environmental Needs to Sustain Wellbeing among Older Adults. *Environment and Behaviour,* 33, p809–829.

Davern, M., Higgs, C., Boulange, C., Arundel, J., Gunn, L., & Roberts, R. (2018). Rail Access Improves Liveability, but All Regional Centres are Not Equal. *The Conversation.* Available online at https://theconversation.com/rail-access-improves-liveability-but-all-regional-centres-are-not-equal-96462. Accessed on 20 June 2018.

Davey, J. A. (2007). Older People and Transport: Coping Without a Car. *Ageing & Society,* 27(1), p49–65.

Diener, E. (2009) Subjective Wellbeing. In E. Diener (Ed.) The Science of Wellbeing: *The Collected Works of Ed Diener* (p11–58). Dordrecht: Springer.

Dolan, P., Peasgood, T., & White, M. (2006). *Review of the Research on the Influences on Personal Wellbeing and Application to Policy Making.* Report to DEFRA, London.

Duarte, A., Garcia, C., Giannarakis, G., Limão, S., Polydoropoulou, A., & Litinas, N. (2010). New Approaches in Transportation Planning: Happiness and Transport Economics. *Netnomics,* 11, p5–32.

Ettema, D., Gärling, T., Olsson, L. E., & Friman, M. (2010). Out-of-Home Activities, Daily Travel, and Subjective Wellbeing. *Transportation Research Part A: Policy and Practice,* 44, p723–732.

Freudendal-Pedersen, M. (2009). *Mobility in Daily Life. Between Freedom and Unfreedom.* Farnham: Ashgate.

Galloway, S., Birkin, N., Hamilton, C., Bell, D., & Petticrew, M. (2006). *Quality of Life and Wellbeing: Measuring the Benefits of Culture and Sport—A Literature Review.* Edinburgh: Scottish Executive. Available online at http://www.scotland.gov.uk/Resource/Doc/89281/0021350.pdf. Accessed on 15 March 2018.

Goffman, E. (1963). *Stigma.* London: Penguin.

Hetherington, K. (1998). *Expressions of Identity: Space, Performance, Politics.* Thousand Oaks, CA: Sage.

Hird, S. (2003). *What Is Wellbeing? A Brief Review of the Literature and Concepts.* Edinburgh: NHS Scotland.

Marks, N., & Thompson, S. (2008). *Measuring Wellbeing in Policy: Issues and Applications.* London: New Economics Foundation.

Marottoli, R. A., Mendes de Leon, C. F., Glass, T. A., & Williams, C. S. (1997). Driving Cessation and Increased Depressive Symptoms: Prospective Evidence from the New Haven EPESE. *Journal of the American Geriatrics Society,* 45, p202–206.

Metz, D. (2000). Mobility of Older People and Their Quality of Life. *Transport Policy,* 7(2), p149–152.

Mollenkopf, H., Hieber, A., & Wahl, H.-W. (2011). Continuity and Change in Older Adults' Perceptions of Out-of-Home Mobility Over Ten Years: A Qualitative-Quantitative Approach. *Ageing & Society,* 31, p782–802.

Mollenkopf, H., Marcellini, F., Ruoppila, I., Széman, Z., & Tacken, M. (2005). *Enhancing Mobility in Later Life: Personal Coping, Environmental Resources and Technical Support. The Out-of-Home Mobility of Older Adults in Urban and Rural Regions of Five European Countries.* Amsterdam: IOS Press.

National Express West Midlands. (2015). Welcome to Platinum. Available online at http://nxbus.co.uk/west-midlands/information/welcome-to-platinum. Accessed on 15 December 2015.

Nordbakke, S., & Schwanen, T. (2014). Wellbeing and Mobility: A Theoretical Framework and Literature Review Focusing on Older People. *Mobilities,* 9(1), p104–129.

Nussbaum, M. (2000). *Women and Human Development: The Capabilities Approach.* Cambridge: Cambridge University Press.

O'Neill, J. (1993). *Ecology Policy and Politics: Human Wellbeing and the Natural World*. London: Routledge.

O'Neill, J. (2006). Citizenship, Wellbeing and Sustainability: Epicurus or Aristotle? *Analyse & Kritik*, 28, p158–172.

Phillips, D. (2006). *Quality of Life: Concept, Policy and Practice*. London: Routledge.

Psarikidou, K. (2018). Towards a 'meaning'-ful analysis of the temporalities of mobility practices: Implications for Sustainability. In A. Hui, R. Day and G. Walker (Eds.). *Demanding energy: Spaces, temporalities and change* (pp. 99–119). Cham: Palgrave MacMillan.

Psarikidou, K. (2020). Em-'powering' niche innovations: Learning from cycling inequalities. *Applied Mobilities*. DOI: https://doi.org/10.1080/23800127.2020.1723386

Ragland, D. R., Satariano, W. A., & MacLeod, K. E. (2005). Driving Cessation and Increased Depressive Symptoms. *The Journals of Gerontology Series A: Biological Sciences and Medical Sciences*, 60, p399–403.

Rapley, M. (2003). *Quality of Life Research: A Critical Introduction*. London: Sage.

Reid, L., & Hunter, C. (2011). *Personal Wellbeing and Interactions with Nature*. BeWEL: Behaviour for Wellbeing, Environment & Life. State of Understanding Report I. Available online at www.esrc.ac.uk. Accessed on 20 March 2018.

Ringen, S. (1995). Wellbeing, Measurement, and Preferences. *Acta Sociologica*, 38, p3–15.

Sayer, A. (2004). *Restoring the Moral Dimension: Acknowledging Lay Normativity*. Research paper, Department of Sociology, Lancaster University.

Sheller, M., & Urry, J. (Eds.). (2006). *Mobile Technologies of the City*. London: Routledge.

Shove, E., Pantzar, M., &Watson, M. (2012). *The Dynamics of Social Practice. Everyday Life and How It Changes*. London: Sage.

Sims, R., Schaeffer, R., Creutzig, F., Cruz-Núñez, X., D'Agosto, M., Dimitriu, D., Figueroa Meza, M. J., Fulton, M. J., Kobayashi, S., Lah, O., McKinnon, A., Newman, P., Ouyang, M., Schauer, J. J., Sperling, D., & Tiwari, G. (2014). Transport. In O. R. Edenhofer Pichs-Madruga, Y. Sokona, E. Farahani, S. Kadner, K. Seyboth, A. Adler, I. Baum, S. Brunner, P. Eickemeier, B. Kriemann, J. Savolainen, S. Schlömer, C. von Stechow, T. Zwickel, & J. C. Minx (Eds.), *Climate Change 2014: Mitigation of Climate Change. Contribution of Working Group III to the Fifth Assessment Report of the Intergovernmental Panel on Climate Change*. Cambridge and New York: Cambridge University Press. Available online at https://www.ipcc.ch/site/assets/uploads/2018/02/ipcc_wg3_ar5_chapter8.pdf. Accessed on 1 October 2017.

Smith, J., Borchelt, M., Maier, H., & Jopp, D. (2002). Health and Wellbeing in the Young Old and Oldest Old. *Journal of Social Issues*, 58 (4), p715–732.

Spinney, J. E. L., Scott, D. M., & Newbold, K. B. (2009). Transport Mobility Benefits and Quality of Life: A Time-Use Perspective of Elderly Canadians. *Transport Policy*, 16, p1–16.

Szerszynski, B. (2005). *Nature, Technology and the Sacred*. Oxford: Blackwell.

The Conversation. (2018). Articles on Liveable Cities. Available online at http://theconversation.com/global/topics/liveable-cities-23433. Accessed on 20 June 2018.

The Economist. (2017). Global Liveability has Improved for the First Time in a Decade. Available online at https://www.economist.com/graphic-detail/2017/08/16/global-liveability-has-improved-for-the-first-time-in-a-decade. Accessed on 20 June 2018.

Urry, J. (2007). *Mobilities*. Cambridge: Polity.

Waldron, S. (2010). *Measuring Subjective Wellbeing in the UK*. Working paper for the Office for National Statistics. Publication Office of Public Sector Information.

Weber, M. (1978). *Economy and Society*. Berkeley, CA: University of California Press.

Ziegler, F., & Schwanen, T. (2011). I Like to Go Out to be Energised by Different People: An Exploratory Analysis of Mobility and Wellbeing in Later Life. *Ageing & Society*, 31, p758–781.

4

TRANSPORT AND WELLBEING IN THE FUTURE CITY

Nick Tyler

The 'Creation of Adam', the centrepiece of Michelangelo's cornucopian ceiling for the Sistine Chapel, and the sculpture 'Paolo and Francesca', Rodin's test-piece for the eventual marble sculpture 'La Baisée', raise a similar question. Each displays a moment in time through the disconnect between two people, but leaves unanswered whether the depicted separation takes place before or after the implied connection. The extended sequence of dissonances in Lotti's 'Crucifixus' has a sense of a single direction, exemplifying Bergson's irreversibility of time (Bergson, 1911), but by delaying the resolution to consonance frustrates the sense of satisfaction of completion until the ultimate cadence. That implication of connective completion – whether a connection has just happened, or if it is about to happen, and the sense of release when this question is finally resolved and the act finally comes to completion – is an important feature of the way in which a human city, and in particular its transport system, works.

For a city is all about connections, and the transport system is the means by which such connections are enabled. Given the complexity of cities as they have evolved, and the costs and complexity of the transport systems we have developed over the past few hundred years, how we may be able to deliver wellbeing in a future city is going to depend on how we understand that relationship between the transport system that connects and the city that is based on separation. At its heart will be the way in which we understand and resolve separation and connection and the role that is played by time, and its perception by the people in the city. Transport not only connects, but also separates: we do not know whether the frisson in Paolo's hand is anticipation of an illicit touch, or the shiver of curtailed contact, yet for us as an observer of the work of art, the outcome is pleasure, enjoyment and satisfaction: is it possible to make a transport system that also provides such senses in the way it resolves that gap between people coming together, or parting their ways? The seeking of wellbeing implies moving above the merely technical service base of a transport system into something that speaks to the higher order of human needs, and, if a future city is to thrive, rather than be just 'liveable', it needs its main means of connection to function at such a higher level. The questions of Michelangelo, Rodin and Lotti need to be answered by the designers of the transport system if such a state of wellbeing is to be achieved.

To explore how the transport system might evolve to create, or at least facilitate, a state of human wellbeing in a city, I will examine the transport for a future city from the perspective of the person, then the city itself and finally the implications of these for the design of the transport system. The transport system is crucial to the city and its people, but it must serve not to dominate; to achieve the objective, it is essential to have a clear view of the people and how they function, how the city serves their function and thus how the transport system could enable both to reach their full potential.

The Person

Of course, cities are people and, by definition, they contain a lot of people. Too often, we consider cities in terms of their overall population and treat the people as simply members of an amorphous crowd. We ask, 'How do we enable millions of people to travel to work and back each day?' without thinking that each of these millions of journeys is made by a single person, with their single needs and single set of constraints. So one place to start thinking about the future city is to understand how a person looks at their world.

A useful model for considering how a person looks at their world is known in neurology as the 'Ecological Brain' (Fuchs, 2018). This is a model of the brain that is based on how the brain functions in the wide world outside the neurological laboratory of brain scanners and abstract tests. In this world, the ecological brain is a summation of the brain itself, with its neurons and synapses, the perceiving person and the environment that they perceive. This is illustrated in Figure 4.1. On the left of this diagram is the 'lived body', which is perceived subjectively by a person, through the lens of their personal history and trajectory of experience over their life until 'this' moment. This also includes how the person sees someone else in a similar role, who has also arrived at 'this' point from their own personal history and experiential trajectory, but who is now enjoying a joint experience with the first person. You can imagine these people as, for example, passengers in a bus or train, in a crowded station, or even just passing each other in the street. Looking at the whole-person in this way is described as a 'Personalistic Attitude'. On the right of the diagram is the 'living body'. This is the composite organism consisting of its physiological structures and processes, as observable by a third

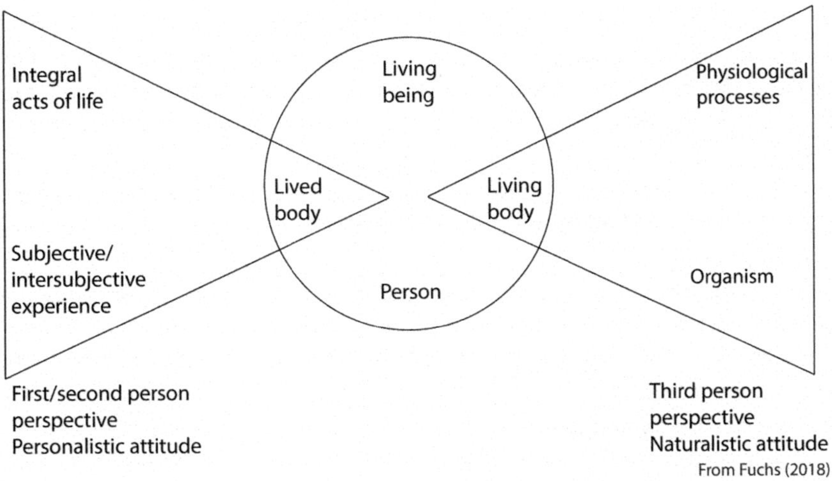

FIGURE 4.1 The dual aspect: personalistic (lived body) vs. naturalistic (living body) perceptions of a person.

Source: Fuchs (2018).

person and is how a person might be seen by someone or something else. This is known as the 'Naturalistic attitude' and characterises the way in which neurologists and others perceive the person. Of course, the actual person is both a lived and living body. For my purposes of considering transport and wellbeing in a future city, I will consider the personalistic, lived body rather than its naturalistic counterpart.

The ecological brain takes the personalistic attitude a stage further and regards the interactions of the person with their environment as being the complete picture of how they perceive the world. This is represented diagrammatically in Figure 4.2. Here, the person is seen as a combination of how they perceive themselves, for example, in a crowd (first or second person), how others see them, for example, an observer of the crowd (third person), and how they perceive and are perceived by the environment (the environment). This consideration of the person is important when thinking about the transport system in the context of wellbeing, because it is this full characterisation of people that we are designing for, including the political element of any intervention that we might choose to make. If there is a disconnect between any of these, we have problems that could be unresolvable, or at least very difficult to solve. For example, poor consideration of the perception between first and second persons could result in anger, frustration and conflicts. The difference in perspective of the third person from the first and second could lead to misinterpretations of intent. Moreover, poor perceptions of the environment could result in malicious treatment of the natural or made world, or in making certain actions, which might be quite legitimate and even desirable, impossible because of environmental constraints (e.g. accessibility issues).

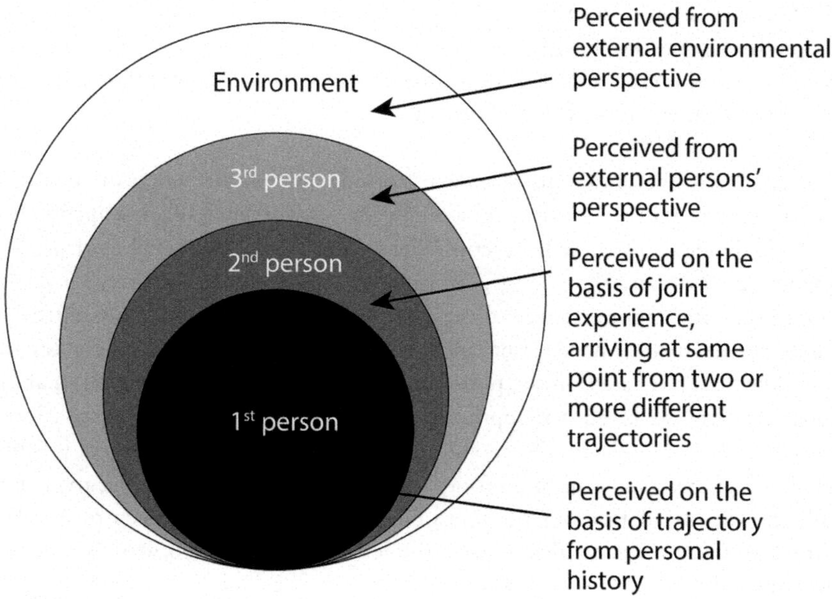

FIGURE 4.2 Ecological brain view of personal perception.
Source: Fuchs (2018).

The City

To understand cities, it is useful to consider examples that have undergone significant changes, where questions of their 'essence' have been raised and approached. One such example is the city of Medellín in Colombia, which has passed from a very difficult period in its history in the 1990s to one of significant success (it won the Lee Kuan Yew World City Prize in 2016). A fuller account of this trajectory and its effect on planning and transport can be found in Dávila et al. (2016). Essentially, Medellín had to shift from a crime-ridden situation, dominated by large-scale drug wars and a civil war, to a city in which people could thrive. We examined this trajectory and encapsulated it in the form of a simple model, which describes five, basic perspectives of a city as a means by which its vision of being a city of, and for, the people could be attained (Tyler, 2013, Ortegon & Tyler, 2015). This can be seen in Figure 4.3. The vision consists of satisfying five perspectives of the city (Ortegon & Tyler, 2018):

1. The city should encourage people to have mutual respect for each other (the 'courteous city')
2. The city should have activities that enable people to thrive and that these should be accessible to everyone (the 'active and inclusive city')
3. The city should have a sense of belonging to its inhabitants and that they should feel responsible for it and its future (the 'public and aesthetic city')

4. The city should promote and deliver health to all its inhabitants and the environment (the 'healthy city')
5. The city should evolve through time to continue to support future generations of inhabitants (the 'evolving city').

The vision described in Figure 4.3 makes considerable requirements on the transport system, and it is interesting to see how the city of Medellín has approached these challenges, which will be considered later in the chapter. For now, it is instructive to discuss the changes brought about by trying to resolve a health issue in one of the poorer areas of the city. This was the issue of poor nutrition, which was deemed to have arisen because of poor access to fresh vegetables and fruit. The area is located on the periphery of the city and, at an altitude of about 2,000 m above sea level, it is approximately 500 m above the main city centre. Following discussions with the people in the area, a collaborative project was initiated, which involved building a footpath ('Camino de la Vida') along an ancient trail, and the installation of a number of buildings (an education centre, a police station) and a series of gardens where the local residents could grow vegetables and fruit. The works were undertaken by the local people with strong support from the city authority, providing training, as well as equipment, so that a future employment track could be developed once the works had been completed. However, the gardens were so successful that more food was grown than could

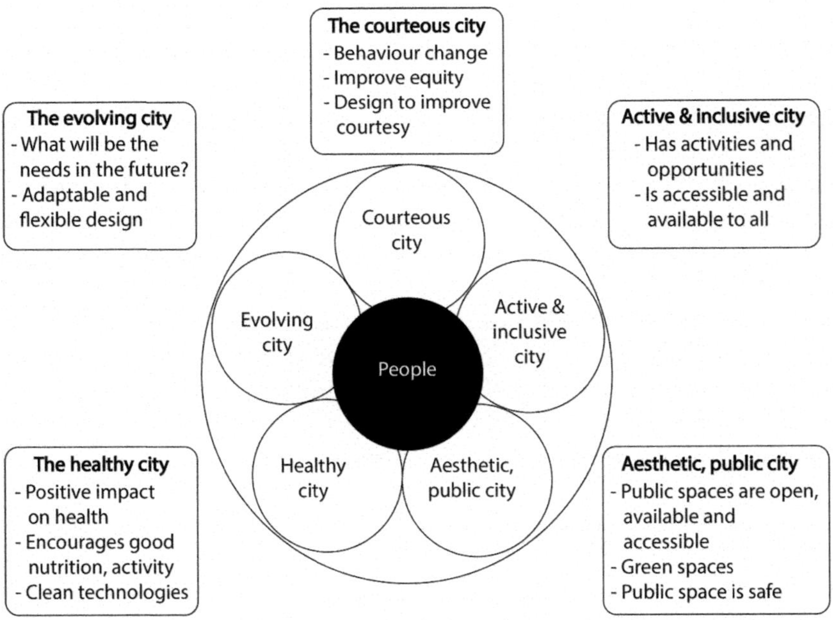

FIGURE 4.3 The five cities model.
Source: Ortegon and Tyler (2018).

be eaten by the local residents, so a project was put in place to make transport to the main city centre easier, in order that the excess food could be sold there. This transport system involved the construction of a cable car for part of the journey and a tramway for the remaining section into the city centre. The tramway was a challenge as it had to be capable of working on a gradient of 13%. In addition, the opportunity was taken to improve the supply of water and sanitation systems to the houses in the area, and to provide the residents with paint and materials, so that they could create a better environmental appearance to suit their wishes.

The tram was conceived to be as much a social space as a means of transport; its technology and capacity are sufficient to enable people to be able to converse. The tram is much quieter than a bus would have been, both for those inside and those outside the vehicle. It was not designed to be an implementation of the ecological brain, but, in fact, it goes quite a long way to showing how this might be applied.

The whole project was fomented on the issue of nutrition, but turned into a consideration of how a personalistic attitude can help understand how people function. This involved thinking about how they perceive themselves and their neighbours (in their homes, in the tram or on the street), which are first- and second-person perspectives; how they are perceived by others, in the sense of the response to the need for casual conversation and what that requires of infrastructure; and how the environment, itself, in the form of artwork and the sense of ownership obtained by passing the decision-making about the artworks to the local people. Although transport is an element of the project, and an important one at that, it is absolutely not a 'transport project'. Regarding this from the perspective of the five cities, we can see the development of improved nutrition (the healthy city); the development of accessible activities, including business, art and walking (active and inclusive city); the increase in the sense of ownership of public space (the aesthetic and public city); the facilitation of casual conversation in and around the tram and cable car system (the courteous city); and the development of a sense of change for the future by enabling education and training, and encouraging involvement in local decision-making (the evolving city). This integration is part and parcel of how a future city needs to evolve and shows how the immersion of transport within a larger perspective of city life leads to an improved sense of wellbeing in the people involved in, and affected by, this investment.

So what can we conclude from this, in terms of the city, its people and transport? The city has people and activities spread around the physical area it occupies. We need to think through how these are connected, not only spatially and temporally, but also functionally. Where people grow their vegetables and fruits and where they can sell them might not be in the same place, so these need to be connected to allow them to conduct their business and to ensure that the opportunity afforded by being able to grow more than they need, can be met. This transition needs to be made available through a transport system. However, the transport system is not just a means of joining A to B. It is a purveyor of public space, able to afford the chance to chat and contribute to the made environment.

The fact is that the city needs to be able to support many things happening at once – the growing and selling of vegetables and other functions of the city coincide in time even though they may happen in different places. That is, they have different needs and these need to be satisfied concurrently. Having said that, it is important that there are spaces between, and away from, the foci of activity – the artwork along the tramway allows for life to pause, people to linger, along the way from growing to selling. The importance of paying attention to the edges of the city is a highly important issue in Medellín, and it is significant that this project took place at the periphery (the drugs cartels made use of the effective absence of city authority in the periphery to impose their own governance over local people and thus gain their footholds on the city and its environs). The sense of continual evolution is delivered in the way in which implementation now has been imbued with education and training for the future, so that the city will evolve well rather than badly and the whole means that one can view the city in many different ways, depending on one's own perspective, time of day, place within the city and activity being undertaken.

Bergson (1911) defined the 'Vital Principle', as a living organism made up of living organisms, where all must be enabled to thrive in order that the organism is able to thrive. For me, the future city needs to be a Vital City, not just liveable, but able to sustain both physical and emotional life and vitality through the ability of all its constituent organisms – organic, physical, sensorial and emotional – to thrive. The need for us to understand how this vitality depends on that frisson between separation and connection is demonstrated in the way we enable people to make those partings and arrivings; thus, how we consider the transport system so that it will be the enabler of the city's vitality. Another take on vitality is to consider the way in which people in a city might thrive and the contribution that the transport system makes to this. Richard Sennett (2018) proposes five 'Open Forms' for a thriving city. A thriving city needs to allow and encourage many things to happen at once ('Synchronous'). It needs to be 'Punctuated', providing a kind of grammar, so that particular places have particular importance for varying reasons. A city must be 'Porous', so that it is alive at the edges and people can pass easily in and out, including not only the physical structures but also sounds and smells. It must be 'Incomplete', allowing for continuous evolution across generations and it must be 'Multiple' in providing many images of the city that can be assembled in different ways.

Putting all this together is really a case of creating a society – the association of all those ecological brains – not only in the public and private spaces of the city, but also while they are on the move, and thus transport lies at the centre of creating that vital city in the future.

Transport

Many cities have grown outwards from an initial centre; as they have done so, they have developed transport systems to cope with the need to connect new places with the old centre. This has reflected technology as time has passed. The City of London was initially essentially a pedestrian city, based on walking, so that the capability of people to turn sharply and change direction is reflected in its street patterns to this day. This network is also good for delivering the chance encounters – these favour businesses based on encounters and it is no surprise that financial transactions became such a strong force in such an environment. To the west of London, in Mayfair, for example, the street network looks very different. This was developed during the seventeenth century, and more particularly the eighteenth century, when the need was to provide access for carriages, so the streets are straighter and the curves more gradual. London has never had the Haussmann effect of a complete, unified, redesign that characterises Paris. There, the street network was redesigned in the late nineteenth century to eradicate the narrow tangle of streets that proved so helpful to the Communards and so difficult for the authorities to deal with them. Wider, straighter streets were harder to barricade and easier for troops and cannons to be moved around. Both cities developed metro systems, and in the case of London, a comprehensive bus network.

In the modern context, the cities have grown, and the transport systems have followed. London is more spread than Paris, but in both cases, radial railways (metros) provide a major transport resource that has stimulated both development and increased commuting opportunities as speeds have increased and the inner city has become overcrowded and/or expensive for many to live. Metros have also been affected by the physical situation, such as ground conditions – why London has hardly any underground metro in the south of the city – but it is often considered that the main function of the transport system of a current 'modern' city is to provide peak-hour access to work. This provides many problems, not least the need to convey large numbers of people from the periphery to the centre within a very limited timeframe: the population of central London increases by around 2.5 million between 7am and 9am every day, and this has a massive effect on the need to provide a high-capacity infrastructure in order to satisfy this apparently insatiable demand. This thinking continues – the investment in Crossrail and the current planning for Crossrail 2 are both responses to relieving congestion on other (mainly rail/metro) lines arising from this demand.

But need this be so in the future? One can certainly ask about the wellbeing of commuters – look at Japan, where all the major cities have extensive metro systems. Japanese culture has a very strong appreciation and value of space. Some of this appreciation is represented behaviourally, in the sense that the space between people is honoured and applied ritualistically in the way people greet each other – typically by bowing. The distance between people is set by the depth of the bow and this is codified and learnt at a very young age. But the Tokyo metro at 8am is characterised by the phenomenon of crowding. Metro trains run with up to seven passengers per square metre (London, e.g. rarely exceeds four passengers per square metre). This has many consequences, but two, in particular, are important here. First, the 'giving up' of the cultural value of personal space ('commuter amnesia') actually means a loss – temporary at the moment – of culture and there has to be a question about the ethics of having a system that requires people to do this every day as part of their daily need to work and survive economically. Second, it is extremely inefficient for the railway to operate in this way. Crowded trains and stations increase the time it takes for people to board and alight trains, and these delays mean that travel times are slower, and more trains are needed to provide the same overall capacity. This is not the way of future wellbeing.

The world of work is changing and the availability of the internet – and in particular, wireless connectivity – means that it is changing. One of the ways it is changing is the location and time of work for many people. This change has still not settled, but in the future we can expect a lot more people to forgo the daily commute and work in different places on different days, according to need or just wanting to be in a different kind of place. This could change several times during a day as well as for different days in the week. Although some work will have to take place at a fixed location, the way in which that is organised could still be very different in terms of when and where people need to travel.

We have seen an interesting shift in the use of cars in recent years. London, Paris and other European cities seem to have seen 'peak car' and now have decreasing levels of car ownership and use. This is an issue raised initially in the work of John Urry (e.g. Lyons & Urry, 2005) and highlighted more recently, for example, by Stapleton et al. (2017) and the work of Peter Jones (2018). However, the rise of cheap gig-economy services, such as Uber and Lyft, are bringing a change in use, especially by younger people, so that journeys previously taken on public mass transport (buses and metros) are now being undertaken in taxi-like services. Some of these journeys would not have happened before the availability of these services. These reflect the fact that a lot of the journeys that people wish to make are not served easily by mass transport, and the concept of aggregation (putting many journeys into one vehicle or service), on which public transport is typically based, is being replaced by a demand that is more diverse in terms of both space and time, which mass transport simply cannot provide.

Added to the 'Uber effect' is the increase in active travel – cycling and walking – that gives freedom of movement for relatively limited distances, but increasingly suited to a more disparate activity base, including in terms of both location and time. So people are prepared to walk or cycle between activities rather than use a vehicle, partly because it is more convenient, partly because it is healthier, partly because it is cheaper and partly because it is more agreeable.

If we look at transport and wellbeing in a future city, it seems clear that the transport paradigm, such as it is, needs to change. This is a real challenge because it is not yet clear just how that change should be effected. The desire for increased spatial and temporal flexibility suggests that massive, high-capacity transport needs to be thought about very carefully indeed so that very expensive investments are not made where they really are not required or desirable. However, current needs for such transport are undoubtedly still there. It leads crucially to the realisation that they key to wellbeing lies in pedestrian activity. It is here that people meet and interact with each other. Designing transport around walking and providing spaces for encounters – small public spaces and parks, good footways, places to sit and chat – provide a strong core on which the other means of transport can build (Tyler, 2015).

It is, therefore, important that we look at what we mean by the future city – and much of this is considered elsewhere in this book – so that we can determine what the transport system should be required to do. However, by looking at our three issues – the person, the city and the transport – we can begin to see what might be needed in the future. The genetic need to socialise has often been lost in the environment of a city, due to the need to deal simultaneously, at a personal level, with many more people than is physiologically possible. The response is to 'switch off' (like the commuter amnesia in Tokyo), often using technology to help us do that – mobile phones, headphones, social media – by freeing us up to choose our own individual 'environment' in which to act, especially during travel. To improve wellbeing, we need to increase the presence of 'weak ties' (e.g. waving to someone on the street one recognises but does not know as a friend or family member), which are known to increase the sense of wellbeing (Joffe & Smith, 2016). We need to increase the sense of lingering (remaining in a place longer than intended), so that people enjoy being in an environment, rather than just moving through it as quickly as possible. We need to provide more opportunities where people are within a relatively small, reachable and accessible area, so that we can reduce the need for movement that, for reasons of distance and convenience, tend to require motorised means of transport. The key is to see people walking in the city as the way to create the interactions that oil the cogs of future society.

We need to think more about accessibility than movement: what and how people can access what they need and want so that needs and desires are met, rather than enforce either non-achievement of what people want and need to do, or the use of complex transport systems in order to achieve them. What are these needs and desires is, of course, an important issue, and these will change for different communities and different times. A useful starting point is to ask people what these are and then work with them to define the priorities in terms of what they need or want access to every day, weekly, monthly, annually, irregularly and so on. It seems to be a good way of creating a transport priority, so that the more frequent needs are met on foot or bicycle, whereas others can be met by a variety of appropriate transport modes, depending on the degree of aggregation available because of multiple, common journeys and the technological constraints of providing this in a sustainable and resilient way.

Overall, this ties into the need for that vision of the city of the future – one in which people are the city – and the infrastructure is needed to enable that is created around them and their needs. Transport is a major enabler of wellbeing, but it can also be a major reducer. We need to view motorised transport as a kind of failure mode: the more we need in order to help people live a higher quality life, the poorer our core society really is. By considering it as a slightly toxic resource, we can invest in a more concentrated way to improve the quality of life and wellbeing for all the inhabitants of a city. Minimising the use of transport will minimise the amount of emissions it generates either at source or elsewhere and we can then concentrate on making the transport system actively work towards improving wellbeing. The Medellín nutrition project is an interesting case where the design was intended to bring a sense of social integration, including making it easier to talk, rest, work and enjoy life, as a major objective of the scheme – and not to see it as a way of moving a large number of people around the city.

An interesting thought to close with is that all the drivers of the tram in Medellín, as well as the drivers of the metro trains and formal buses, are university students. Why? The idea is that these students will be future leaders – in engineering, law, business, medicine, education and so forth – of the city. While they are learning their disciplinary skills and knowledge, they can, by driving the trains, trams and buses, and see and feel the importance of people coming together in the city. 'These people will be my patients', one metro driver (a second-year medical student) told me. The transport system taking us to a sense of wellbeing is one in which we learn about society. Seeing at first hand the importance and value of bringing people together is a strong lesson to learn about a city that only one generation before was a byword for violence, murders and fear. How we can make the transport system become an educational formation of society for the future through the way in which it interacts with the people today is a major challenge, but one we need to address.

Therefore, those questions of connections and separations, of suspensions and resolutions, with which we started this chapter are to be answered by embodying each person's desire and predilection for temporal and spatial connection in the context of their daily life within the city. Transport systems in the future city need to start with a full understanding of people, from the way they perceive and interact individually and collectively with others and the environment around them, and the way in which the city, as an outside observer, perceives them. Then building those connections and easing the separations helps to create that sense of society, the sense of belonging and the way of acting within the city to generate wellbeing. To achieve this, at its heart the city needs people to interact with each other. Transport can contribute to that by building its systems around people walking. This is the easiest way to achieve those weak ties, the interactions and the conversations that will drive wellbeing in the future city.

References

Bergson H. (1911) *Creative Evolution*, Dover Publications (1998), p225–226.

Fuchs T. (2018) *Ecology of the Brain*, Oxford University Press, p79.

Joffe H., Smith N. (2016) City dweller aspirations for cities of the future: How do environmental and personal wellbeing feature? *Cities*, 59, p102–112.

Lyons G., Urry J. (2005) Travel tie use in the digital age, *Transportation Research A*, 39 (2–3), p257–276.

Ortegon A., Tyler N. (2015) Constructing a vision for an 'ideal' future city: A conceptual model for transformative urban planning, *Transportation Research Procedia*, 13, p6–17.

Ortegon A., Tyler N. (2018) *The Little Book of City Principles and Practice,* ImaginationLancaster.

Sennett R. (2018) *Building and Dwelling: The Ethics for the City*, Allen Lane, p205.

Stapleton L., Sorrell S., Schwanen T. (2017) Peak car and increasing rebound: A closer look at car travel trends in Great Britain, *Transportation Research D,* 53, p217–233.

Tyler N. (2013) A vision for cities the 5-city model, *ARGNote,* 1 (5), https://tinyurl.com/5citymodel

Tyler N. (2015) *Accessibility and the Bus System (2nd Edition): Transforming the World*, ICE Publishing.

5

NATURE'S CONTRIBUTION TO HEALTH AND WELLBEING IN THE CITY

Philip James, Konstantinos Tzoulas and Matthew Dennis

Introduction

Biodiverse, vegetation-rich, greenspaces are important in the context of public health in urban environments. Links between residential proximity and equitable access to natural environments have been made with cardiometabolic disorders and emotional wellbeing. Also, there is evidence to support the notion that spending time in nature improves cognitive restoration, decreases oxidative stress and lowers markers of stress physiology and low-grade inflammation.

While the main focus of this chapter will be on the outdoor environment, it must not be overlooked that contact with nature indoors also influences human health. Today, some architects and designers include spaces for luxuriant indoor planting schemes as part of the facilities provided for those who work in or are visiting a building.

Many of the ills affecting urbanites in the beginning of the twenty-first century – cancer, diabetes, obesity and depression – may be explained by an emergent central theory. This theory posits that chronic, low-level inflammation is at the root of the problem and is, in part, a direct consequence of the environment in which people live. This raises the important question of what could be done to improve urban environments.

Emerging from the discussion in this chapter is the view that if the health benefits attributable to contact with nature are to be realised, there needs to be a change in the framing of nature within urban environments. The incorporation of greenspaces for urban environments needs to be repositioned in policy and practice. In this chapter, the discourse around that challenge and a suggested reframing are set out.

Nature

Nature, a noun, is defined as 'the phenomena of the physical world collectively, including plants, animals, the landscape, and other features and products of the earth, as opposed to humans and human creations' (OED, 1998; p. 1235). This definition might appear to present a problem when considering nature in cities; cities are human creations and, by the definition stated here, not included within nature. Such a view is overly simplistic. Nature is to be found between, on and within the buildings and infrastructure that humans create and which form cities. Nature is all pervasive within cities. For example, plants and animals can be found in areas that are remnants of the landscape before the city was constructed; alongside public parks and domestic gardens; growing and living on roofs and walls, and under buildings; and in abandoned, derelict areas.

Long-term modification of nature involves replacing one ecosystem with another (e.g. from wetlands to suburbs; Beichler et al., 2017). Short-term human inputs to nature refer to regular maintenance activities (e.g. pesticides, planting; Beichler et al., 2017). Based on the amounts of human input and modification, nature in cities could be understood as natural (i.e. least human input and modification), managed (e.g. parks, gardens), overbuilt (e.g. grass pavers) or constructed (e.g. green roofs, canals; Beichler et al., 2017).

Health and Wellbeing

Today, health is frequently defined in three ways: the absence of any disease or impairment; a state that allows the individual to adequately cope with all the demands of daily life; and as a state of equilibrium that individuals have established within themselves and with their social and physical environment (Satorius, 2006). The consequences of adopting each definition are considerable. The first definition implies that the medical profession is the only one that can declare an individual free from disease or impairment and, hence, healthy. How an individual feels about his or her state – feeling unwell as a result of an un-diagnosed illness, for example – does not feature in this medical model of health. In the second definition the concept of coping is introduced and with that, one must recognise that there is a wide range regarding coping: some individuals cope with a disease of infirmity very well; others, with no discernible symptoms, cope very poorly. The third definition is focussed on the individual and their internal equilibrium that allows them to get the most from life despite the presence of an illness or infirmity (Satorius, 2006).

The concept of wellbeing is central in concepts of health. Wellbeing can be defined by social, economic or psychological factors, or any combination of such factors (Rioux, 2005). Connectedness to nature is also considered an aspect of wellbeing (Mayer & McPherson-Frantz, 2004). The Millennium Ecosystem Assessment defined wellbeing as the outcome of five interrelated factors:

1. Security – personal safety, secure access to resources and security from disasters;
2. Basic material for a good life – adequate livelihoods, sufficient nutritious food, shelter, access to goods;
3. Health – strength, feeling well, access to clean air and water;
4. Good social relationships – social cohesion, mutual respect, ability to help others;
5. Freedom of choice and action – opportunity to be able to achieve what an individual values doing and being (Millennium Ecosystem Assessment, 2003).

This multi-faceted definition illustrates the range of issues that are brought together within the concept of wellbeing and indicates that many factors need to be addressed in order to promote wellbeing within cities.

Linking Nature with Health and Wellbeing

So far, we have examined the concepts of nature, health and wellbeing separately. It is time now to draw these together and explore how nature affects the health and wellbeing of those living and working in cities (Sandifer et al., 2015). Rather than seeing these as two separate systems, with nature set apart from human health and wellbeing, it is possible to conceptualise the two elements together as part of a social-ecological system (McGinnis & Ostrom, 2014). Within such a system, ecosystems provide services and disservices which benefit or are detrimental to humans (Döhren & Haase, 2015). According to this conceptualisation, the concept of ecosystem services becomes central to integrating the social and ecological aspects of human health and wellbeing.

Within the Millennium Ecosystem Assessment (2003) a clear link is established between ecosystem services and constituents of wellbeing. Within that report, for example, it is pointed out how flood regulation (an ecosystem service) affects security, basic materials for a good life and health (three constituents of wellbeing). Similarly, the provision of fresh water affects security and basic material for a good life. Many other examples could be given of these links, examples which would serve to indicate the integration of social-ecological systems whereby ecosystem (dis-)services affect humans who, in turn, affect the ecosystem services.

Ecosystem services can be delivered by passive, or indirect, and active, or direct routes (Berman et al., 2008; Bolund & Hunhammer, 1999; Bowler et al., 2010; Dallimer et al., 2012; Fuller et al., 2007; Larson et al., 2014; McPherson, 1994; Mitchell, 2013; Shanahan et al., 2015) (Table 5.1).

Greenspace within cities is an example of an ecosystem service that can be delivered, and benefits humans, in different ways. First, it improves individuals' short-term psychological health, cognitive functioning and stress levels. Over a longer-term, these beneficial health impacts may translate to greenspace

TABLE 5.1 Passive/direct and active/indirect ecosystem services associated with domestic greenspace

	Description	*Examples*
Passive or indirect ecosystem services	Can be delivered via pathways that do not require people to engage actively with the natural environment – services provided even when a person is not in the greenspace.	Climate regulation Privacy Noise reduction Screening from unwanted views Flood mitigation
Active or direct ecosystem services	Delivered via pathways requiring people to actively engage with the natural environment. This requires people to spend time in the greenspace, and experiences and benefits derived are dependent on the behavioural patterns of a person and the characteristics of the vegetation.	Gardening activities Sitting in the greenspace Play activities

Based on McPherson (1994), Fuller et al. (2007); Berman et al. (2008), Bowler et al. (2010), Dallimer et al. (2012), Mitchell (2013), Larson et al. (2014), Shanahan et al. (2015).

Source: Authors.

reducing chronic disease and illness. Empirical, theoretical and anecdotal evidence demonstrates positive impacts on blood pressure, cholesterol, outlook on life and stress reduction (Hartig et al., 1991; Kaplan, 1992; Kaplan & Kaplan, 1989; Leather et al., 1998; Lewis, 1996; Moore, 1981; Parsons et al., 1998; Rohde & Kendle, 1994; Ulrich et al., 1991). Second, the reduced crime, promotion of social cohesion and regeneration of local economies that are associated with greenspace revitalise communities. Third, greenspace, directly and indirectly, supports healthy ecosystem functioning, and, in turn, human and societal health and wellbeing. Finally, both the presence and lack of greenspace can encourage pro-environmental behaviour and stewardship from local communities, which often increases the ecosystem functioning and, in turn, ecosystem services provided back to communities (Dennis et al., 2016; James, 2018).

Cities are not isolated from their surrounds in terms of ecosystem services. This applies equally to the way that people use both urban and non-urban environments; for example, people may take day-trips or long excursions into the countryside to go walking. There is also a movement of waste products – waste energy as heat, the products of combustion of carbon-based products, including fuel, solid waste, chemicals and particles in water and air – out of urban environments (Figure 5.1). Hence, some ecosystem services are derived from areas outside the urban boundary while others come from both the surroundings and the urban area. Yet others come from just the urban area (Sadler et al., 2018).

Despite the theoretical attractiveness of the notion of ecosystem services, the very broad and fundamental way in which nature supports conditions vital to

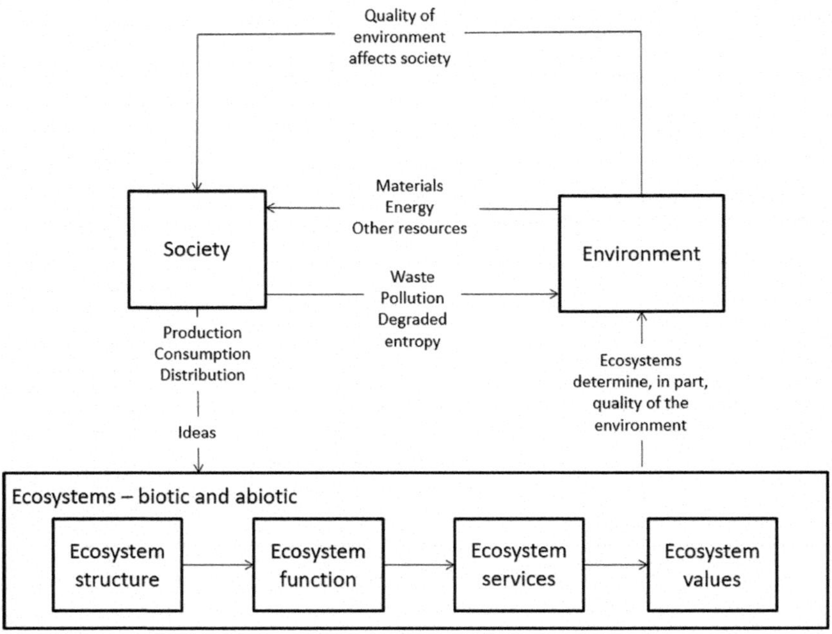

FIGURE 5.1 Conceptual diagram of a social-ecological system in cities.
Source: Authors.

human health is reflected in the equally broad attempts to describe the influence of ecosystem services on health. It is largely agreed that the degradation of global ecosystems has led to a reduction in ecological functioning, which affects human wellbeing through a range of natural, economic and political processes (Millennium Ecosystem Assessment, 2003; Watts et al., 2012). Described at these scales of operation (i.e. from regional to global), the processes that lead to a worsening in human wellbeing are complex and mediated by coupled socio-economic and environmental inequalities. This renders the establishing of clear associations between ecosystem functions and individual health outcomes particularly challenging. In order to facilitate a clearer view of how ecological conditions affect processes that directly influence human wellbeing, models have been developed that attempt to offer intermediary stages in the pathway, leading from biophysical features or processes to end-point benefits to humans. Examples of such models that have received much attention, and subsequent development, are the notions of ecosystem service 'cascades' and service-providing units (SPUs).

The Cascade Model and Service-Providing Units

The ecosystem services cascade model (Haines-Young & Potschin, 2010) appeared several years following the largest global assessment of the condition and use of natural systems, the Millennium Ecosystem Assessment. Within that time, the notion of ecosystem services and an acknowledgement of the theoretical advantages of adopting a utilitarian approach to ecosystem management and nature conservation had gained political and academic support within the field of ecological economics (e.g. Costanza et al., 1997; Fisher et al., 2008; UK NEA, 2011). However, despite the increasing popularity of ecosystem services as the environmental unit of measurement *de rigeur*, confusion over exactly how to quantify the end-usage of such services, how to trace them to their ecological functions of origin and how to distinguish between them has remained a challenge for the scientific community. This has resulted in the wide, but inconsistent, use of terminology on the topic of ecosystem services (Jax, 2007); the ecosystem services cascade model was developed in an attempt to remediate such inconsistency. The principal tenet of the cascade model is one of a production chain-like flow of energy. The chain charts the journey made by any given, nature-derived benefit to human wellbeing. This originates with the living organisms that comprise natural habitats (e.g. woodlands), proceeds to the capacity of such habitats to carry out important ecological functions (e.g. slowing and filtration of water), then to individual services relevant to human health (e.g. flood prevention) and finally to the benefits as perceived by humans (e.g. willingness to pay for forest management and protection). Note that the benefit described, as has often been the case in the literature on ecosystem services, takes on an economic mode of expression – the result of attempts to make natural habitats more visible in market-based transactions that so often lead to environmental degradation. Therefore, although the cascade model has contributed to an understanding of the relationships, and distinctions, between ecosystems, their functions and related services, such models still stop short of providing clear links between those services and human health outcomes.

The idea of service-providing units (SPUs) has similarly emerged from a utilitarian approach to nature conservation, grouping individual or groups of organisms according to the benefits (ecosystem services) that their unique or collective functional traits provide. This has allowed for the development of pragmatic approaches to ecosystem management and allowed for the reduction of much ecological complexity through an anthropocentric rendering of ecological groups and their interactions (Andersson et al., 2015). Again, however, in the case of SPUs, emphasis has been placed on the links between organisms and the services they provide, rather than on clarification of the subsequent pathways linking individual services and human health.

Two reasons why evidence on the links between ecosystem services and human health has not been forthcoming relate to the scale at which the ecological processes determining ecosystem service production have been considered and the spatial distribution of the recipients of such services. Ecosystems (and their functional components) operate and interact across scales. In addition, end users and beneficiaries are often located at large, spatial and temporal distances from those ecosystems. As a result, benefits to humans derived from large-scale, natural processes, such as carbon sequestration, water regulation, provision of food and medicines and pollination, are difficult to quantify at the local spatial and temporal scales at which benefits to wellbeing are experienced. The situation becomes even more complex in light of the increasingly urban nature of today's global population, which sees highly dense populations relying on spatially and culturally distant, regional-to-global ecological functions.

However, as we have observed earlier in this chapter, the increasing rural-to-urban migration and the parallel rise in chronic health conditions affecting urban populations has led to increasing interest in the role of the natural environment on the health of urbanites (i.e. the majority of humans today). Much of the evidence on this relationship stems from the public health disciplines, and the mechanisms already discussed have been offered as potential causal pathways. Notably, very little research within public health, and none of the mechanisms identified in this chapter, takes recourse to the notion of ecosystem services. Rather, the presence of nature and biodiversity itself is often treated as a fundamental component directly influencing human health. In contrast, biodiversity is presented in ecosystem services models as generating and supporting (cascading) ecological functions, via service-providing units, and subsequent benefits to human wellbeing. In this way, these two modes of describing the health benefits to humans stemming from the natural environment (one, from a public health perspective and the other, from an ecological perspective) are characterised by their contrasting emphasis on biodiversity. That is to say, public health researchers tend to view biodiversity as something that may directly affect the biological, social and emotional mechanisms that regulate human health, regardless of intermediate functions, products, goods or services that may be involved. Conversely, ecologists – at least those promoting a utilitarian approach to nature conservation – tend to see biodiversity as that which allows the existence of ecosystems and their various functions to be beneficial to human wellbeing.

However, these two perspectives need not be irreconcilable and, especially in an urban context, there exists both the need and the opportunity to explore links between ecosystem services and health. As we have seen, the urban environment has received much attention as a context for public health research, but has equally been the focus of much work within the ecological sciences. The latter has sought to better understand this unique environment and its implications for land-use change, nature conservation and human wellbeing. One of the key concepts to emerge from research on urban ecosystems is that of urban green infrastructure (UGI). The use of UGI – 'an interconnected network of greenspaces that conserves natural ecosystem values and functions and provides associated benefits to human populations' (Benedict & McMahon, 2002), stems back to the 1980s. More recently, it has been used to denote the biophysical features within the urban environment from which ecosystem services are derived at the city-scale (Hansen & Pauleit, 2014). An important premise in the promotion of an urban green infrastructure approach is that, although fundamental benefits to human livelihoods are derived from distant ecosystems, important ecosystem services are delivered within urban environments at the neighbourhood-to-city scale by the presence of natural surface cover. Subsequently, evidence is forthcoming at increasingly local scales on the influence of local urban nature on topics relevant to health, such as access to greenspace (Benedict & McMahon, 2002), air quality (Pugh et al., 2012), neighbourhood walkability (Wolch et al., 2014), crime levels and social inclusion (Kuo & Sullivan, 2001). Many of these characteristics are critical to quality of life in urban areas, and their related well-being outcomes can be described through recourse to mechanisms identified in the public health literature. Therefore, given the current body of evidence, there is scope to integrate knowledge from research into urban green infrastructure and public health. Table 5.2 presents an example of how, drawing on the relevant literature, health outcomes for urban residents can be charted from types of urban green infrastructure to the ecosystem services they provide to the health benefits received by humans via relevant pathways.

Although such an undertaking may provide some conceptual clarity, the assigning of unique health outcomes to individual green infrastructure types is not

TABLE 5.2 Urban green infrastructure, ecosystem services and potential mechanisms affecting human health

UGI	*Ecosystem Service Category (Millennium Ecosystem Assessment (MEA))*	*Ecosystem Service*	*Benefit*	*Mechanism*
Protected areas	Supporting	Habitat for wildlife	Sense of place/heritage	Connectedness with nature
Urban wetlands	Provisioning	Water filtration/ purification	Clean water	Alleviate stress caused by pollutants
Street trees	Regulating	Capture of ultra-fine particles from traffic	Reduced cardiovascular disorders	Alleviate oxidative stress
Riparian habitat		Flood prevention/ management	Lower risk to people and property associated with extreme weather events	Hydrological filtration
Urban parks		Evapotranspiration and shading	Reduction of heat stress	Physical/ physiological
Playing fields/ recreational grounds	Cultural	Recreation/exercise	Lower obesity levels	Physical activity
Neighbourhood greenery		Amenity/aesthetic	Hedonic uplift	Increased life satisfaction
Community gardens		Social interactions	Improved social ties	Participation

Source: Authors.

without its problems. For example, much of the evidence linking greenspaces to health comes from cross-sectional studies and causality cannot be established through such methods where latent variables may be at work. Moreover, many of the outcomes described in Table 5.2 could be linked to an increase or decrease in the experience of stress. This suggests that, although types of urban green infrastructure may be more or less closely linked to certain ecosystem services and related health mechanisms, the regulation of stress within may comprise a central pathway through which urban ecosystems influence human health.

Contact with Nature in Cities

Contact with nature has been tied to health and wellbeing in many studies. Links, through correlational studies, have been made to measurable human positive benefits in terms of physical health, psychological wellbeing and social cohesion. The modernisation theory posits that social-economic development expands the resource base and is the driving force of political mobilisation. This is often used to explain the emergence of the environmental movement in advanced industrial societies.

The hygiene hypothesis postulates that a reduced exposure to environmental microbes and harmless infections, which is linked to increased economic wealth, leads to an increased prevalence of allergic reactions. Reduced exposure to environmental bacteria in early life, growing up in an urban environment, and less contact with people and animals are associated with an increased risk of developing allergies and asthma in later life (Jatzlauk et al., 2017). Exposure to the microbiota associated with pets alters the gut microbial composition of infants, a putative pathway by which exposure to pets can reduce these health risks. The absence of pets, for example, from homes reduces the early-life exposure to microorganisms and contributes to the increased prevalence of allergies and asthma (Tun et al., 2017). These authors reported that following exposure to pets, there was increased abundance of two bacteria in the gut flora (*Ruminococcus* and *Oscillospira*). Both of these bacteria have been negatively associated with childhood atopy (a predisposition to developing certain hypersensitivity reactions) and obesity. The range of specific health outcomes linked to contact with nature is wide and includes diabetes mellitus, various infectious diseases, cancer, obesity, birth outcomes, cardiovascular disease, musculoskeletal complaints, migraines and respiratory disease.

Theoretical Frameworks Linking Nature and Human Health and Wellbeing

There are a variety of disciplinary traditions in understanding the contributions of nature to health and wellbeing. These include the main disciplines in health and wellbeing, such as medicine, public health, epidemiology, environmental sciences, geography, sociology and environmental psychology. Furthermore, research in biology, physical activity, ecology, urban planning, economics, leisure and recreation also contribute to knowledge in the area of health and wellbeing. This variety of disciplinary traditions has resulted in a range of theoretical frameworks for explaining the contributions of nature to health and wellbeing. Frameworks explain the contributions of nature to health and wellbeing by emphasising different biological, social, economic, ecological or environmental factors or mechanisms that link environmental influence, internal processes and health and wellbeing outcomes.

Nine mechanisms, five starting intrinsic and four extrinsic, emerge that underpin the theoretical frameworks. These mechanisms are outlined below.

Mechanisms Starting with Internal Intrinsic Processes

The stress reduction mechanism is based on the emotional functioning of the brain. This mechanism asserts that contact with nature stimulates psycho-evolutionary emotions, which, in turn, reduce or increase stress. This mechanism starts in the emotional part of the brain. For example, Kellert (1996) reported that citizens of suburban and urban areas tend to place a much higher value on species conservation than those living in rural areas. Kellert suggested that this was because those living in urban and suburban areas perceive biodiversity as a cultural ecosystem service, one that links them to the natural world, and provides an aesthetic and stress-reducing function rather than a provisioning service. The latter, particularly the provision of food, may be a more prevalent view in rural areas where natural resources are more closely associated with provisioning ecosystem services.

The attention restoration mechanism is based on the cognitive functioning of the brain. This mechanism asserts that contact with nature restores involuntary attention, which, in turn, restores voluntary attention. This mechanism starts in the cognitive part of the brain. The cultivation of local biodiversity, which brings with it a need to focus on certain activities and, hence, is a cognitive activity, has been shown to provide psychological benefits for people (Fuller et al., 2007).

The built environment mechanism is based on sensory arousal. The assertion here is that increasing complexity of the environment is the cause of overstimulated brain functions, which, in turn, causes stress. This mechanism starts in the cognitive part of the brain. The 'extinction of experience' to use a phrase coined by Miller (2005) that comes about as a result of the disconnection from nature, felt by many people living in urban environments, can have a negative impact on humans as wellbeing.

The physical activity mechanisms are based on the biophysical functioning of the body. The assertion is that infections, disease, injury, pollution or inactivity produce hormones, which, in turn, affect the immune and other systems. These mechanisms start in the endocrine system. Physical activity has been shown to be a major contributor to health. Intuitively, greenspace is associated with physical activity; however, this relationship is empirically inconsistent and may hold only under certain conditions and for certain populations. While greener residential areas do not consistently predict physical activity, they do consistently predict lower rates of obesity. This suggests that the pathway between nature and obesity may depend less on nature's effects on physical activity and more on its effects on adiponectin, stress and impulse control.

The self-perception mechanism is based on the concept of actualisation. This mechanism asserts that progressively fulfilling physiological, safety and psychological needs underpins the actualisation of self-potential, that is to say, that one fulfils one's potential. This mechanism starts in the physiological needs: the need for food, clean drinking water and shelter (appropriate housing). Then, it moves to the need to feel safe from natural disasters and from attack by animals or other humans. The third step is for meaningful relationships with others who are part of the community. This hypothesis states that it is only when one's needs at all three of these levels are met that one can move on to develop one's full potential: learning new skills and achieving something above meeting one's basic requirements for life.

Mechanisms Starting with Extrinsic Processes

The place identity mechanism is based on cultural conditions and norms. Here, the assertion is that culture preconditions people for what parts of nature are liked or disliked, or seen as good, bad, moral, immoral, healthy or unhealthy. This mechanism starts in cultural norms. Citizens of urban areas may support innovative initiatives that are framed as addressing the needs of people as much as the needs of wildlife, such as landscaping green roofs, and the cultivation of native plants. People assign and express diverse values and meanings to nature and their experience of it based on individual experiences and cultural backgrounds; hence, perceptions, context, and culture determine the number and types of cultural ecosystem services experienced that are shaped by difference in attitude and belief (Bertram & Rehdanz, 2015; Buchel & Frantzeskaki, 2015; Camps-Calvet et al., 2016; Voigt & Wurster, 2015). The link to health is that if one assigns negative values to the place in which one lives and/or works, that will have a detrimental effect on one's health. As these values are based on individual and cultural norms, it means that two people with different life experiences and different cultural norms will assign different values to the same place. In the extreme, while one person may be unhappy and possibly depressed due to the negative values they assign to a particular place, to another person, this same place may be one in which they feel comfortable due to the positive values they assign to the community of that place or as a result of a life time of memories built up in that place.

The community mechanism is based on social interactions. This mechanism asserts that social isolation, exclusion and disadvantage cause ill health and poor wellbeing because humans need social ties and other group dynamics. This mechanism starts in social interactions between individuals. A well-educated public, alignment with voluntary organisations, leisure time to devote to political activism and attention to post-material goods also have been related to high levels of activism (Dalton, 2005). Opportunities for community-based, environmental protesters to translate concerns into activism are facilitated by social interactions characterised by dense communication structures, mass education, urbanisation and high degrees of social mobility that characterise advanced industrial societies.

The care provision mechanisms are based on institutional settings. These mechanisms assert that health and wellbeing are the outcomes of appropriate institutions providing prevention, treatment, care and management of disease. These mechanisms start in institutional settings.

Finally, the ecological mechanisms are based on interdependencies between factors. The assertion is that air, land, water, biodiversity, social and economic determinants affect personal, physical and psychological determinants of health. These mechanisms start in the broad environment. Long-term, positive health and wellbeing outcomes have been linked with time spent in and around urban greenspace – tree-lined streets, gardens, parks, and forested and agricultural lands. The greener a person's surroundings, the lower is the risk of morbidity and mortality, even after accounting for confounding variables.

A Central Mechanism Linking Nature to Health and Wellbeing

Stress has significant effects on human biology and appears to be a central factor in the external and internal mechanisms of health and wellbeing. There are two major hormonal stress systems. First, the autonomic nervous system controls the release of noradrenaline and adrenaline. These hormones are released within milliseconds and prepare the body to 'fight or flight' in response to a perceived threat (Adli, 2011). Second, the hypothalamus-pituitary-adrenocortical system releases hormones that control digestion, the immune system, mood and emotions, sexuality, and energy storage and expenditure (Spencer & Hutchison, 1999). Under chronic stress, this system continuously produces cortisol (the stress hormone). Too much cortisol antagonises insulin and other hormones, leading to suppressed immune system, inhibited physiological and psychological functions, and toxic effects on neurons in certain brain regions.

The effects of low-level chronic stress can be seen physiologically at the cellular level. Under low-level chronic stress, cells are damaged by free radicals, lose their regeneration capacity and ultimately die. The result is premature ageing (Adli, 2011). As cells die, they release chemicals that cause inflammation. In order to deal with the inflammation, the body's immune system is switched on and remains so until the cause of the stress is addressed. Inflammation caused in this way is recognised as 'the cause of causes' leading to arthritis, cancers, cardiovascular disease, diabetes, anxiety and depression, obesity and the decline of the brain and its abilities that collectively are described as dementia (Epel et al., 2009; Hazel et al., 2005; Kuo, 2015; Manoli et al., 2007).

Drawing all the mechanisms together this theory posits that chronic, low-level inflammation is at the root of ill health and is, in large part, a direct consequence

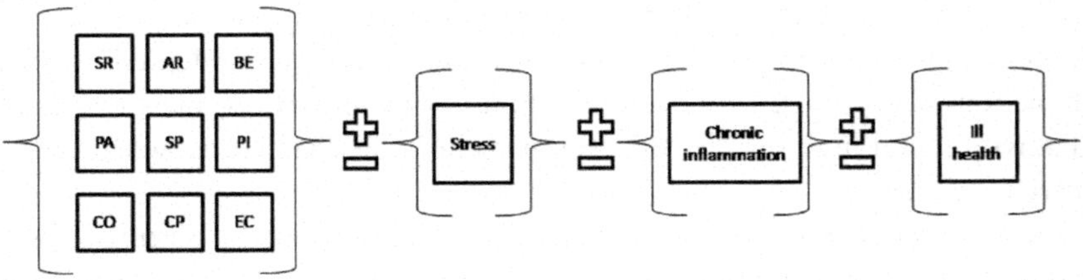

FIGURE 5.2 Links between mechanisms determining health and wellbeing and ill health.

Note. Mechanisms - SR, Stress Reduction; AR, Attention Restoration; BE, Built Environment; PA, Physical Activity; SP, Self-perception; PI, Place Identity; CO, Community; CP, Care Provision; EC, Ecological.

Source: Authors.

of the environment in which people live. Many current urban settings cause low-level stress. Low-level stress causes physiological and psychological changes. Physiological and psychological changes are manifested as ill health and poor wellbeing (Figure 5.2).

Conclusion

Nature within cities forms part of a complex social-ecological system. The ecological components of the system produce ecosystem services and disservices that influence the health and wellbeing of people living and working in cities. Both health and wellbeing are complex, multi-faceted concepts that have been studied by many and diverse disciplines. With an accompanying diversity of approaches there are a wide range of models explaining different aspects of the links between nature in cities and health and wellbeing. The unifying feature of all these models is that there is a tangible link and that people benefit from there being nature in cities. If these benefits are to be exploited in order to address the health concerns of the early twenty-first century, then four areas need further development. First, the theoretical gaps need addressing, for example, there is much to be done to determine the potential health and wellbeing benefits that arise from contact with nature for a range of population groups (e.g. for an ageing population and those with dementia). Second, preventative or therapeutic outcomes need clarity, for example, clear links established with, for example, reductions in the rates of obesity, cardiovascular disease, type II diabetes, certain cancers and mental ill health (e.g. depression and anxiety). Third, passive and active contact with nature needs promoting, so that preventive 'upstream' health interventions are developed and delivered. This will require changes in the way in which health and wellbeing are managed by the health professions and by individuals. In turn, this will necessitate the design and delivery of health and wellbeing interventions that are based on contact with nature. Fourth, appropriate architectural and urban designs need implementing. In order to achieve the maximum benefits, it will be necessary to design towns and cities in such a way that contact with nature is both possible and encouraged as part of everyday living. The challenge for the designer is to set aside ideas that see nature apart from people in cities but which integrates nature into all elements of the fabric of cities. Ideally, from the moment someone opens their bedroom curtains in the morning to drawing them in the evening, they should be able to see some form of greenery – a park, a green façade on the building opposite or a green roof visible to those living in high-rise buildings – at all times of the day.

References

Adli, M. (2011). *Urban Stress and Mental Health*. LSECities Retrieved from https://lsecities.net/media/objects/articles/urban-stress-and-mental-health/en-gb

Andersson, E., McPhearson, T., Kremer, P., Gomez-Baggethun, E., Haase, D., Tuvendal, M. & Wurster, D. (2015). Scale and context dependence of ecosystem service providing units. *Ecosystem Services*, 12, 157–164. doi: 10.1016/j.ecoser.2014.08.001

Beichler, S. A., Bastian, O., Haase, D., Heiland, S., Kabisch, N. & Müller, F. (2017). Does the ecosystem service concept reach its limits in urban environments? *Landscape Online*, 51, 1–21. doi: 10.3097/LO.201751

Benedict, M. A. & McMahon, E. T. (2002). Green infrastructure: smart conservation for the 21st century. *Renewable Resources Journal*, 20(3), 12–17.

Berman, M. G., Jonides, J. & Kaplan, S. (2008). The cognitive benefits of interacting with nature. *Psychological Science*, 19(12), 1207–1212. doi: 10.1111/j.1467–9280.2008.02225.x

Bertram, C. & Rehdanz, K. (2015). Preferences for cultural urban ecosystem services: comparing attitudes, perception, and use. *Ecosystem Services*, 12, 187–199. doi: 10.1016/j.ecoser.2014.12.011

Bolund, P. & Hunhammar, S. (1999). Ecosystem services in urban areas. *Ecological Economics*, 29(2), 293–301. doi: 10.1016/S0921-8009(99)00013-0

Bowler, D. E., Buyung-Ali, L., Knight, T. M. & Pullin, A. S. (2010). Urban greening to cool towns and cities: a systematic review of the empirical evidence. *Landscape and Urban Planning*, 97(3), 147–155. doi: 10.1016/j.landurbplan.2010.05.006

Buchel, S. & Frantzeskaki, N. (2015). Citizens' voice: a case study about perceived ecosystem services by urban park users in Rotterdam, The Netherlands. *Ecosystem Services*, 12, 169–177. doi: 10.1016/j.ecoser.2014.11.014

Camps-Calvet, M., Langemeyer, J., Calvet-Mir, L. & Gómez-Baggethun, E. (2016). Ecosystem services provided by urban gardens in Barcelona: Spain, insights for policy and planning. *Environmental Science and Policy*, 62, 14–23. doi: 10.1016/j.envsci.2016.01.007

Costanza, R., d'Arge, R., De Groot, R., Farber, S., Grasso, M., Hannon, B. ... & Raskin, R. G. (1997). The value of the world's ecosystem services and natural capital. *Nature*, 387, 253–260.

Dallimer, M., Irvine, K. N., Skinner, A. M., Davies, Z. G., Rouquette, J. R., Maltby, L. L. ... & Gaston, K. J. (2012). Biodiversity and the feel-good factor: understanding associations between self-reported human wellbeing and species richness. *BioScience*, 62(1), 47–55. doi: 10.1525/bio.2012.62.1.9

Dalton, R. J. (2005). The greening of the globe? Cross-national levels of environmental group membership. *Environmental Politics*, 14(4), 441–459. doi: 10.1080/ 09644010500175783

Dennis, M., Armitage, R. P. & James, P. (2016). Social-ecological innovation: adaptive responses to urban environmental conditions. *Urban Ecosystems* 19(3), 1063–1082. doi: 10.1007/s11252-016-0551-3

Döhren, P. & Haase, D. (2015). Ecosystem disservices research: a review of the state of the art with a focus on cities. *Ecological Indicators*, 52, 490–497. doi:10.1016/j.ecolind.2014.12.027

Epel, E., Daubenmier, J., Moskowitz, J. T., Folkman, S. & Blackburn, E. (2009). Can meditation slow rate of cellular aging? Cognitive stress, mindfulness, and telomeres. *Annals of the New York Academy of Sciences*, 1172, 34–53. doi:10.1111/j.1749–6632.2009.04414.x

Fisher, B., Turner, K., Zylstra, M., Brouwer, R., De Groot, R., Farber, S. ... & Balmford, A. (2008). Ecosystem services and economic theory: integration for policy-relevant research. *Ecological Applications*, 18(8), 2050–2067. doi: 10.1890/07–1537.1

Fuller, R. A., Irvine, K. N., Devine-Wright, P., Warren, P. H. & Gaston, K. J. (2007). Psychological benefits of greenspace increase with biodiversity. *Biology Letters*, 3(4), 390–394. doi: 10.1098/rsbl.2007.0149

Haines-Young, R. & Potschin, M. (2010). The links between biodiversity, ecosystem services and human wellbeing. In D. G. Raffaelli & C. L. J. Frid (Eds.), *Ecosystem Ecology: A New Synthesis* (110–139). Cambridge: Cambridge University Press, British Ecological Society.

Hansen, R. & Pauleit, S. (2014). From multifunctionality to multiple ecosystem services? A conceptual framework for multifunctionality in green infrastructure planning for urban areas. *Ambio*, 43(4), 516–529. doi: 10.1007/s13280-014-0510–2

Hartig, T., Mang, M. & Evans, G. W. (1991). Restorative effects of natural environment experiences. *Environment and Behavior*, 23, 3–26. doi: 10.1177/0013916591231001

Hazel A. F., Bardeesy, N. & Maser, R. S. (2005). Telomere induced senescence: end game signalling. *Current Molecular Medicine*, 5(2), 145–152.

James, P. (2018). *The Biology of Urban Environments*. Oxford: Oxford University Press.

Jatzlauk, G., Bartel, S., Heine, H., Schloter, M. & Krauss-Etschmann, S. (2017). Influences of environmental bacteria and their metabolites on allergies, asthma and host microbiota. *Allergy*. doi: 10.1111/all.13220

Jax, K. (2007). Can we define ecosystems? On the confusion between definition and description of ecological concepts. *Acta Biotheoretica*, 55(4), 341–355. doi: 10.1007/s10441-007-9024–7

Kaplan, R. (1992). The psychological benefits of nearby nature. In D. Relf (Ed.), *Role of Horticulture in Human Wellbeing and Social Development: A National Symposium* (125–133). Arlington, VA: Timber Press.

Kaplan, R. & Kaplan, S. (1989). *The Experience of Nature: A Psychological Perspective*. Cambridge: Cambridge University Press.

Kellert, S. R. (1996). *The Value of Life*. Washington, DC: Island Press.

Kuo, F. E. & Sullivan, W. C. (2001). Environment and crime in the inner city: does vegetation reduce crime? *Environment and Behavior*, 33(3), 343–367.

Kuo, M. (2015). How might contact with nature promote human health? Promising mechanisms and a possible central pathway. *Frontiers in Psychology*, 6, 1093. doi: 10.3389/fpsyg.2015.01093

Larson, L. R., Whiting, J. W., Green, G. T. & Bowker, J. M. (2014). Physical activity locations in Georgia: frequency of use by socio-demographic groups. *Journal of Outdoor Recreation and Tourism*, 5, 68–72. doi: 10.1016/j.jort.2013.11.001

Leather, P., Pyrgas, M., Beale, D. & Lawrence, C. (1998). Windows in the workplace. *Environment and Behavior*, 30, 739–763.

Lewis, C. A. (1996). *Green Nature/Human Nature: The Meaning of Plants in Our Lives*. Chicago: University of Illinois Press.

Manoli, I., Alesci, S., Blackman, M. R., Su, Y. A., Rennert, O. & Chrousos, G. P. (2007). Mitochondria as a key component of the stress response. *Trends in Endocrinology and Metabolism*, 18(5), 190–198. doi: 10.1016/j.tem.2007.04.004

Mayer, F. S. & McPherson-Frantz, I. (2004). The connectedness to nature scale: a measure of individuals' feeling in community with nature. *Journal of Environmental Psychology*, 24, 503–515. doi: 10.1016/j.jenvp.2004.10.001

McGinnis, M. D. & Ostrom, E. (2014) Social-ecological system framework: initial changes and continuing challenges. *Ecology and Society,* 19(2): 30. doi: 10.5751?ES-06387–190230

McPherson, E. (1994). Cooling urban heat islands with sustainable landscapes. In R. H. Platt, R. A. Rowntree & P. C. Muick (Eds.), *The ecological city: Preserving and restoring urban biodiversity* (151–171). Boston: University of Massachusetts Press.

Millennium Ecosystem Assessment. (2003). *Ecosystems and Human Wellbeing.* Washington, DC: Island Press.

Miller, J. R. (2005). Biodiversity conservation and the extinction of experience. *Trends in Ecology and Evolution,* 20, 430–434. doi:10.1016/j.tree.2005.05.013

Mitchell, R. (2013). Is physical activity in natural environments better for mental health than physical activity in other environments? *Social Science & Medicine*, 91, 130–134. doi: 10.1016/j.socscimed.2012.04.012

Moore, E. O. (1981). A prison environment's effect on health care service demands. *Journal of Environmental Systems*, 11, 17–34.

OED. (1998). *The New Oxford Dictionary of English.* Oxford: Oxford University Press.

Parsons, R., Tassinary, L. G., Ulrich, R. S., Hebl, M. R. & Grossman-Alexander, M. (1998). The view from the road: implications for stress recovery and immunization. *Journal of Environmental Psychology*, 18, 113–140.

Pugh, T. A., MacKenzie, A. R., Whyatt, J. D. & Hewitt, C. N. (2012). Effectiveness of green infrastructure for improvement of air quality in urban street canyons. *Environmental Science & Technology*, 46(14), 7692–7699. doi: 10.1021/es300826w

Rioux, L. (2005). The wellbeing of ageing people living in their own homes. *Journal of. Environmental Psychology,* 25, 231–243. doi: 10.1016/j.jenvp.2005.05.001

Rohde, C. L. E. & Kendle, A. D. (1994). *Report to English Nature—Human Wellbeing, Natural Landscapes and Wildlife in Urban Areas: A Review.* Bath: Department of Horticulture and Landscape and the Research Institute for the Care of the Elderly, University of Reading.

Sadler, J., Grayson, N., Hale, J., Locret-Collet, M., Hunt, D., Bouch, C. & Rogers, C. (2018). *The Little Book of Ecosystem Services in the City.* Lancaster, PA: Imagination.

Sandifer, P. A., Sutton-Grier, A. E. & Ward, B. P. (2015) Exploring connections among nature, biodiversity, ecosystem services, and human health and wellbeing: opportunities to enhance health and biodiversity conservation. *Ecosystem Services,* 12, 1–15.

Satorius, N. (2006). The meanings of health and its promotion. *Croatian Medical Journal,* 47(4): 662–664.

Shanahan, D. F., Lin, B. B., Gaston, K., Bush, R. & Fuller, R. A. (2015). What is the role of trees and remnant vegetation in attracting people to urban parks? *Landscape Ecology,* 30, 153–165. doi: 10.1007/s10980-014-0113-0

Spencer, R. L. & Hutchison, K. E. (1999). Alcohol, aging, and the stress response. *Alcohol Research and Health,* 23(4), 272–283. PMID 10890824.

Tun, H. M., Konya, T., Takaro, T. K., Brook, J. R., Chari, R., Field, C. J. … the CHILD Study Investigators. (2017). Exposure to household furry pets influences the gut microbiota of infants at 3–4 months following various birth scenarios. *Microbiome*, 5, 40. doi: 10.1186/s40168-017-0254-x

UK NEA (United Kingdom National Ecosystem Assessment). (2011). *UK National Ecosystem Assessment: Understanding Nature's Value to Society.* London: UK NEA.

Ulrich, R. S., Dimberg, U. & Driver, B. L. (1991). Psychophysiological indicators of leisure benefits. In B. L. Driver, L. R., Brown & G. L. Peterson (Eds.), *Benefits of Leisure* (73–89). State College, PA: Venture Publishing.

Ulrich, R. S., Simons, R. F., Losito, B. D., Fiorito, E., Miles, M. A. & Zelson, M. (1991). Stress recovery during exposure to natural and urban environments. *Journal of Environmental Psychology*, 11, 231–248.

Voigt, A. & Wurster, D. (2015). Does diversity matter? The experience of urban nature's diversity: case study and cultural concept. *Ecosystem Services*, 12, 200–208. doi:10.1016/j.ecoser.2014.12.005.

Watts, N., Maiero, M., Olson, S., Hales, J., Miller, C., Campbell, K. … & Cooper, D. (2012). *Our Planet, Our Health, Our Future. Human Health and the Rio Conventions: Biological Diversity, Climate Change and Desertification*. Geneva: World Health Organization.

Wolch, J. R., Byrne, J. & Newell, J. P. (2014). Urban green space, public health, and environmental justice: the challenge of making cities 'just green enough'. *Landscape and Urban Planning*, 125, 234–244. doi: 10.1016/j.landurbplan.2014.01.017

6

ENERGY, WELLBEING AND CITIES

AbuBakr S. Bahaj, Luke Blunden, Leonidas Bourikas, Milena Büchs, Patrick James and Yue Wu

Introduction

For cities to be low carbon, what is required is not only a radical transformation of current infrastructures, technologies and services, but also of people's daily practices to be geared towards reducing fossil fuel consumption. In the UK, for example, urbanisation and economic growth of cities have put housing and transport at the top of the political agenda (HM Treasury, 2017; HM Treasury & Hammond, 2018). This set of policy priorities often affects available land resources with a direct impact on the size and quality of greenspace and the form of the public realm. Energy use in cities, and people's wellbeing and health, have a symbiotic relationship; to date, though, little research has been carried out to understand these links. This is partly because datasets concerning health and wellbeing are often not linked to data on energy and public open space use. This is especially important, as there may be synergies between access to greenspace, health, wellbeing and energy use. For instance, if people are able to walk or cycle in good-quality public space, they may choose these modes of transport instead of using their car for other city journeys. However, there may be negative health and wellbeing implications of reducing energy use. For example, if temperatures inside the home fall below a level that is healthy and comfortable due to limited heating, this may result in damp and mould becoming established. In contrast, if money were no object, then most people would not worry about leaving their windows open for fresh air whilst having the heating on continuously to provide the warmth required in their homes. Clearly, this is undesirable from a sustainability point of view. Therefore, it is important to explore the relationships between income, energy use, health status and wellbeing, and access to greenspace. In particular, it would be helpful for policy makers to know how interdependent these are and how they can be optimised so fewer resources are used whilst providing better wellbeing for citizens of low-carbon cities. Insight into these relationships was attained through a longitudinal study surveying over 200 households in Southampton. The study was designed to provide initial understanding of: (a) any relationship between the choices of transport, urban greenspace and people's health and happiness; (b) wellbeing in cities related to energy usage and how lifestyle choices affect energy consumption; (c) how important is economic growth to achieving wellbeing and; (d) what are the implications of energy-related policies to health and wellbeing as a whole.

Case Study: Southampton, UK

Southampton is a major port city on the south coast of the UK, which is approximately 121 km southwest of London. It is the second largest container port and largest cruise terminal in the UK. Alongside the port, major employers in the city include the University of Southampton, Southampton Solent University, Southampton Airport, BBC South, NHS, Carnival UK (Cruise ships) and Ordnance Survey.

During the Second World War, the city was heavily bombed and much of the city centre was damaged. Large areas of the city's post-war regeneration are now being replaced with new developments in the city, such as West Quay and the Cultural Quarter. As of 2011, the city's population was around 250,000 with the surrounding areas forming the sixth largest built-up area in the UK, with a population of 855,000.

Greenspace covers 20% of the city's area (Southampton City Council, 2008) due to the high number of formal parks including, Victorian Park and the Common, a large area of historical pasture-turned-park in the city. While Southampton is a port city, it is surprisingly disconnected from the water and its medieval city core has been somewhat overwhelmed by post-war redevelopment. In recent years, these weaknesses have been recognised and city regeneration has been undertaken to reconnect the city with the sea (James et al., 2017).

Figure 6.1 shows the major phases of Southampton's expansion (Landmap; The GeoInformation Group, 2014). The city is constrained at the south by the estuary, but it has a radial sprawl towards the north, west and east. The largest periods of expansion happened in the early part of the twentieth century before the Second World War, reflecting the city's increasing importance as a major port, and then later from 1965 to 1979 when car-friendly housing estates were constructed around the periphery of the city.

Methods

Field Study Surveys

The aim of the field study was to see if a soft intervention – giving personalized, energy-saving advice – could affect transport and home energy use while improving or maintaining perceptions of wellbeing. The study was focussed on a geographical area of the city where a high proportion of people were known to

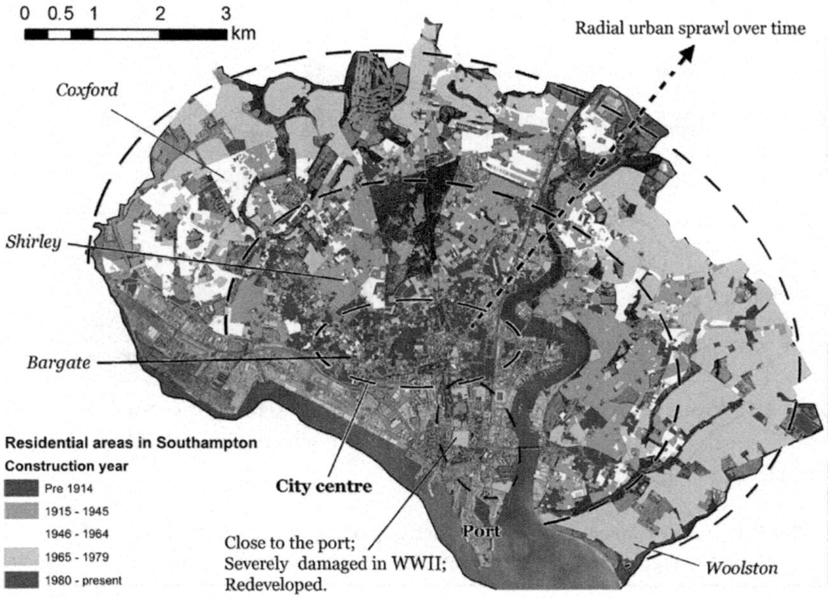

FIGURE 6.1 The city of Southampton and the different phases of urban expansion through its history.

Source: Landmap; The GeoInformation Group (2014).

own two or more cars. The total number of dwellings (identified by addresses) in the Output Area Classification Type 2 (Vickers & Reeves, 2007) was around 28,000. Of these, 6,000 households were invited to participate via post, selected using a random sample with the constraint that each type of building must be separated from each other by a minimum distance (which was allowed to vary globally to maintain sample size). This was done to reduce the likelihood of households being neighbours and of buildings being of very similar form and aspect to one another. A combination of Gazetteer, LIDAR and Ordnance Survey datasets in conjunction with geographical information system (GIS) and other software were used for this process. Out of the 6,000 invitations, 384 households responded and 218 were accepted following initial screening. Figure 6.2 shows the relative proportion of accepted responses in different building categories compared with those invited and those in the overall population.

The field study consisted of two sets of surveys, each conducted on a three-monthly basis from 2014 to 2016 (Büchs et al., 2018a). The first was a survey on home energy use and vehicle mileage ('household' survey; HH), which was completed by a self-identified household representative. The second was a survey on travel behaviour, attitudes, health and wellbeing ('individual' survey; IND), completed by all adult participants of the study households. In total, there were eight survey rounds. Table 6.1 shows the time periods and the number of responses for each survey round. HH and IND surveys were launched simultaneously.

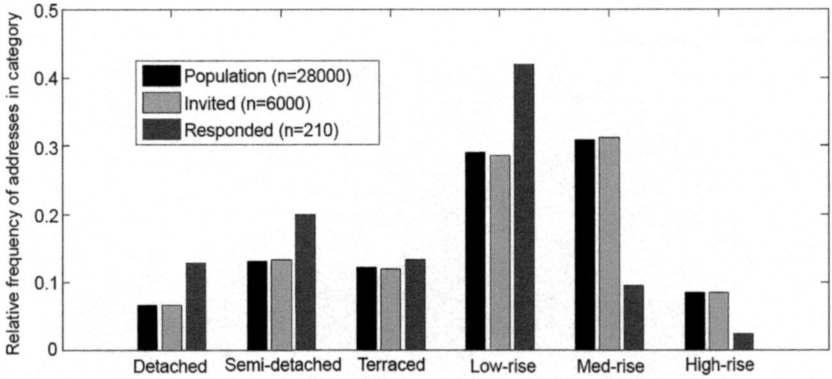

FIGURE 6.2 Proportion of addresses in different building categories for OAC Supergroup 2 population, invited and finally selected households.

Source: ONS.

TABLE 6.1 Periods of survey rounds, number of participants in each survey and percentage of responses received

Round	*Period*	*Household (HH) participants*	*Response (%)*	*Individual (IND) Participants*	*Response %*
1	Jul 14–Nov 14	218		336	
2	Oct 14–Jan 15	198	90.8	306	91.3
3	Jan 15–Apr 15	200	91.7	307	91.6
4	Apr 15–Jun 15	199	91.3	303	90.4
Intervention	Carbon calculator interviews May 15–Jun/Jul 15	95		143	
5	Jul 15–Oct 15	196	89.9	301	89.9
6	Oct 15–Jan 16	184	84.4	283	84.5
7	Jan 16–Mar 16	187	85.8	285	85.1
8	May 16–Jul 16	192	88.1	291	86.9

Source: Büchs et al. (2018a).

The Household (HH) survey had the format of a face-to-face interview. Survey Rounds 1–4 were considered as the base case. Between Rounds 4 and 5, the households in the study were randomly assigned to an 'intervention' and a 'control' group. This enabled us to test whether an intervention, which is only given to half of the participants, made a significant difference to their attitudes and/or behaviour, compared to a control group, which did not receive the intervention. The 'intervention' group comprised 95 of these households (143 individuals); the remainder were in the 'control' group (Büchs et al., 2018a).

The 'intervention' was a face-to-face interview with the use of a carbon calculator tool, which was created by the Centre for Alternative Technology in collaboration with the Carbon Conversations initiative (Carbon Conversations, 2018). The 'individual' survey also included subjective questions that tried to assess the perceptions of urban dwellers regarding their health and city environment. The results from the 'household' and the 'individual' surveys are discussed in the 'Results from Field Study' section.

In addition to the two questionnaire surveys, a bespoke environmental monitoring system was used to collect observations of temperature (T), relative humidity (RH), carbon dioxide levels (CO_2) and electricity consumption from the households in the HH survey sample.

Greenspace Analysis

Recent studies have shown that green spaces have a positive impact on the physical and psychological wellbeing of residents living in adjacent areas (Jones et al., 2009; Lee et al., 2015; Morris, 2003; Ward Thompson et al., 2012; Wood et al., 2017). The concept of 'greenspace' has been used in the literature with several different definitions. In general, the term refers to the natural environment of cities and to urban vegetation (Taylor & Hochuli, 2017). Different types of greenspace in cities are usually defined by their main use. Southampton City Council (SCC) specifies open spaces as parks, sports grounds, churchyards and cemeteries, local/neighbourhood/city parks, allotments, school grounds, civic or public realm spaces and so forth. Focussing on the greenspace, this study selected seven categories of open spaces (Table 6.2) and includes the quantity (Qty), the mean, minimum and maximum sizes in hectares for these seven categories in Southampton. The total area of the greenspace listed is 844 hectares, which accounts for 15% of the land area of Southampton City. The aim was to investigate the proximity of greenspace to the participants of the household survey in order to examine its impact on participants' health and wellbeing.

Figure 6.3 shows the approximate location of participant household locations in the context of the areas of greenspace identified in Table 6.2.

Two types of spatial analysis were carried out to ascertain participants' access to greenspace: (i) identification of the nearest greenspace and the distance to each participant's home, and (ii) estimation of the greenspace available within 5 and 15 minutes walking distance from each home along roads and footpaths. Analysis of the ease of accessing green spaces was conducted to reveal any relations to a range of socio-economic factors. In addition, a new travel-time model was developed for use with a geographical information system (GIS) tool, ArcGIS. This model was used to estimate the distance and the walking time required to reach the nearest greenspace from each participant's home. Roads and footpaths had been mapped using datasets from UK Ordnance Survey (Crown Copyright and Database Right 2017. Ordnance Survey (Digimap Licence)). All participants were assumed to walk at a constant speed of 1.2 m/s and their speed was not affected by any elevation changes or other factors.

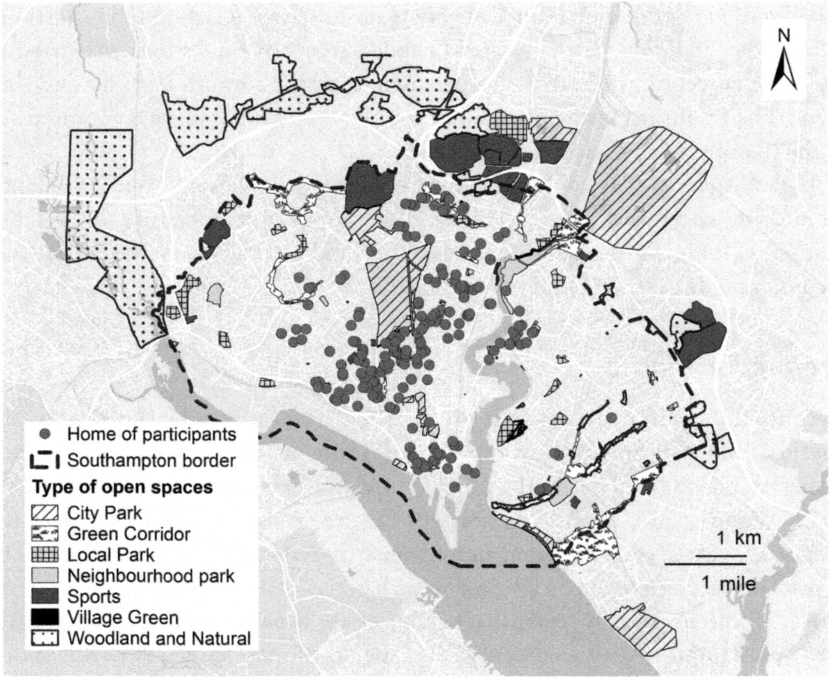

FIGURE 6.3 The approximate location of the households in the survey (bullet points) and their proximity to different types of urban greenspace.
Source: Southampton City Council.

TABLE 6.2 Types of urban greenspace in Southampton selected for this study

Type	*Qty*	*Mean size (ha)*	*Min (ha)*	*Max (ha)*	*Sum*
Village green	3	4.00	0.17	7.22	12.01
Green corridor	18	16.46	0.28	76.17	296.20
Woodland and natural	20	2.73	0.02	7.90	54.62
Sports	17	6.43	0.04	68.07	109.23
Local park	45	2.49	0.01	14.99	111.97
City park	19	10.97	0.02	108.47	208.35
Neighbourhood park	5	10.38	1.70	18.89	51.92
Overall	127	6.65	0.01	108.47	844.30

Source: Authors.

Figure 6.4 shows an example for a random house location in Southampton and the shaded area shows the five-minute walking range from the sample house (asterisk). The dotted lines denote various route options a participant can take. The possible 'entrance(s)' to the nearest greenspace was identified (grey circles in Figure 6.4). Entrances were defined as junctions (intersection points) between outlines of greenspace and footpaths.

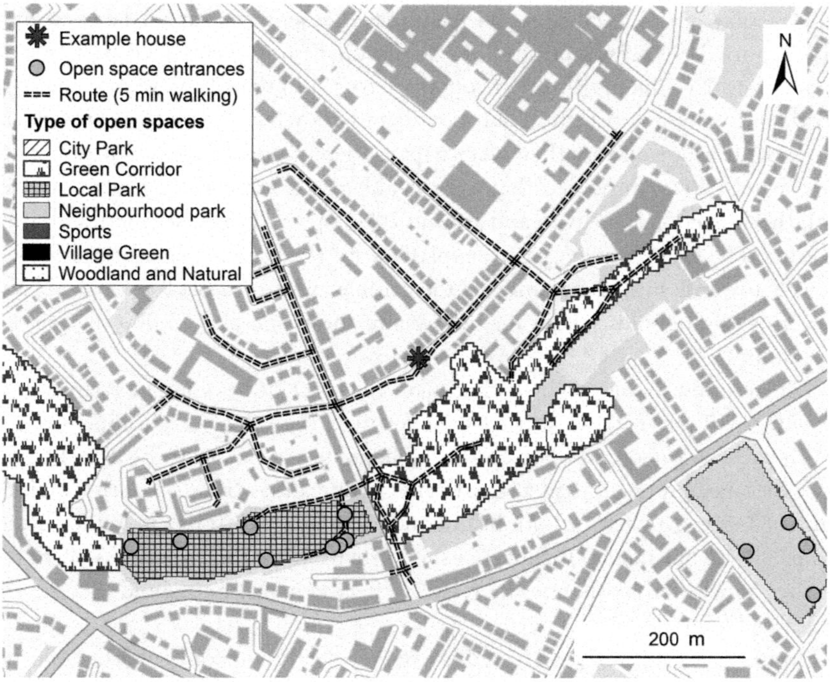

FIGURE 6.4 Distance travelled (dotted lines) on foot within five minutes from the example house location (asterisk).

Source: Crown Copyright and Database Right 2017. Ordnance Survey (Digimap Licence).

Secondary Data Analysis

A parallel analysis of secondary data ('national' study) from the UK Understanding Society dataset (University of Essex, 2017) was conducted to gain an insight into the attitudes of the UK public towards their living environment and their wellbeing (Büchs et al., 2018b). The findings from this study were compared with the HH and IND survey results to investigate if there were similar trends and critically evaluate any differences.

Results and Discussion

The following sections provide detailed results and discussion related to components of the field surveys and the secondary data analysis.

Income, Health and Happiness

Results from Field Study

Previous research has shown that, at the individual level, income and health status are important factors for people's happiness (Gu & Wei, 2018; Natali et al., 2018;

Subramanian et al., 2005). Here we examine whether our sampled data and analysis support these presumptions. The 'individual' survey collected participants' perception of wellbeing through responses to a number of questions regarding health and income satisfaction and how happy they feel. More than 90% of the respondents reported that they were happy ('happy' to 'completely happy'); approximately 70% considered that their health was good and they were satisfied with this aspect of their lives; and around 70% appeared to be satisfied with their income. The latter can be partly explained by the income distribution that is skewed towards higher incomes in the sample, where 55% of the participants were from households whose income was in the range of £35,000 to £45,000 per annum.

The responses from each of the quarterly IND surveys (eight rounds conducted, see Table 6.1) were used to determine the effect of age, income and health satisfaction on the perception of happiness as a measure of wellbeing. Both income and health had a statistically significant association with happiness (rounds 2–8: $p \leq 0.001$ for both health and income, wave 1: $p = 0.009$ for health and $p = 0.002$ for income). Table 6.4 shows the results of the goodness-of-fit test for the model used to analyse the relations between age, household income and health and happiness.

Dummy variables were created to recode health, income satisfaction and happiness from a five-level scale to a three-level scale that groups responses into negative (dissatisfied), neutral (neither satisfied nor dissatisfied) and positive (satisfied). This transformation was necessary in order to satisfy basic regression assumptions and ensure a representative sample size per response category. Table 6.3 includes the detailed results from the regression models for each round. The

TABLE 6.3 Overall goodness-of-fit for the ordinal logistic regression model of age, household income and health satisfaction on the self-perception of happiness from the IND survey responses

Variables	*Household income satisfaction*	*Health satisfaction*	*Age*
Round 1	$\chi^2(2) = 12.526$ [p = 0.002]	$\chi^2(2) = 9.372$ [p = 0.009]	$\chi^2(1) = 0.640$ [p = 0.424]
Round 2	$\chi^2(2) = 21.825$ [p < 0.001]	$\chi^2(2) = 32.998$ [p < 0.001]	$\chi^2(1) = 1.421$ [p = 0.233]
Round 3	$\chi^2(2) = 21.337$ [p < 0.001]	$\chi^2(2) = 42.405$ [p < 0.001]	$\chi^2(1) = 0.164$ [p = 0.685]
Round 4	$\chi^2(2) = 17.460$ [p < 0.001]	$\chi^2(2) = 32.423$ [p < 0.001]	$\chi^2(1) = 6.516$ [p = 0.011]
Round 5	$\chi^2(2) = 14.878$ [p = 0.001]	$\chi^2(2) = 25.616$ [p < 0.001]	$\chi^2(1) = 0.459$ [p = 0.498]
Round 6	$\chi^2(2) = 13.453$ [p = 0.001]	$\chi^2(2) = 27.347$ [p < 0.001]	$\chi^2(1) = 0.014$ [p = 0.906]
Round 7	$\chi^2(2) = 17.024$ [p < 0.001]	$\chi^2(2) = 19.209$ [p < 0.001]	$\chi^2(1) = 0.503$ [p = 0.478]
Round 8	$\chi^2(2) = 30.603$ [p < 0.001]	$\chi^2(2) = 30.615$ [p < 0.001]	$\chi^2(1) = 0.002$ [p = 0.965]

Ordinal logistic regression // *Dependent variable: Overall Happiness; Wald Chi-Square (df) and [Significance].*

The p-value shows the statistical significance of a test. A p-value smaller than 0.001 denotes a 99.9% probability that these results could not occur if the null hypothesis (health and income do not affect happiness) is true.

Source: Authors.

results show the calculated parameter for each variable, the standard error in parentheses and the statistical significance in square brackets. The last category of each variable was considered to be the reference. The negative sign of the parameters can be interpreted as a reduction in likelihood of somebody to be happy in comparison with the people in the reference category. For example, in Round 1, the odds of participants being more happy if they are satisfied with their health compared to the odds of being more happy if they are dissatisfied with their health was in a ratio of 3 to 1 (exp(1.16)).

In general, people satisfied with their health and income were much more likely to feel happier than people who were less satisfied with these two aspects of their lives (Table 6.4). It should be noted that the results have been checked for co-linearity; that is, the relationships between health satisfaction and happiness, and income satisfaction and happiness, are sufficiently independent of each other. In the IND survey, both income and health have a comparable effect, while the impact of age on happiness is not statistically significant (Table 6.4).

TABLE 6.4 Results from the ordinal logistic regression of age, household income and health satisfaction on the self-perception of happiness from the IND survey responses

	Health (Exp)			*Income (Exp)*			
	Dissatisfied	*Neutral*	*Satisfied*	*Dissatisfied*	*Neutral*	*Satisfied*	*Age*
Round 1 (N = 328)	*−1.16 (0.38) [***]*	*−0.68 (0.64) [p > 0.1]*	*Reference category*	*−1.33 (0.38) [***]*	*−0.62 (0.59) [p > 0.1]*	*Reference category*	*0.01 (0.01) [p > 0.1]*
Round 2 (N = 297)	*−1.75 (0.31) [***]*	*−1.12 (0.62) [*]*		*−1.29 (0.32) [***]*	*−1.68 (0.49) [***]*		*0.01 (0.01) [p>0.1]*
Round 3 (N = 298)	*−2.15 (0.35) [***]*	*−1.88 (0.45) [***]*		*−1.44 (0.35) [***]*	*−1.61 (0.52) [***]*		*−0.004 (0.01) [p > 0.1]*
Round 4 (N = 295)	*−2.03 (0.37) [***]*	*−1.80 (0.60) [***]*		*−1.08 (0.38) [***]*	*−1.88 (0.50) [***]*		*0.027 (0.01) [**]*
Round 5 (N = 291)	*−1.69 (0.34) [***]*	*−1.16 (0.49) [**]*		*−1.24 (0.36) [***]*	*−1.10 (0.43) [**]*		*0.006 (0.01) [p > 0.1]*
Round 6 (N = 274)	*−1.47 (0.35) [***]*	*−2.45 (0.60) [***]*		*−1.31 (0.38) [***]*	*−1.10 (0.46) [**]*		*0.001 (0.01) [p > 0.1]*
Round 7 (N = 277)	*−1.42 (0.33) [***]*	*−1.18 (0.57) [**]*		*−1.24 (0.35) [***]*	*−1.5 (0.53) [***]*		*0.006 (0.01) [p > 0.1]*
Round 8 (N = 285)	−1.99 (0.36) [***]	*−1.3 (0.61) [**]*		*−1.94 (0.38) [***]*	*−2.1 (0.55) [***]*		*0 (0.01) [p > 0.1]*

Ordinal logistic regression // *Dependent variable: Overall Happiness; (Std. Error); [Significance]*: *** $p < 0.01$, ** $p < 0.05$, * $p < 0.1$. N shows the number of valid individual responses.

Source: Authors.

Secondary Data Analysis

The analysis of the UK Understanding Society dataset in the 'national' study showed a similar trend with the IND survey findings. Health status in the 'national' study was positively associated with household income (Büchs et al., 2018b). 'Healthy' households (those listed as 'very good' in health) were earning on average 80% more than households reported with 'poor' health (Büchs et al., 2018b). The differences in income were also significant between neighbouring health categories (i.e. 1 – Very good, 2 – Good, 3 – Fair, 4 – Poor), depicting this positive correlation between households' heath and income. From a policy perspective, it can be assumed that household health is strongly related to education status. This may be a consequent result as it is expected that education will have an impact on income and it has been shown in previous surveys that higher incomes are associated with better health. In particular, at the 'national' study, it was found that 30% of the people who responded as having 'very good' health had gained a higher education qualification in comparison with 9% in the 'poor' health group (Büchs et al., 2018b).

Health, Energy and Travel Choices

Results from Field Study

The relationship between health, energy and mobility was also part of this analysis using the responses from HH and IND surveys covering walking and cycling habits. This analysis was based on Round 1 of the surveys only, which constituted the largest sample (see Table 6.5).

The findings indicate that an increase of one level in health score decreases electricity consumption by 15% ($\exp(-0.16) - 1$; $p < 0.05$) and gas consumption by 63%; however, for gas usage, the result is not statistically significant with a p-value above 0.05. At the same time, better health is associated with choosing to walk for short journeys ($p < 0.01$) as well as an increase in the number of flights taken ($p < 0.05$) and train destinations travelled to ($p < 0.05$). This result indicates that people in the 'healthy' households are more mobile and spend more time away from home. Nonetheless, cycling is negatively associated with age, indicating that as people grow older, they are less likely to cycle.

The association of health status and car travel was not statistically significant, but there was a strong, positive correlation between household size ($p < 0.01$), household income ($p < 0.05$) and miles driven per day. The use of the private car proved to be one of the three things (others being air travel and eating habits) that most participants were reluctant to change (Büchs et al., 2018a). In particular, participants were asked in what area they felt it would be hardest to make any changes. It was clear from their replies that changing travel mode away from private car use is very complex and challenging. Car use was associated with commuting, efficient use of time, practicality, privacy and financial benefits compared with expensive, peak-hour train transport systems. The main barrier to any changes in participants' modes of travel was related to availability of convenient public infrastructure, cost and its service quality. By contrast, however, the barriers to change towards less carbon-intensive air travel and food choices were mainly due to lifestyle considerations (Büchs et al., 2018a). These outcomes and perceptions show the complex nature and interdependencies between health, energy and mobility, and imply that a range of policies will be required to tackle carbon emissions in these sectors effectively.

TABLE 6.5 Table of results from the cross-sectional analysis of associations between HH and IND surveys variables.

	Gas kWh/day OLS	*Elec KWh/day (log)* OLS	*Miles/day (log)* OLS	*Number of flights* Poisson	*Number of train destinations* Poisson	*Number of bus destinations* Poisson	*Walking shorter distances (scale)* OLS	*Engage in cycling* Logistic
Health status	−0.37★	−0.16★★	0.13★	0.13★★	0.31★★	0.19★	0.26★★★	0.28★
	(0.19)	(0.08)	(0.07)	(0.06)	(0.12)	(0.10)	(0.09)	(0.17)
Age	0.00	−0.00	−0.00	−0.01★★	−0.01★	0.03★★★	−0.01	−0.04★★★
	(0.01)	(0.00)	(0.00)	(0.00)	(0.01)	(0.01)	(0.01)	(0.01)
HH size	0.18	0.08	0.14★★★	−0.18★★★	−0.14★★	0.01	−0.17★★	0.10
	(0.13)	(0.05)	(0.05)	(0.04)	(0.06)	(0.07)	(0.07)	(0.14)
Property: house (vs. flat)	1.75★★★	0.34★★	0.14	−0.01	0.16	−0.22	0.02	1.04★★★
	(0.35)	(0.14)	(0.13)	(0.10)	(0.17)	(0.16)	(0.18)	(0.33)
Renting (vs. owner-occ.)	−0.10	−0.03	0.10	−0.73★★★	−0.39★	0.11	−0.01	−0.34
	(0.39)	(0.15)	(0.14)	(0.12)	(0.21)	(0.19)	(0.18)	(0.34)
HH income	0.06	0.07★★★	0.06★★	0.12★★★	0.10★★	−0.07★★	−0.10★★★	0.04
	(0.07)	(0.03)	(0.03)	(0.02)	(0.04)	(0.03)	(0.04)	(0.07)
University education	0.27	0.00	−0.13	0.19★★	0.45★★★	0.23	0.22	0.30
	(0.28)	(0.12)	(0.11)	(0.09)	(0.15)	(0.15)	(0.14)	(0.26)
Employed/student vs. retired/UE	0.27	−0.00	0.27★	−0.08	0.17	−0.10	0.13	0.07
	(0.38)	(0.16)	(0.16)	(0.13)	(0.22)	(0.20)	(0.20)	(0.36)
Female	−0.57★★	−0.26★★	−0.07	−0.05	0.04	0.37★★★	−0.38★★★	−0.64★★
	(0.26)	(0.10)	(0.11)	(0.08)	(0.14)	(0.14)	(0.14)	(0.25)
Climate change interest	−0.14	0.01	−0.10	0.02	−0.01	0.13★	0.14★	0.27★
	(0.16)	(0.06)	(0.07)	(0.05)	(0.08)	(0.08)	(0.08)	(0.15)
Constant	2.50★	1.88★★★	2.01★★★	0.46	−1.97★★	−2.65★★★	3.29★★★	−1.23
	(1.30)	(0.52)	(0.52)	(0.43)	(0.78)	(0.68)	(0.67)	(1.26)
Observations	126	121	173	212	283	283	325	325
R-squared / pseudo R2	0.39	0.31	0.29				0.14	

Standard errors in parentheses, Significance: ★★★ $p < 0.01$, ★★ $p < 0.05$, ★ $p < 0.1$.

Secondary Data Analysis

The 'national' study on the UK Understanding Society dataset shows a similar trend to the findings of the HH and IND surveys regarding the relation of health to energy and travel choices (Büchs et al., 2018a). Most importantly, the 'national' study indicated that poor health is associated with higher energy usage at home. It was also shown that reduced mobility due to health issues restricts the travel mode choices and limits the time spent for travelling (Büchs et al., 2018b).

Greenspace, Health and Happiness

Table 6.6 shows the results for the time required for the 216 participants to walk to the nearest green space. The table gives the mean and maximum time of walking required. On average, survey participants have walking access to greenspace within seven minutes from their homes. Further detailed analysis is given in Figure 6.5. This shows that ten of the households are located very near to greenspace with an estimated journey time of less than one minute. Furthermore, the majority of the households are located within a 15-minute walking distance to greenspace and only three households are outside this walking time range.

From the analysis conducted, it is clear that 35% of the households could reach some type of greenspace within a five-minute walk and 80% within a ten-minute walk from their homes. Unfortunately, there is no currently agreed framework for rating the quality of a particular greenspace. Our intention is to develop this work further by creating greenspace quality maps that could help in providing a better understanding of the links been greenspace and wellbeing.

An ordinal logistic regression model was used to determine the effect of: (a) visits to greenspace; (b) health satisfaction and (c) age on the self-perception of happiness as an indicator of wellbeing. The deviance goodness-of-fit test (χ^2 (461) = 236.11, p = 0.512) indicated that the model was a good fit to the observed data, and the final model statistically predicted the dependent variable 'Overall Happiness' (χ^2 (7) = 31.53, p = 0.001). In general, the results in Table 6.7 show that a change from visiting greenspace once a month or less to visiting greenspace several times a week is very likely to be associated with an increase in happiness but the effect is not statistically significant. Satisfaction with health had a more prominent effect, as has already been discussed in the 'Health, Energy and Travel Choices' section.

TABLE 6.6 Time in minutes needed for survey participants to walk to the nearest greenspace available.

	Min	*Max*	*Mean*	*Median*	*Std. dev.*
n = 216	**0**	**19**	**7**	**6**	**3.5**

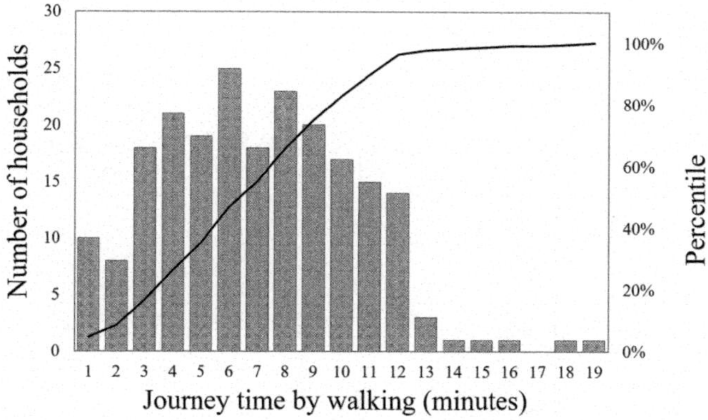

FIGURE 6.5 Proximity of survey households to greenspace by walking. The cumulative percentage is shown with the black line.

Energy Consumption and Environmental Conditions in Households

A strong, positive correlation was found between household size ($p < 0.01$), household income ($p < 0.05$) and miles driven per day (Table 6.5). In particular, household income is positively correlated with daily electricity usage and this link is statistically significant ($p < 0.01$). However, household size, which would be expected to have a direct impact on energy use, does not seem to have a significant effect on gas and electricity consumption. One important finding with significant relevance to policy making is the association of property type with energy use. Houses in the HH survey sample consume 1.75 times more gas ($p < 0.01$) and 1.4 times (exp(0.34), $p < 0.05$) more electricity than flats.

In this section, we provide sample results of bespoke, environmental monitoring systems deployed at participants' houses to measure temperature (T), relative humidity (RH), carbon dioxide levels (CO_2) and electricity consumption.

Figure 6.6 shows the observations from a randomly chosen household on 23 January 2017 during the UK heating season. On the night of Monday, 23 January 2017, the mean ambient temperature in Southampton was -0.8 °C. Figure 6.6a shows the readings from four sensors: CO_2 concentration in the living room, living room temperature and relative humidity, and boiler's case temperature (as an indication of its operation). Three distinct periods can be identified regarding heating (indicated by an arrow in Figure 6.6a): a long heating period during the morning and afternoon and two shorter heating periods between 5pm and 11pm when the occupants would have been back home. This profile is further justified by the carbon dioxide concentration and the relative humidity levels in the living room that follow a similar trend. Note that the following day, the timing of the heating period changed, even though it was also a weekday. This indicates manual control of the boiler by the occupants.

TABLE 6.7 Results from the ordinal logistic regression of age, greenspace visits frequency and health satisfaction on the self-perception of happiness from the IND survey responses.

	Greenspace visits frequency (Exp)					*Health satisfaction (Exp)*			
	Everyday	*Not everyday but several times a week*	*Once a week*	*Less than once a week but several times in a month*	*Once a month or less*	*Health – Dissatisfied*	*Health – Neutral*	*Health – Satisfied*	*Age*
Round 1 (N = 327)	*0.35 (0.66) [p>0.1]*	*−0.47 (0.51) [p>0.1]*	*−0.51 (0.56) [p>0.1]*	*−0.76 (0.58) [p>0.1]*	*Reference category*	*−1.72 (0.34) [***]*	*−1.16 (0.62) [*]*	*Reference category*	*0.01 (0.01) [p>0.1]*
Round 2 (N = 297)	*0.07 (0.54) [p>0.1]*	*0.04 (0.36) [p>0.1]*	*0.25 (0.46) [p>0.1]*	*-0.27 (0.40) [p>0.1]*		*−2.11 (0.30) [***]*	*−1.40 (0.60) [**]*		*0.01 (0.01) [*]*
Round 3 (N = 298)	*1.74 (0.73) [**]*	*0.50 (0.40) [p>0.1]*	*0.33 (0.46) [p>0.1]*	*0.08 (0.40) [p>0.1]*		*−2.51 (0.35) [***]*	*−2.39 (0.44) [***]*		*0.01 (0.01) [p>0.1]*
Round 4 (N = 296)	*0.74 (0.59) [p>0.1]*	*0.69 (0.45) [p>0.1]*	*0.10 (0.46) [p>0.1]*	*0.65 (0.48) [p>0.1]*		*−2.43 (0.35) [***]*	*−1.86 (0.58) [***]*		*0.03 (0.01) [***]*
Round 5 (N = 291)	*0.84 (0.57) [p>0.1]*	*0.54 (0.42) [p>0.1]*	*0.58 (0.44) [p>0.1]*	*−0.01 (0.40) [p>0.1]*		*−2.01 (0.33) [***]*	*−1.34 (0.47) [***]*		*0.02 (0.01) [p>0.1]*
Round 6 (N = 275)	*0.68 (0.60) [p>0.1]*	*0.27 (0.40) [p>0.1]*	*0.04 (0.44) [p>0.1]*	*0.21 (0.42) [p>0.1]*		*−1.95 (0.32) [***]*	*−2.75 (0.60) [***]*		*0.01 (0.01) [p>0.1]*
Round 7 (N = 277)	*0.47 (0.57) [p>0.1]*	*0.98 (0.38) [**]*	*0.89 (0.44) [**]*	*0.08 (0.41) [p>0.1]*		*−1.95 (0.31) [***]*	*−1.97 (0.56) [***]*		*0.02 (0.01) [*]*
Round 8 (N = 285)	0.90 (0.62) *[p>0.1]*	*0.35 (0.40) [p>0.1]*	*0.58 (0.50) [p>0.1]*	*0.13 (0.47) [p>0.1]*		*−2.50 (0.34) [***]*	*−2.26 (0.57) [***]*		*0.02 (0.01) [*]*

Ordinal logistic regression // Dependent variable: Overall Happiness; (Std. Error); [Significance]: ***$p < 0.01$, **$p < 0.05$, *$p < 0.1$.

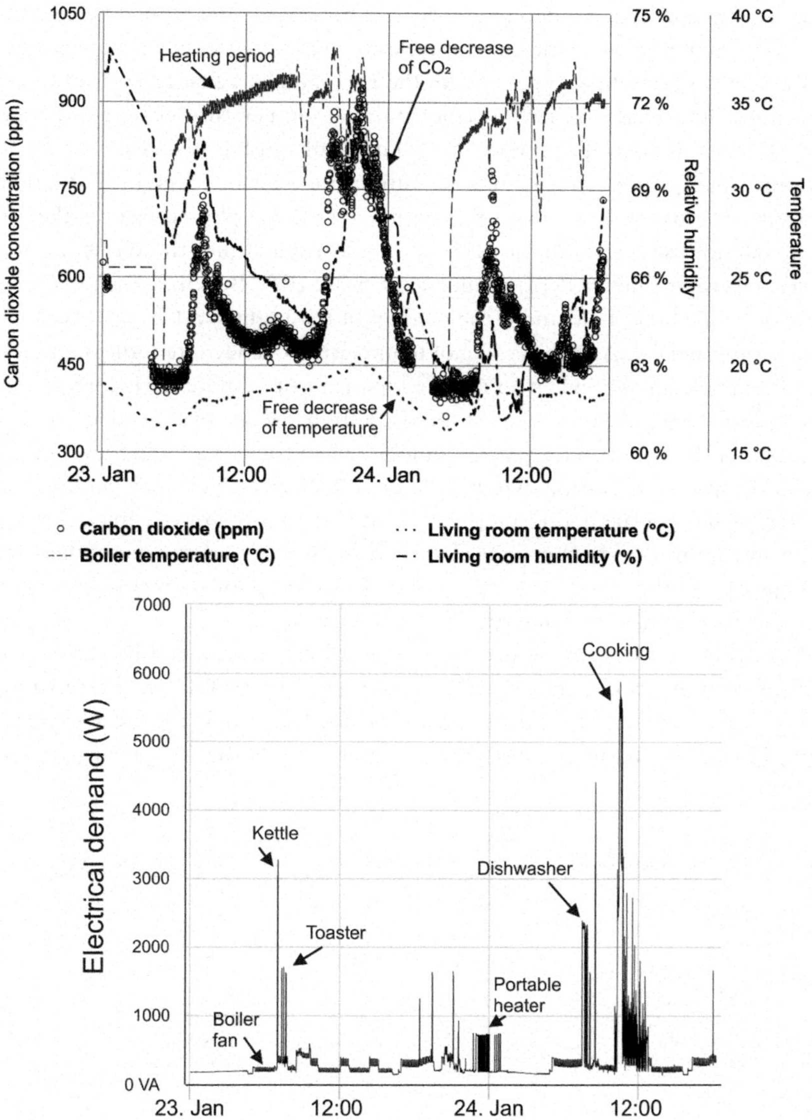

FIGURE 6.6 House environmental conditions ((a); carbon dioxide, air temperature and relative humidity) and the electric load ((b) monitored in one house from the HH survey sample).

Figure 6.6b shows the electric load of the household during the day, depicting the various appliances and their use. Household appliances can usually be recognised by their electricity consumption profiles. Different appliances will have certain ranges of power rating and will work for specific period of time. For example, as shown in Figure 6.6b, the kettle is expected to have a constant power load in the 2 kW–3 kW range that last for a few minutes only. However, a dishwasher and cooking appliances operate for longer periods of time and their load profile changes in relation to the cycle and temperature they are operating at.

In terms of household types within the HH sample, a first analysis of the observations show that flats have smaller internal temperature changes compared with different house types (Figure 6.7). The results in Figure 6.7 show the temperature change rate (internal temperature change for one Kelvin of difference between internal and external temperature, per hour) plotted against the CO_2 decay rate for the houses in the HH survey, distributed into three categories according to their Energy Performance Certificate (EPC[1]) rating. Each data point represents one household and is the median of the nightly values over the 2016-2017 winter period. A higher value of temperature change rate indicates that the dwelling cools quickly when an external temperature difference is applied, or in other words is poorly insulated. Similarly, a higher value of CO_2 decay rate indicates that the concentration drops quickly when there is a higher level of CO_2 inside compared to outside, which is to say it is 'leaky'. Note that both of these inferences rely on the main living space not being heated or occupied during at least some hours during the night. This may be the reason for some of the scatter in Figure 6.7; other sources of scatter include building form (exposed area compared to internal volume) and drift in CO_2 sensors.

Normally, it would be expected that dwellings with low EPC ratings and a lot of openings and exposed walls would have bigger CO_2 and temperature changes. Figure 6.7 indeed does show that, for low-rated (i.e. less energy efficient) houses, the temperature change is greater while the CO_2 change is more

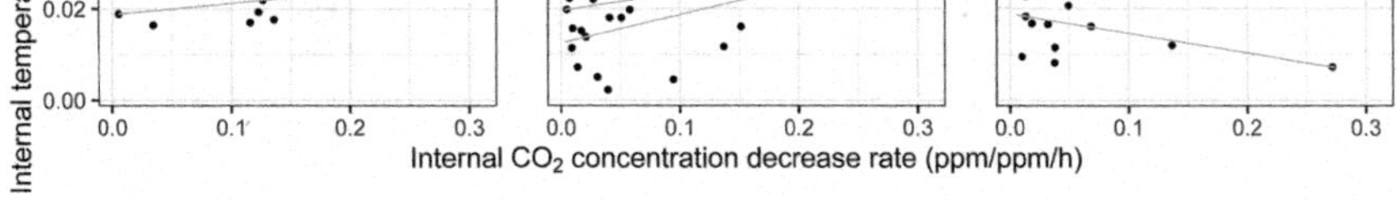

FIGURE 6.7 Relationship between free decrease in temperature versus decrease in carbon dioxide concentration overnight between 00:00 and 06:00 for the main living area in each of the households in the study during the winter of 2016–2017 (01-Oct-2016 to 31-Mar-2017). Each data point represents the median of nightly values for that household. Temperature decrease rate normalized by average difference between internal and external temperature; carbon dioxide decrease normalized by average difference between internal and ambient (assumed 400 ppm). Quantile regression lines for 25th, 50th and 75th percentiles are plotted for each of three categories of Energy Performance Certificate (EPC) rating.

spread and higher compared with the high EPC rated buildings. However, the link between 'leakiness' and temperature change is not very strong, as indicated by the quantile regression lines on the plots (25th, 50th and 75th percentiles). In general, this pattern shows that low-rated EPC houses may not be heated to high temperatures while concomitantly being much leakier compared with the higher rated EPC categories (Figure 6.7) (Bahaj et al., 2018). Most of the flats score high in EPC rating due to their age – flats are usually newer than houses – and small heat loss area compared to volume (Bahaj et al., 2018).

Conclusions: City Growth, Energy and Wellbeing

This study suggests that the two most important linkages to happiness are health and income (Table 6.4, 'national' study). Interestingly, the health of the households also was strongly associated with education. For the energy future of cities, it is important to note that any increase in health has a significant association with electricity consumption, resulting in approximately a 15% decrease in consumption. In addition, people with better health are more likely to walk for short distances. However, good health is also linked to high mobility, with more flights taken and train journeys made than people with poor health. Moreover, poor health was associated with higher energy usage at home but reduced mobility and hence energy for travelling. This relation of health and energy usage is of particular importance to policy makers, as any policy targeting domestic energy consumption could inevitably affect people with low income and poor health. These people tend to have large, home energy consumption because they lack alternative options.

The most important variables relating to travel behaviours and associated energy usage were household size, household income and miles driven per day, all strongly positively related as expected. There might be opportunities to intervene and break the link between car mileage and household income, especially through stricter air quality measures and policies to incentivise the use of public transport and restrict car access to city centres. However, private car use, travel and eating habits will be very challenging to change, as most of the people are reluctant to change their behaviour and their lifestyle (Büchs et al., 2018a). This has been confirmed by the comparison between the periods before and after the intervention with the carbon footprint calculator tool that did not show noticeable reductions in energy use and the carbon emissions associated with it (Büchs et al., 2018a).

Previously, we indicated that urban growth and land utilisation place pressure on public open spaces and greenspaces in particular. From the analysis, it is clear that Southampton does not have a problem with the amount of greenspace available. However, when considering the use of greenspaces, it is clear that future work needs to focus on the quality of the greenspaces and their connectivity to households and other destinations in the city. In the 'Greenspace, Health and Happiness' section, it was shown that more frequent visits to greenspace are highly likely to be associated with an increase in wellbeing, but this effect was not statistically significant.

The results of the environmental and electricity monitoring in the houses (see Figure 6.7) showed that low-performing houses are leaky and they might not be heated up to an adequately high temperature. This outcome, in combination with the results regarding health, income and home energy usage, points out the complexity of the problem of energy reduction in a city. At the same time, it is apparent that any measures and policy will need to approach these issues with care, making sure that the poor and vulnerable who have limited choices and options are not going to be disproportionally affected. Daily electricity usage was positively correlated with income but household size was not found to have an effect. When different house types were examined, the results indicate that residents in houses in the study consume 1.75 times more gas and 1.5 times more electricity compared to those living in flats.

A 'happy' city will need to satisfy the requirements for high-quality health and income. Health and education have a prominent role to play as they can stimulate economic growth and the results indicate that good health can lead to reductions of domestic electricity demand. Future cities should be designed to accommodate active dwellers. The design of liveable, healthy cities needs to provide diverse options of mobility and housing that ensure inclusivity and energy efficiency. At the same time, the design of cities should not disregard peoples' aspirations for affordable, spacious homes with good indoor air quality and access to greenspace. Interestingly, the positive correlation of electricity consumption with income shows the importance that lifestyle has on future decisions regarding energy policy and the shape of the urban realm. Effective interventions should promote certain lifestyle choices that are 'equal', less polluting alternatives of the current practice; for example, making affordable, low (or zero)-emission cars instead of banning private cars. It is also important that policy makers protect vulnerable people and that any new energy policy does not disproportionally affect people with poor health and low income as these are highly likely to have high home energy consumption without alternative options to upgrade their home, or leave – that is stuck at home!

It has been said that, 'Money can't buy happiness… but … rather be miserable with than without',[2] and this study indicated that satisfaction with income along with health are indeed important indicators for people's happiness. In addition, it is important to examine the quality of the public realm and design open spaces in ways that increase their positive impacts on wellbeing. Finally, while economic growth is associated with increased consumption of resources, it does enable people to find satisfactory jobs and hence income, which is strongly linked to their wellbeing.

Acknowledgements

This work is part of the research theme on Energy and Cities conducted by the Sustainable Energy Research Group (SERG) and the Energy and Climate Change Division within the Faculty of Engineering and Physical Sciences at the

University of Southampton (www.energy.soton.ac.uk). Funding for this work is through the UK's Engineering and Physical Science Research Council (EPSRC) under grant EP/J017698/1.

Notes

1 Energy Performance Certificate, rated from 1 (Band G; least efficient) to 100 (Band A; most efficient).
2 Dean Martin and Jerry Lewis, 'Money Song' (1948).

References

Bahaj, A. S., Blunden, L., Bourikas, L., Büchs, M., James, P. A. B., & Wu, Y. (2018). Household survey : Energy use and interaction of occupants with building systems. Retrieved from http://www.energy.soton.ac.uk/liveable-cities-case-studies/

Büchs, M., Bahaj, A. S., Blunden, L., Bourikas, L., Falkingham, J., James, P., Kamanda, M., & Wu, Y. (2018b). Sick and stuck at home – how poor health increases electricity consumption and reduces opportunities for environmentally-friendly travel in the United Kingdom. *Energy Research and Social Science, 44*, 250–259.

Büchs, M., Bahaj, A. S., Blunden, L., Bourikas, L., Falkingham, J., James, P., Kamanda, M., & Wu, Y. (2018a). Promoting low carbon behaviours through personalised information? Long-term evaluation of a carbon calculator interview. *Energy Policy, 120*, 284–293.

Carbon Conversations. (2018). Retrieved August 8, 2018, from http://www.carbonconversations.co.uk/

Gu, Y., & Wei, H.-L. (2018). Significant indicators and determinants of happiness: Evidence from a UK survey and revealed by a data-driven systems modelling approach. *Social Sciences,* 7 (4), 53.

HM Treasury. (2017). Autumn Budget 2017: 25 things you need to know. Retrieved December 7, 2018, from https://www.gov.uk/government/news/autumn-budget-2017-25-things-you-need-to-know

HM Treasury, & Hammond, P. (2018). Budget 2018: 24 things you need to know. Retrieved from https://www.gov.uk/government/news/budget-2018-24-things-you-need-to-know

James, P., Atehortua, V., Herbert, L., Bahaj, A., Bourikas, L., Blunden, L., & Wu, Y. (2017). *The Little Book Of Rezoning*. Lancaster: Lancaster University.

Jones, A., Hillsdon, M., & Coombes, E. (2009). Greenspace access, use, and physical activity: Understanding the effects of area deprivation. *Preventive Medicine, 49* (6), 500–505.

Landmap; The GeoInformation Group. (2012). Building class database. Retrieved from http://learningzone.rspsoc.org.uk/index.php/Datasets/Building_Class/

Landmap; The GeoInformation Group. (2014). UK building blocks.

Lee, A. C. K., Jordan, H. C., & Horsley, J. (2015). Value of urban green spaces in promoting healthy living and wellbeing: Prospects for planning. *Risk Management and Healthcare Policy, 8,* 131–137.

Morris, N. (2003). *Health, Wellbeing and Open Space: Literature Review.* Edinburgh: Edinburgh College of Art and Heriot-Watt University.

Natali, L., Handa, S., Peterman, A., Seidenfeld, D., & Tembo, G. (2018). Does money buy happiness? Evidence from an unconditional cash transfer in Zambia. *SSM - Population Health.* https://doi.org/10.1016/j.ssmph.2018.02.002

Office of the National Statistics. (n.d.). 2001 Area classifications. Retrieved December 7, 2018, from https://webarchive.nationalarchives.gov.uk/20160112013445/http://www.ons.gov.uk/ons/guide-method/geography/products/area-classifications/ns-area-classifications/index/index.html

Ordnance Survey. (n.d.). AddressBase Plus. Retrieved December 7, 2018, from https://www.ordnancesurvey.co.uk/business-and-government/products/addressbase-plus.html

Southampton City Council. (n.d.). Where i live-mapsouthampton. Retrieved from https://www.southampton.gov.uk/whereilive/mapsouthampton.aspx

Southampton City Council. (2008). *Green spaces great places Southampton's Green Space Strategy Summary and Action Plan Information from Southampton City Council about Southampton's Parks and Green Spaces.* Retrieved from https://www.southampton.gov.uk/policies/green space strategy summary and action plan_tcm63–363566.pdf

Subramanian, S. V., Kim, D., & Kawachi, I. (2005). Covariation in the socioeconomic determinants of self rated health and happiness: A multivariate multilevel analysis of individuals and communities in the USA. *Journal of Epidemiology and Community Health, 59* (8), 664–669.

Taylor, L., & Hochuli, D. F. (2017). Defining greenspace: Multiple uses across multiple disciplines. *Landscape and Urban Planning, 158*, 25–38. https://doi.org/10.1016/j.landurbplan.2016.09.024

University of Essex. (2017). Understanding Society: Waves 1–7, 2009–2016 and Harmonised BHPS: Waves 1–18, 1991–2009. https://doi.org/http://doi.org/10.5255/UKDA-SN-6614-10

Ward Thompson, C., Roe, J., Aspinall, P., Mitchell, R., Clow, A., & Miller, D. (2012). More green space is linked to less stress in deprived communities: Evidence from salivary cortisol patterns. *Landscape and Urban Planning, 105* (3), 221–229.

Wood, L., Hooper, P., Foster, S., & Bull, F. (2017). Public green spaces and positive mental health – investigating the relationship between access, quantity and types of parks and mental wellbeing. *Health and Place, 48,* 63–71.

7

DESIGN FOR FOOD AND WELLBEING IN FUTURE CITIES

Stephen Clune and Serena Pollastri

Introduction

While this chapter is focussed on food wellbeing and cities, it may be first appropriate to acknowledge that in a vast majority of contemporary cities, examples can be found of what may be considered food ill-being. As a starting point, what 'well' is may be defined as the polar opposite to what 'ill' is. Unfortunately, you do not have to search too hard for statistics in the UK, the US and Australia that indicates food-related ill-being is prevalent. For example:

- Fifty-four per cent of adult Australians were overweight or obese in 2004–2005, rising to 63% in 2011–2012 (ABS, 2013); it is suggested that 62% of adults in England are overweight or obese (Public Health England, 2016). The economic costs of obesity globally are estimated to amount to two trillion dollars (Dobbs et al., 2014). In England, the direct cost sustained by the National Healthcare System (NHS) for treating overweight or obese people grew from £479 million in 1998 to £4.2 billion in 2007 (National Obesity Observatory, 2010).
- Obesity and malnutrition negatively affect quality of life by increasing the risk of contracting serious conditions that are life-altering, such as diabetes, and often life-threatening, such as heart and vascular diseases and several types of cancers (GBD, 2015; Obesity Collaborators, 2017).
- An estimated 30% of food purchased for home consumption is not eaten and wasted (FAO, 2013), so much so that if all food waste was its own country, it would rank as the third largest global greenhouse gas emitter.
- A significant proportion of a person's overall greenhouse gas impact is attributed to food consumption (Dey et al., 2007), accounting for 20% of an individual's CO2e footprint globally (Hertwich & Peters, 2009); agricultural production is responsible for 19%–29% of global anthropogenic greenhouse gas emissions (Vermeulen et al., 2012).

These elements of food ill-being on individual health and planet are interrelated, according to the WWF. Their Livewell report suggested that a healthy diet is also a more sustainable one (Macdiarmid et al., 2011), recommending a reduction in fats (predominately from overeating meat) and sugars (increasingly added to processed foods), and an increase in plant-based protein. The gravity of the situation should not be underestimated, given that 'no country has yet managed a successful, sustained reduction in the prevalence of overweight and obesity, despite health and medical research' (NHMRC, 2014, p. 1).

Design Contribution to Food Ill-being

A legacy exists today, as past designs continue to script and influence the way designers design. This phenomenon may be explained through the concept of ontological design. Heidegger's (1971) claim that we make our locations but we are also made by them illustrates the central argument of ontological design in that as we design, the things we design also design us: thus, design designs (*things have the capacity to thing*).

> The designs produced by designers come from their worlding as designers, the objects or systems that come from these designings in turn become parts of worlds and thus enter into worlding, this in ways in which as things they thing.
>
> *(A. M. Willis, 2006, p. 91).*

This perspective prompts us to consider how might design, and the design of cities, have contributed to food-related ill-being.

At the domestic level, the microwave, freezer, packaging, supermarket and car are perhaps some of the most recognisable examples to explain 'things, capacity to thing' and impact upon the food system. This is significant, given that in Australia, 72% of meals are cooked in the home. The microwave allows food to be prepared quicker; the freezer allows you to cook on Saturday so you can store food to be quickly reheated with a reduced preparation time through out the week. The proliferation of single-serve microwave meals and associated 'microwave safe' packaging also has a symbiotic relationship with the freezer and frozen meals. Packaging and longer shelf lives may enable less frequent shopping and the supermarket to thrive. The associated, innovative plastic packaging removes our dependency on fresh produce and what is locally and seasonally available, removing us further from the production supply chain and direct engagement with what sustains us. Plastics have been well covered as ontologically transformative (i.e. Tonkinwise, 1998), suggesting that plastics changed our disposition to the material world by making disposability a new possibility. Manzini (2003) critiques designers continuing to design for convenience as a remedial approach that does not address the root cause of the problem.

Henry Ford's 'car for the masses' did far more than enable people with the opportunity to drive. Individual mobility afforded by the car equally altered the 'planning of cities, suburbs, urban design, rural life, retail shopping, tourism, leisure and more' (Fry, 2009, p. 39). Once the car was viewed as a dominant transport mode, a range of services were designed that rely on the car. For example, many supermarkets in Australia and the US would not survive without the car. The dominance of the supermarkets may have led to the decline of local shops and alterations to the practice of shopping (Clarke, 2000). On the extremes, car dependency could be seen as a contributing factor to an obesogenic urban environment, a double whammy of suburbs designed with poor access to wholefoods, and car-dependent neighbourhoods that limit the ease at which active travel and exercise can take place.

At a macro level, most Western cities have decreased food production within the city and outsourced production. For example, areas of Western Sydney are built upon the rich, fertile soil that was once the food bowl for the city. If we map out the food system, we see the enormous impact industrialisation has had on the food system, from farm-to-fork. Mechanised farming matching the increasing need for efficiency in production leads to fewer, larger farms. Quantum leaps in road, transport and logistics enable ease for international trade, facilitated by advancements in packaging that enable us to store food for extended periods of time. Larger, centralised, supermarket buying power influence the supply of food available to purchase, and where (and often how) we have to go to purchase such food (see Millstone and Lang, 2003 for an excellent overview of the evolution of agricultural technology and diet).

In the UK, an historical review of the last 60 years of retail shows just how radically the way in which food is purchased has changed, and how rapidly these changes have happened as a consequence of design and policy decisions. Until the Second World War, women – for the most part responsible for their family's grocery shopping – used to shop every day in local stores, where customers were served from across the counter by shop assistants. In the 1950s self-service shopping, where customers are given a basket and chose products arranged in aisles, became increasingly popular. In the first 'supermarkets' as we know them now, branding, advertisement and product placement were carefully planned to influence shoppers, and particularly to enhance 'impulse buys'. For the first time, processed and packaged food became more appealing to customers than fresh food.

The first out-of-town retailer was opened in Britain in 1964, and was designed, according to its chief executive, as a 'one-stop discount stores for the motorised shopper' (Whysall, 2005). In the 1970s, the first wave of retail decentralisation was indeed led by out-of-town food stores (Schiller, 1988). Following the American model, in just over 20 years, food went from being a matter of planning, daily shopping and labour-intensive preparation to being increasingly about taste and impulse, accumulation and storage, and convenience. The weekly grocery shopping, which privileges easy-to-store, lasting food over fresh produce and infrastructure-promoting car dependency and social changes in the family – including more women at work – resulted in radical changes in how food is sold, processed and prepared.

The industrialised systems and factory farming has led to the ease at which we can eat what once may have been considered luxury items in sweets, as well as meats. This system brings the effortless distribution of affordable food, often with a high global warming potential. For example, Figure 7.1 illustrates the limited correlation between the cost of food and global warming potential.

It could be reasonable to expect that the abundance, convenience and availability of food that industrialised countries like the UK, the US and Australia came to enjoy in the last few decades would have brought higher levels of wellbeing. Indeed, economist Tim Harford (2017a) includes ready meals among the 'Fifty Things that Shaped Modern Economy', noting how industrialised food processing (and the already-mentioned new home appliances, such as fridge, freezer and microwave) dramatically reduced the time that had to be spent for food planning and preparation: from two to three hours every day to an average of 15–45 minutes. This shortening in time is a direct function of the availability of processed food: affordability if produced at a large scale, and readily available for purchase at supermarkets or fast food chains. For the most part, food preparation has always been responsibility of women; Harford (2017a)

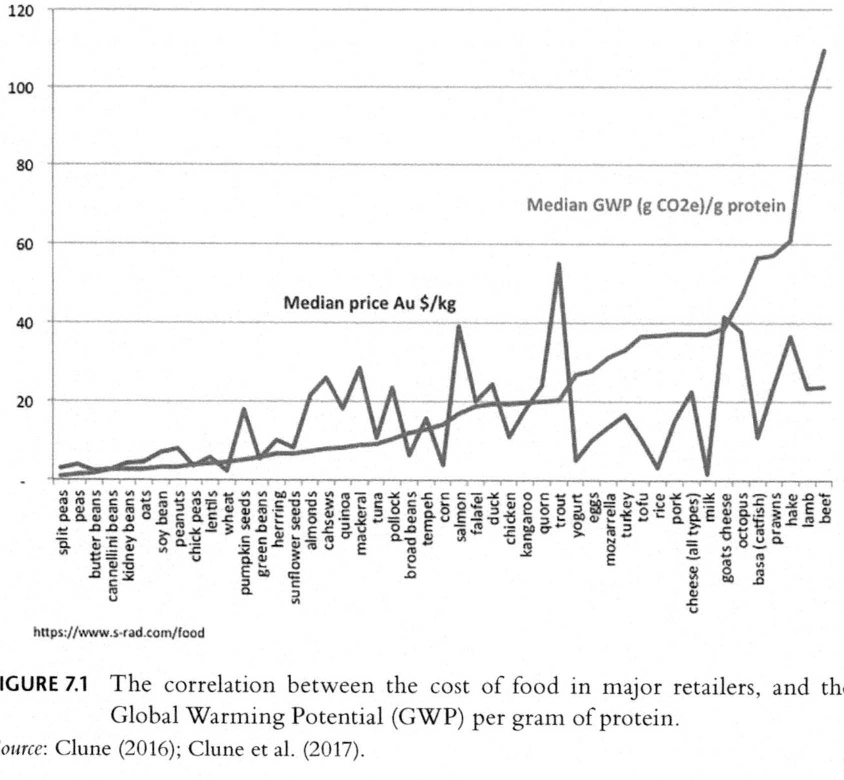

FIGURE 7.1 The correlation between the cost of food in major retailers, and the Global Warming Potential (GWP) per gram of protein.

Source: Clune (2016); Clune et al. (2017).

also makes the case that ready meals contributed to their emancipation, and their ability to enter the workforce full time.

However, convenience food also has undeniable side effects, and has been directly linked to the increase in obesity rates (Butland et al., 2007). As Harford notes:

> experiments by behavioural scientists show that we make very different decisions about what to eat depending on how far away the meal is. A long-planned meal is likely to be nutritious, but when we make more impulsive decisions, our snacks are more likely to be junk food than something nourishing.
>
> *(Harford, 2017b)*

And the out-of-town food stores that can be seen as islands of food abundance also created, on the flip side, food deserts: urban areas where fresh food is now difficult to find, and where the only affordable options are often take-away restaurants or convenience stores (Steel, 2013). In a book chapter reflecting on the importance for designers to 'listen' to people and contexts, Roberta Tassi, a design researcher working on a new insulin pump with design consultancy *frog*, recounted her experience during an ethnographic study with diabetes patients in a deprived urban area of Atlanta (US). During the study, members of the research group found themselves unable to maintain a healthy diet, as the only food options that were close to her accommodation were roadside, take-away shops. Through this direct experience, the group of design researchers understood the systemic ramification of what originally was framed as a product design project (Tassi & Valsecchi, 2016).

The way in which *design designs* – or at least heavily influences – our behaviours around food is evident in the impacts of urban design, retail design, (car-based) infrastructures, packaging and product design. Of course, there are many other factors shaping food and the way we eat, but those highlighted here are intended to show the huge responsibility of design when it comes to food and wellbeing.

From Ill-being to a More Nuanced Understanding of Wellbeing and a Rich Food Culture

While showing just how systemic and complex the issue is, the examples presented above have been void of the cultural significance of food and the relationship to a holistic notion of wellbeing, which is the focus of the chapter. As the World Health Organization's early report on wellbeing stated in 1948 'health is not the mere absence of diseases… a state of complete physical, mental and social wellbeing' (WHO, 1948, p. 16). Wellbeing is as much about how we feel at a *personal* level – happy, satisfied, good quality of life, healthy – as it is about ensuring that the *people and places around us* are doing well (Boyko et al., 2018). Jan Gehl, an expert in liveable cities and public places, advocates for comfortable places to sit within the city, enabling people to eat, read, people-watch and socialise (Gehl, 2010).

While the chapter so far has focussed on the effects of ill-being of food, the positive effects of food on wellbeing are just as evident. Food can often evoke positive memories of childhood, or meaningful moments spent with others. Eating certain dishes when ill or unhappy can provide comfort, and help us feel better at a chemical as well as psychological level. As food preferences and acquired habits are extremely personal, what we eat and how we eat matters beyond the simple act of fuelling our body. In its broader sense, food is meaningful to people, cultures and societies (Counihan & Van Esterik, 2012). Anyone who has travelled may have come across places and locales that may be considered to have a rich food culture, with a celebration of food, joy in cultivation, preparation, and eating together. This is true not only in small, idyllic villages where traditions have resisted unchanged for centuries, but also – and perhaps more significantly – in diverse and evolving urban neighbourhoods, where different communities coexist. Here, food is often one of the markers of cultural and social identity. It is the way in which social groups build ties and define themselves as separate from other groups, or build new, shared identities by mixing and innovating cooking traditions and practices (Bonnerjee et al., 2012). All of this transcends the issue of whether the food that brings us joy, cultural meaning and connection is healthy for us or the planet.

Whether we value it or not, we all have a deep and intimate connection with food. Food is, after all, the only product that we all consume and which becomes, through this act of consumption, part of our body. Similar to attempts to map the systemic ways in which *design designs*, the way we eat can help unveil the causes of urban food ill-being. However, any design action aimed at improving human and planetary wellbeing through the design *of* or *for* food must move away from a purely solutionist and rational approach to optimise healthy and sustainable food systems, and embrace their deeply personal and cultural aspects.

Indeed, the exploration of diversity of food practices and traditions can help us discover novel ways of addressing challenges related to human and planetary wellbeing. For example, by learning from, and celebrating others' culinary culture, such as from the Indian or Central American extensive use of pulses and beans or East and South-East Asian seaweed dishes, we can envisage creative and meaningful ways of moving towards diets with far lower carbon footprints.

Design Approaches to Change

Design can have a redirecting and transformative effect on urban food systems through the rethinking of places, services, products or infrastructures. In recent years, designers who would normally work in other areas have rediscovered an interest in food and food futures (Celi & Rudkin, 2016; DiSalvo, 2012; Zampollo, 2013), and often provided radical visions of alternative scenarios of food in cities. For example, in 'Food City', architect and urbanist C. J. Lim looked at cities through the lenses of food, and proposed an alternative food infrastructure for London (Lim, 2014). The Centre for Genomic Gastronomy (http://genomicgastronomy.com/) has prototyped critical artefacts, such as 'smog meringues', that act as provocations in broader discussions. In 'Spectacles and Tropes: Speculative Design and Contemporary Food Cultures', DiSalvo (2012) collected a series of case studies showing how food issues have been explored in speculative design.

What food and design have in common is the central role of culture, pleasure and aesthetic (Maffei & Parini, 2011). Future-focussed, design-led approaches can support the development of radical visions of possible urban food futures that prioritise wellbeing and the emotional qualities of food. These approaches include: nowcasting, backcasting, forecasting and design orienting scenarios.

Nowcasting

'Now-casting' (Burns, 2016, p. 27) identifies contemporary best practice that exists in the present from a social and a technical perspective. It then attempts to amplify and normalise best practices, with designers assisting to 'upscale' or 'multiply' the promising ones. John Thackara (2008) also advocates this simple approach, of looking around the community you live in, identifying what is fundamentally positive and saying, 'Hi, I am a designer. How can I help?' Despite the damning statistics, it is possible to walk around almost every city and identify a plethora of initiatives that may be representative of a positive food future. This also avoids a solutionist approach (i.e. just telling people to eat less, and avoid processed food in order to fix the obesity issue), in favour of a respectful approach that takes into consideration the economic, environmental, social, cultural contexts within which the issue of food and well/ill-being is situated.

For example, a surprising result of two workshops completed in Birmingham and Lancaster was the numerous, grassroots examples identified in relation to food, including spaces, places, gardens, cafés, food and chickens (Boyko et al., 2017). Many of these initiatives were run via word of mouth, often informally or without economic exchange. Groups involved in these projects were passionate about, and proud of, the positive results that they were seeing, but also acknowledged some difficulties in involving people outside their communities. Designers could work with these groups to develop solutions to amplify their impact. For example, Perth City Council in Australia, relaxed red tape for planting edible plants when insurers wanted volunteers to do an induction course, have their work checked and a logbook kept of their hours. The council went back and 'explained to the insurers that these reserves are generally zoned for recreational purposes...Gardening is recreational so it's not volunteering for the city, it is utilising the land for the purpose which it is zoned for' (Wynne, 2018, p. 1).

Forecasting and Backcasting

Forecasting techniques of forecasting and backcasting are used to create pathways for sustainable innovations:

> The future is never empty, never a blank space to be filled with the output of human activity It is already colonised by what the past and present have sent to it. Without this comprehension of what is finite, what limits reign we have little knowledge of futures, either those we need to destroy, or those we need to create.
>
> *(Fry, 1999, p. 11–12)*

Fry's above quote is useful on several fronts, in that it states that when considering the future, we are not simply dreaming up utopian, Sci-fi scenarios, but responding to what the past and present have already predetermined to a large extent. Forecasting and backcasting techniques envisage the range of possible futures (forecasting) or what steps would lead to any of these futures (backcasting) (Quist & Vergragt, 2006).

Strategic forecasting projects the trajectories of the past into the future, by gathering data on emerging trends, analysing the potential of those trends in relation to each other and creating pictures that speculate possible worlds based on this analysis. This process may often present us with a 'business as usual' scenario where historical events are extrapolated forward into the future. The trajectories of practices can be extrapolated forward and read together to enable speculation on possible futures. This understanding is critical for strategic forecasting as it enables a response by working with the trends that are occurring to creating desirable futures. These futures may upscale (amplify) social or technical innovations, or consider what social or technical innovations are needed to actively discourage or disrupt from occurring.

In Backcasting (Robinson, 1990), you take time to develop what would be a desirable, long-term, future scenario, and then attempt to map out the steps that would need to be taken to make that future happen.

Scenario Planning

A probabilistic approach to forecasting often involves the development of sets of scenarios that are used to describe the main characteristics of possible futures. Developing scenarios is a way of taking into account the complexities and uncertainties of thinking about futures. For this reason, scenario building is one of the most used techniques in the field of future studies (Börjeson et al., 2006; Schwartz, 1996).

Scenario planning is slightly different to strategic forecasting in that the scenarios generated are not meant to be accurate predictions of the future; rather, 'they are a means to project likely future circumstances in order to reflect on these and to inform action to be taken' (A.-M. Willis, 2014, p. 2). Scenarios can be predictive (*what will happen if?*), explorative (*what if?*) or normative (*how can we?*) (Börjeson et al., 2006; Quist & Vergragt, 2006). This means that scenarios could be used to plan and react (predictive or explorative scenarios) as well as to design (normative scenarios).

Normative scenarios are commonly used in design as a way of describing stories of possible futures that design solutions could engender. They are particularly important in design for sustainability, where they are used to describe the systemic impact of discrete or coordinated design actions.

Evans (2014) defines scenarios in the design fields as 'descriptive visions of the future communicated through a narrative structure outlining how certain dynamics of change occur over time' (p. 195). Manzini and Jégou call these types of scenarios design orienting scenarios, and describe them as probable hypotheses that are brought up for discussion (2003). If desirable, those with a vested interest could choose to make the scenarios happen. Design orienting scenarios have a strong, human element in that the scenarios are rooted in, and trying to, present a quality to everyday life that enhances liveability and wellbeing, rather than viewing humans as merely passive consumers to be waited on. Design orienting scenarios are often speculative in nature, and describe ideas that are 'realistic enough to make us question our own lifestyle, but sufficiently open-ended for us to adapt them to our own lives' (Jegou, 2008).

Exploring futures of urban eating through design orienting scenarios could be a way of creating spaces for conversations in which various ideas can be co-created and discussed by various actors. This would give space to radical solutions based on social and cultural values to emerge within the context of a low-carbon meta-narrative (see, e.g. Moy & Ryan, 2011). Our research has developed a set of co-designed cards to assist in facilitating such conversations, by encouraging an engagement in the contextual complexity of designing food systems for personal and planetary wellbeing in future cities.

Conversation Cards for Wellbeing: An Intelligent Guide for Critical Conversations

The conversation cards (Clune et al., 2016) were developed to assist in scenario planning by translating ideas from lifecycle analysis, social practice theory, and design for behavioural change into palatable prompts. These prompts encourage users to think about how their current food environment may have been designed, and suggests design approaches that may need to be considered to reorient the food environment.

For example, a card may be asking how design may have mediated the available choices in what you ate yesterday. As a counterpoint, a card then asks you what a guilt-free, sustainable and healthy food environment would be like. This is based on the concept of choice architecture from the design for behavioural change literature (Niedderer et al., 2017), suggesting that the default options presented to us could be more sustainable and healthy (see Figure 7.2).

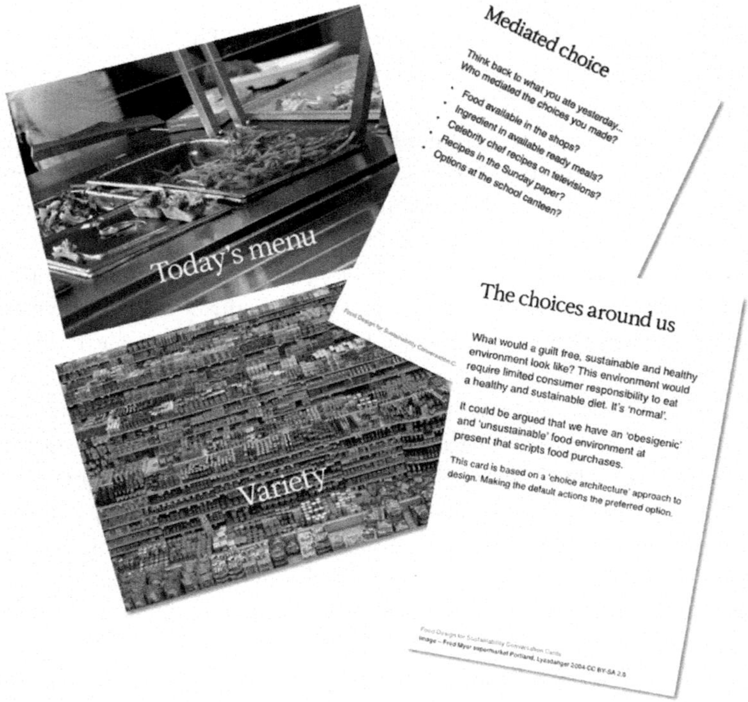
Today's menu
Variety
Mediated choice
Think back to what you ate yesterday...
Who mediated the choices you made?
• Food available in the shops?
• Ingredient in available ready meals?
• Celebrity chef recipes on televisions?
• Recipes in the Sunday paper?
• Options at the school canteen?
The choices around us
What would a guilt free, sustainable and healthy environment look like? This environment would require limited consumer responsibility to eat a healthy and sustainable diet. It's 'normal'.
It could be argued that we have an 'obesigenic' and 'unsustainable' food environment at present that scripts food purchases.
This card is based on a 'choice architecture' approach to design. Making the default actions the preferred option.

FIGURE 7.2 Food design for sustainability conversation cards mediated choice, and the choices around us.

Source: Authors.

Other cards may seek to reflect on concrete examples of change in others, and oneself (see Figure 7.3). This reflection is explored against a framework from social practice theory to map out various elements that may have supported this change.

The cards, when used in co-design design sessions, have enhanced participants' understanding of planetary and personal wellbeing in relation to food, enabling more targeted ideation.

Conclusions

There is no shying away from the complexity of the situation. Only two strategies have proven to be successful for losing weight: moving more and eating less (or better), yet no country has managed to reverse the trend of obesity, even without the additional complexity of any concern for the planet. This chapter has illustrated the necessity of reorientating ill-being for wellbeing in future cities, by identifying how design has contributed to the problem of ill-being, and offering several tools for envisioning promising food futures that enhance personal and planetary wellbeing in cities.

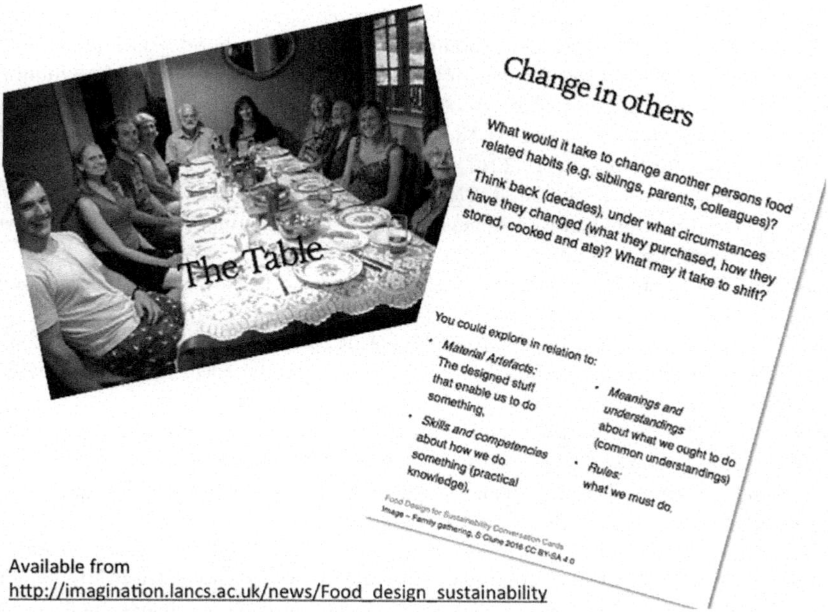

FIGURE 7.3 Food design for sustainability conversation cards change in others.
Source: Authors.

References

ABS. (2013). 4338.0-Profiles of Health, Australia, 2011–13. Retrieved from Canberra: http://www.abs.gov.au/ausstats/abs@.nsf/Lookup/by Subject/4338.0~2011–13~MainFeatures~Overweight and obesity~10007

Bonnerjee, J., Blunt, A., McIlwaine, C., & Pereira, C. (2012). *Connected Communities: Diaspora and Transnationality*. London: Queen Mary University.

Börjeson, L., Höjer, M., Dreborg, K.-H., Ekvall, T., & Finnveden, G. (2006). Scenario Types and Techniques: Towards a User's Guide. *Futures*, 38(7), 723–739. https://doi.org/10.1016/j.futures.2005.12.002

Boyko, C. T., Clune, S. J., Cooper, R. F., Coulton, C. J., Dunn, N. S., Pollastri, S., … De Laurentiis, V. (2017). How Sharing can Contribute to More Sustainable Cities. *Sustainability, 9*(5), 701.

Boyko, C. T., Coulton, C. J., Gomez, A. S., & Cooper, R. F. (2017). *The Little Book of Wellbeing: A Guide to Wellbeing in Urban Environments*. Lancaster: Imagination.

Burns, B. (2016). Daring to be Ordinary on a Finite Planet and How the Centre for Design Is Helping. *RMIT Design Archives Journal, 6* (1), 20–31.

Butland, B., Jebb, S., Kopelman, P., McPherson, K., Thomas, S., Mardell, J., & Parry, V. (2007). *Tackling Obesities: Future Choices (Foresight)*. London: Government Office for Science. Retrieved from https://www.gov.uk/government/publications/reducing-obesity-future-choices

Celi, M., & Rudkin, J. (2016). Drawing Food Trends: Design Potential in Shaping Food Future. *Futures, 83,* 112–121.

Clarke, I. (2000). Retail Power, Competition and Local Consumer Choice in the UK Grocery Sector. *European Journal of Marketing, 34*(8), 975–1002.

Clune, S. (2016). Protein versus Global Warming Potential – A Meta-Analysis of the Global Warming Potential and Protein Ratios for Human Food. Paper presented at the 10th International Conference on Life Cycle Assessment of Food 2016, Dublin.

Clune, S., Crossin, E., & Verghese, K. (2017). Systematic Review of Greenhouse Gas Emissions for Different Fresh Food Categories. *Journal Cleaner Production, 140*(2), 766–783. doi:10.1016/j.jclepro.2016.04.082

Clune, S., Friday, A., & Whitham, R. (2016, 27–30 June 2016). Food Design for Sustainability Conversation Cards. Retrieved from http://imagination.lancs.ac.uk/news/Food_design_sustainability

Counihan, C., & Van Esterik, P. (Eds.). (2012). *Food and Culture: A Reader.* Abingdon: Routledge.

Dey, C., Berger, C., Foran, B., Foran, M., Joske, R., Lenzen, M., & Wood, R. (2007). *Household Environmental Pressure from Consumption: An Australian Environmental Atlas.* Sydney University Press.

DiSalvo, C. (2012). Spectacles and Tropes: Speculative Design and Contemporary Food Cultures | Fibreculture Journal. *Fibreculture Journal,* 20. Retrieved from http://twenty.fibreculturejournal.org/2012/06/19/fcj-142-spectacles-and-tropes-speculative-design-and-contemporary-food-cultures/

Dobbs, R., Sawers, C., Thompson, F., Manyika, J., Woetzel, J., Child, P., & Spatharou, A. (2014). Overcoming Obesity: An Initial Economic Analysis. Retrieved from http://www.mckinsey.com/insights/economic_studies/how_the_world_could_better_fight_obesity

Evans, M. (2014). Researching the Future by Design. In P. Rodgers & J. Yee (Eds.), *The Routledge Companion to Design Research* (206–218). New York: Routledge.

FAO. (2013). Food Wastage Footprint. Impacts on Natural Resources. Summary Report. Retrieved from Rome: http://www.fao.org/docrep/018/i3347e/i3347e.pdf

Fry, T. (2009). *Design Futuring: Sustainability, Ethics and New Practice.* Oxford: Berg Publishing.

GBD 2015 Obesity Collaborators. (2017). Health Effects of Overweight and Obesity in 195 Countries over 25 Years. *New England Journal of Medicine, 377*(1), 13–27.

Gehl, J. (2010). *Cities for People.* Washington, DC: Island Press.

Harford, T. (2017a). *Fifty Things that Made the Modern Economy.* London: Little, Brown.

Harford, T. (2017b, May 15). The Hidden Cost of the Processed Food Revolution. BBC News. Retrieved from http://www.bbc.co.uk/news/business-39490182

Heidegger, M. (1971). *Poetry, Language, Thought,* translated by Albert Hofstadter. New York: Harper Colophon Books.

Hertwich, E. G., & Peters, G. P. (2009). Carbon Footprint of Nations: A Global, Trade-Linked Analysis. *Environment Science and Technology, 43*(16), 6414–6420.

Jegou, F. (2008, December 7). City Eco Lab: "Hybrid Reality Story Scripts" about Creative Communities. Retrieved October 30, 2015, from http://www.doorsofperception.com/city-eco-lab/city-eco-lab-hybrid-reality-story-scripts-about-creative-communities/

Lang, T. (2009). Reshaping the Food System for Ecological Public Health. *Journal of Hunger and Environmental Nutrition, 4*(3), 315–335.

Lim, C. J. (2014). *Food City.* New York: Routledge.

Macdiarmid, J., Kyle, J., Horgan, G., Loe, J., Fyfe, C., Johnstone, A., & McNeill, G. (2011). Livewell: A Balance of Healthy and Sustainable Food Choices. Retrieved from Aberdeen: http://www.businessnz.org.nz/file/2054/Livewell_ A balance of healthy and sustainable food choices - WWF%5B2%5D.pdf

Maffei, S., & Parini, B. (2011). *Food Mood.* Milan and Woodbridge: Electa Mondadori.

Manzini, E. (2003). Scenarios of Sustainable Wellbeing. *Design Philosophy Papers* (1), 5–21.

Manzini, E., & Jégou, F. (2003). *Sustainable Everyday, Scenarios of Urban Life*. Milan: Edizioni Ambiente srl.

Millstone, E., & Lang, T. (2003). The Atlas of Food. *Appropriate Technology, 30*(2), 63.

Moy, D., & Ryan, C. (2011). Using Scenarios to Explore System Change: VEIL, Local Food Depot. In A. Meroni & D. Sangiorgi (Eds.), *Design for Services* (193–205). London: Gower.

National Obesity Observatory. (2010). *Briefing Note: Obesity and Life Expectancy*. Oxford: National Obesity Observatory.

NHMRC. (2014). CEO Roundtable: New Insights into the Biology of Obesity. Retrieved from Canberrá: http://faculty.nhmrc.gov.au/_files_nhmrc/file/media/events/2014/obesity_ceo_rountable_140617.pdf

Niedderer, K., Clune, S., & Ludden, G. (Eds.). (2017). *Design for Behavioural Change, Theories and Practices of Designing for Change*. London: Routledge.

Public Health England. (2016). Health Matters: Obesity and the Food Environment. Retrieved February 15, 2019, from https://www.gov.uk/government/publications/health-matters-obesity-and-the-food-environment/health-matters-obesity-and-the-food-environment--2

Quist, J., & Vergragt, P. (2006). Past and Future of Backcasting: The Shift to Stakeholder Participation and a Proposal for a Methodological Framework. *Futures, 38*(9), 1027–1045.

Robinson, J. B. (1990). Futures Under Glass: A Recipe for People Who Hate to Predict. *Futures, 22*(8), 820–842.

Schiller, R. (1988). Retail Decentralization. A Property View. *The Geographical Journal, 154*(1), 17–19.

Schwartz, P. (1996). *The Art of the Long View: Planning for the Future in an Uncertain World* (Reprint edition). Sydney: Currency Doubleday.

Steel, C. (2013). *Hungry City: How Food Shapes Our Lives*. London: Vintage. Retrieved from http://www.randomhouse.co.uk/editions/9780099531685

Tassi, R., & Valsecchi, F. (2016). The Listening Capability: Three Insights Around and about a Design Way to Storytelling. In Bertolotti, E., Daam, H., Piredda, F., Tassinari, V., *The Pearl Diver. The Designer as Storyteller* (Vol. 1; 34–49). Milan: DESIS Network, Dipartimento di Design, Politecnico di Milano.

Thackara, J. (2008). Keynote. Changing the Change Design, Visions, Proposals and Tools. Politecnico di Milano, Turin, Italy, 10–12 July 2008

Tonkinwise, C. (1998). Everywhere and Nowhere: An Introduction to Plastics. Information Ecology Newsletter. Retrieved March 8, 2019, from http://www.changedesign.org/Resources/EDFPublications/Articles/ArticlesMenuMain.htm

Vermeulen, S. J., Campbell, B. M., & Ingram, J. S. (2012). Climate Change and Food Systems. *Annual Review of Environment and Resources, 37*, 195–222.

WHO. (1948). Official Records of the World Health Organization No. 2 Summary Report on Proceedings Minutes and Final Acts of the International Health Conference Held in New York from 19 June to 22 July 1946. Retrieved from New York: http://apps.who.int/iris/bitstream/handle/10665/85573/Official_record2_eng.pdf;jsessionid=5E2F79DF0FEB4B6F065B265509ABEDC1?sequence=1

Whysall, P. (2005). GEM, 1964–1966: Britain's First Out-of-Town Retailer. *The International Review of Retail, Distribution and Consumer Research, 15*(2), 111–124. https://doi.org/10.1080/09593960500049183

Willis, A. M. (2006). Ontological Designing. *Design Philosophy Papers, 4*(2), 69–92.

Willis, A.-M. (2014). Designing Back from the Future. *Design Philosophy Papers, 12*(2), 151–160.

Wynne, E. (2018). Perth Council Cuts Red Tape to Allow Residents to Plant Fruit and Veg in Public Parks. ABC Radio Perth. Retrieved from http://www.abc.net.au/news/2018-02-08/bayswater-council-opens-up-parks-to-resident-food-planting/9404394

York, H. (2009). Food and Climate Change. Retrieved from http://www.circleofresponsibility.com/page/350/food-and-climate-change.htm

Zampollo, F. (2013). Food and Design: Space, Place and Experience. *Hospitality & Society, 3*(3), 181–187.

8

FUTURE-PROOFING RESIDENTIAL ENVIRONMENTS FOR CHILDREN'S WELLBEING

A Review of Evidence and Design Implications

Marcella Ucci

Introduction: Housing Dimensions for Children's Health and Wellbeing

Several aspects of the home environment are critical for health and wellbeing across the life course. Poor housing has often been the focus of public health interventions and, indeed, the nineteenth century's focus on poor sanitation and infectious diseases has resulted in dramatic improvements of basic housing conditions in middle- and high-income countries. In more recent decades, however, the burden of disease in these countries has increasingly been dominated by chronic conditions, some of which, like asthma, can be exacerbated by poor indoor air quality, to which children can be particularly vulnerable. Therefore, housing design and policy approaches must consider how best to address current and emerging health challenges at the population level. However, there is much evidence on the role played by housing in all spheres of children's health and wellbeing – spanning from physical and mental health, behaviour, cognitive development, educational achievement and life chances. Much evidence is emerging of the lasting effects that exposure to poor housing conditions during childhood can have over the life course. In part, these effects are due to the complex nature of the relationship between housing itself and other factors, which directly and indirectly affect health and wellbeing, as well as housing itself. Within this context, it is imperative to evaluate the nature of existing evidence to establish key design principles for 'healthy' housing and evaluate how these impact on city-scale issues.

Although housing affects children's wellbeing through several and interconnected pathways, for the purposes of clarity, it is useful to identify key domains. In particular in this chapter, the discussion is articulated across three dimensions that represent key mechanisms through which housing impacts upon health and wellbeing:

1 *Physical Hazards*: these include a variety of aspects pertaining to indoor environmental quality, as well as aspects related to the dwelling's overall

state of repair and upkeep. Generally, these hazards have most impact on physical health and/or can cause morbidity or even mortality through accidents. However, some aspects of mental health can also be affected.

2 *Fit to Needs*: this pertains to how well a dwelling's layout, space availability and design features match residents' needs. Key examples include overcrowding and lack of space for socialising or studying. This dimension also includes how well the dwelling meets the needs of children and/or families with special needs, such as those with restricted mobility – however this is a fairly specific aspect, which is not covered in this chapter.
3 *Security and Stability*: this dimension relates to having access to a place which one can consider a 'home' for a reasonable amount of time, and includes issues, such as homelessness and temporary accommodation.

While it is acknowledged that these three dimensions are a convenient way of summarising the main, direct pathways through which housing affects wellbeing, they are also interconnected. For example, overcrowding is technically a manifestation of a dwelling being too small and thus could fit within the 'Fit to Needs' category. However, some of the ways in which overcrowding affects health is via greater risk of infectious diseases, which could also be relevant to the 'Physical Hazards' domain. Figure 8.1 illustrates these three dimensions, highlighting some key overlaps and drivers.

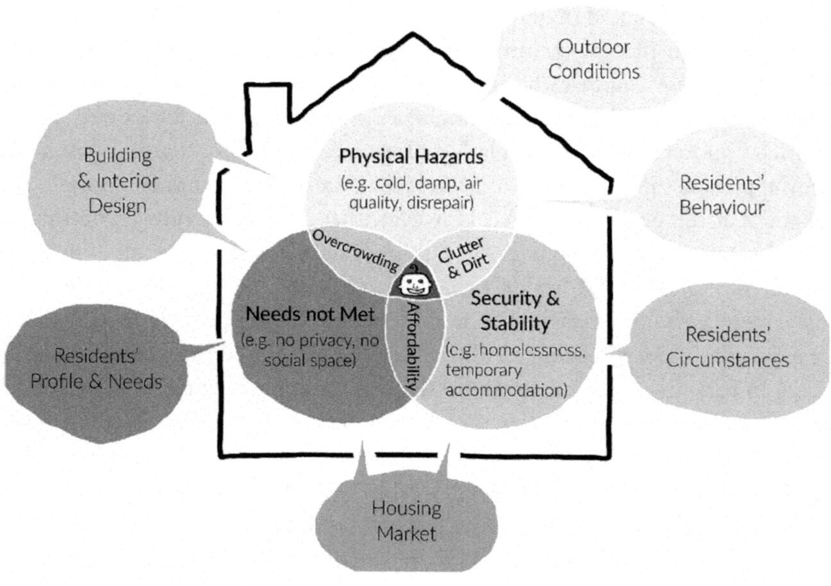

FIGURE 8.1 Three dimensions representing key pathways through which housing impacts on children's wellbeing, with overlapping aspects, and important external drivers.

Source: Ramon Mendoza (graphic) and Marcella Ucci (idea).

This chapter presents the latest evidence and knowledge gaps on the impact of housing on children's health and wellbeing, reflecting upon the role of various, interconnected factors and on design implications at the building and urban scale. The focus is primarily on evidence relevant to middle- and high-income countries, with examples taken mainly from North America and Western Europe. Given the breadth of the topic, this chapter only focusses on general housing and the general population, although the importance of addressing specific needs via inclusive design and specialist/supported housing is important. Whilst evidence was sought based on a broad definition of 'health and wellbeing' spanning across physical, mental and social dimensions, much of the literature encountered addresses their negative dimensions of 'ill-health' and 'ill-being', and focusses especially on low-income and disadvantaged groups. Therefore, most of the evidence can help us understand how to avoid factors that negatively impact on children's' wellbeing and especially in the most disadvantaged groups, with limited evidence on how to enhance wellbeing via housing design across different groups.

Exploring the Evidence through the Three Housing Dimensions

Physical Hazards

Several, indoor environmental factors in the home affect children's health and wellbeing: these include thermal and moisture conditions, light, air quality and noise. Although this dimension also includes home disrepair, which can lead to accidents and fatalities, it is not covered extensively below.

Thermal and Moisture Conditions

Evidence suggests that exposure to excessively low, indoor temperatures can have negative impacts on physical health in the general population, especially in terms of cardiovascular and respiratory outcomes, with older people and those with pre-existing cardiovascular and respiratory conditions being especially vulnerable. Some mental and social health effects have also been widely reported. Jevons et al. (2016) note that while there is limited, specific evidence on the impacts on children, they suggest a minimum threshold of 18 °C (65 °F) in homes during winter, considered to pose minimal risks for a sedentary person wearing suitable clothing. They also remark that, 'Although not strongly evidence based, there is currently a "general consensus" in that rooms in which infants sleep should be heated to between 16 °C and 20 °C and many professional groups and organisations use this range' (p. 8). Excessively high, indoor temperatures also pose a risk to health. Whilst most research on heat waves and health refers to measurements of outdoor temperatures with limited measurements of indoor environments, there is ground for concerns associated with overheating risks in dwellings even in relatively cool climates, such as the UK (Lomas & Porritt, 2016). This is due to a combination of projected climatic changes (i.e. increase in ambient temperatures) and overheating risks associated with poor or inadequate residential design, in part due to the combined effects of insulation and reduced ventilation driven by energy efficiency measures. Infants and young children can be especially vulnerable to heat, since they produce more metabolic heat, have a reduced ability to sweat and have core temperatures that rise faster with dehydration (Public Health England, 2015).

Excessively high, and to some extent, excessively low, moisture indoors can also lead to adverse health effects, either directly through impacts on thermal comfort and through allergens produced by organisms thriving in moist environments (e.g. house dust mites, moulds), or indirectly through degradation of building materials. The WHO has long acknowledged the importance of avoiding dampness in buildings (WHO, 2009), indicating that occupants of damp or mouldy buildings are at increased risk of respiratory symptoms, respiratory infections and exacerbations of asthma. A meta-analysis of dampness and mould in homes and respiratory health effects suggested that risks can be somewhat greater in children (Fisk et al., 2007). However, the WHO also highlighted that there is limited evidence on the dose-response relationships, and it is thus not possible to suggest evidence-based safety thresholds of exposure.

Light

The effects of light on health can be distinguished between visual and non-visual. In relation to building design, most light and lighting research has focussed on understanding the visual effects of lighting, and in particular how buildings can be designed to support performance and every-day functioning. This is important, and it is especially important for those with visual impairments or needs. Aspects, such as how well surfaces and objects are lit, avoidance of glare and colour rendering, are key issues in light and lighting design. However, there are also non-visual effects of light – notably exposure to sunlight is required for UVB-induced vitamin D production. More recently, evidence is emerging of other non-visual effects and especially of the impact of light quality on circadian rhythms, which can help regulate sleep and alertness (Figueiro et al., 2018). Evidence of the non-visual effects of light on children – and of 'light pollution' – is also emerging. For example, exposure to evening bright light in preschool age children was found to suppress melatonin production in an intervention study with ten children (Akacem et al., 2018). Previously, a study on bedtime and evening light exposure on in-home dim-light melatonin onset (DLMO) assessment of 21 children aged 4.5–5 years found that, 'Bedtime explained 37.3% of the variance in the timing of DLMO, and evening light exposure accounted for an additional 13.3% of the variance' (Akacem at al., 2016, p. 27). Overall, however, there is still limited evidence to understand the dose-response relationships, including amount and duration of exposures, for these non-visual effects of light.

Air Quality

The impacts of poor air quality are wide-ranging. While the effects on respiratory and cardiovascular health are well established, more and more evidence is emerging on other widely and long-lasting impacts. These are perhaps best outlined using the words of the Royal College of Physicians' (RCP) report on the lifelong impact of air pollution:

> There is no doubt that air pollution can affect the fetus, either indirectly through the health of the mother, or directly by affecting developing fetal organs and systems. These effects can have a permanent influence on growth and health throughout life. Exposure of the young child to air pollution can produce definite harm and even increase the risk of death from lung infections. There is evidence that it may produce deleterious effects on growth, intelligence and neurological development.
>
> *(RCP, 2016, p. 46)*

It should be emphasised that health outcomes vary across different types of pollutants, including indoor sources, for example, through cooking. Although there is less data on indoor exposures generally, monitoring of 'personal exposure' is emerging, which will enable better characterisation of exposures associated with health effects. Some pollutants are more relevant to indoor sources, such as those included in consumer products, building materials, furniture and finishes. For example, the RCP (2016) report mentioned earlier lists a number of pollutants emitted from indoor sources. However, for many of these pollutants it is difficult to establish an exclusive source, which can make avoidance through housing design or other strategies especially difficult. For example, studies suggest foetal and childhood exposure to some phthalates may perturb normal development, with several studies consistently reporting increased risk of allergic diseases (Braun et al., 2013). While phthalates are included in a range of building materials and finishes, a wide range of sources exist that make it difficult to link this issue with housing specifically. Despite evidence of health effects of poor air quality becoming more and more compelling, in some countries such as the UK, there is still a dearth of data on the prevalence of indoor, domestic exposure to key pollutants. This makes it very difficult to correctly evaluate the risks arising from poor air quality in housing, and it is very likely that these risks are currently being underestimated. Furthermore, whilst it is possible that staying indoors (at home or elsewhere) during episodes of outdoor pollution may reduce exposure to some pollutants, very little is known on how this may relate to greater exposure to indoor pollutants and on whether specific dwelling characteristics or parental behaviours (e.g. smoking indoors) may partly offset health benefits. Poor air quality is truly a 'wicked problem', due to the complexity of understanding the trade-offs between outdoor and indoor air, combined with the lack of individual control over pollution sources and the current drive for airtight buildings for energy efficiency purposes.

Noise

Exposures to loud noise can cause damage to hearing, which could be reversible – however these exposures are relatively rare. The impact of noise pollution on children's health and wellbeing has been investigated primarily by considering ambient noise levels outside the home or the school environment generated by road or air traffic. Most studies found an effect on cardiovascular factors (e.g. blood pressure) and on stress-related factors. For example, a cross-sectional study on night-time exposure to urban road traffic noise in Belgrade (Serbia) found a correlation between noise exposure and preschool children's systolic pressure (Belojevic et al., 2008). Another cross-sectional study of 8–14-year-old children in Germany found that the highest blood pressure readings were found in the group where children's rooms faced a street with 'high or extremely high' traffic volume (Babisch et al., 2009). However, noise pollution has been implicated along with other wellbeing aspects including stress responses (Stansfeld & Clark, 2015) and cognition, such as reading comprehension (Clark et al., 2006). It should also be mentioned that some children can be especially susceptible to sounds, such as children with auditory processing disorder or children on the autistic spectrum. Regarding housing design specifically, there is limited evidence on the modifying effect of housing characteristics on noise exposure and wellbeing outcomes. Noise insulation measures can be applied for dwellings in areas with high levels of noise pollution; however, they may have knock-on effects elsewhere (e.g. risking overheating if not wanting to open a window to reduce outdoor noise). Moreover, children would still be affected when playing outdoors, or in the school environment.

Finally, it must be noted that children may be especially vulnerable to poor, indoor environmental quality because they do not necessarily have control over their environment.

Fit to Needs

One of the major aspects surrounding this dimension is the issue of overcrowding. In simple terms, this can be defined as too little space in relation to the number of residents – although the number of rooms, especially bedrooms and toilets, and availability/size of a space for socialising is also relevant. A specific effect of overcrowding is the greater risk of exposure to infectious diseases such as tuberculosis (Clark et al., 2002), and other respiratory problems in children (ODPM, 2004). However, it is not always possible to disentangle the effects of overcrowding on respiratory health from the role played by exposure to dampness, mould and dust mites, and more generally by poor air quality, which could be a symptom of poor housing quality. On the other hand, overcrowding could be partly responsible for dampness in dwellings, due to greater moisture concentrations because of residents' moisture production and comparatively small room volumes.

Besides the direct effects on physical health, the effects of overcrowding are reportedly wide-spanning, including: children's mental health; social and emotional development (possibly due to lack of privacy, sleep and general stress induced on the family by overcrowding); and educational attainment, either directly – due to lack of quiet space for studying – or indirectly – due to days lost at school because of sickness associated with overcrowding. However, it can be difficult to disentangle the effects of overcrowding from other accompanying issues, such as low socio-economic status, overall poor housing quality and parents' stress arising from these aspects. However, some studies did find an independent effect of the home environment. For example, a study using a longitudinal, nationally representative survey of individuals and families in the US, as well as data from the Los Angeles Family and Neighbourhood Survey, examined the impact of housing crowding, defined as a continuous measure of persons per room, using five, child wellbeing outcomes: two measures of educational achievement (test-based); two measures of child behaviour problems (self-reported by primary caregiver); a measure of child's general health. The analysis, which controlled for demographic and socio-economic variables, revealed an independent, negative effect of crowding on all child wellbeing outcomes (with some differences between the two data sources). Although the effects were not as big as the impact of other factors, such as primary caregiver's education or income, the authors also remarked that, 'the living environment, net of socio-economic status, is an area that can contribute to the intergenerational transmission of social inequality' (Solari & Mare, 2012, p. 474).

Security and Stability

Residential mobility (frequency of moving home) during childhood can have short-term effects on children and adolescent's school achievement and functioning (Leventhal & Newman, 2010). It can also increase the risk of poor, overall health, psychological distress and health behaviours in adolescence and adulthood, after adjusting for socio-demographic characteristics and school moves. Physical health measures are not necessarily associated with childhood mobility (Brown et al., 2012). This could be because moving frequently does not necessarily imply moving to poor-quality housing; indeed, the opposite might be true. However, if families with children live in temporary accommodation and especially for prolonged period of times, this can negatively affect children's wellbeing, including their educational attainment. In these cases, it is not always easy to disentangle the effects of the temporary nature of the housing arrangements, versus the poor housing conditions often accompanying such arrangements. This can include a range of physical hazards and disrepair, and also clutter due to the temporary and/or inadequate nature of the accommodation. The next section discusses the interconnections between these aspects further.

Double or Triple Jeopardy

As previously mentioned, the distinction between the three dimensions presented in Figure 8.1 is, to some extent, artificial. It is not uncommon to find, for example, that temporary accommodation is also overcrowded and presenting a range of physical hazards. Some studies have examined the impact of broadly defined 'poor housing' on children. For example, Schmeer and Yoon (2016) used data from the Los Angeles Family and Neighbourhood Survey, considering how poor home physical environment affects inflammation (measured by C-reactive protein, CRP) in children aged 3–18 years. In the study, poor home environment was defined as: no yard or patio, unsafe inside, unsafe outside, dark or minimally lit, little or monotonous décor, crowded, cluttered and unclean. All these measures were observed by the interviewer, except the no patio/yard, which was reported by the primary caregiver. The outcome of interest was chronic, low-grade inflammation as a measure of physiological stress response in children. The findings indicated that children in poor-quality homes had a higher inflammation and that this effect was more pronounced in younger children. Also the greater the number of poor-quality indicators, the greater the effect: those in a home environment with three or more poor housing indicators had 62% higher CRP than those in homes with two or less indicators. Child obesity was found to be a mediator of this effect.

Another study considered the duration of 'bad housing' and living standards on children's wellbeing, using five waves of data from the Families and Children Study, a representative longitudinal study of families with children (0–18 years old) in Britain (Barnes et al., 2010). The wellbeing outcome measure corresponds to the then Government's 'Every Child Matters' framework. This includes five outcomes: be healthy; stay safe; enjoy and achieve; make a positive contribution; and achieve economic wellbeing. Three housing issues were considered: overcrowding, poor state of repair (incl. condensation, damp and mould), and inadequately heating. Data on specific measures corresponding to the wellbeing outcomes and housing conditions was self-reported. After controlling for socio-demographic and economic factors, the study found that living in persistent bad housing is negatively associated with each child wellbeing outcome, and increased duration is associated with higher odds of disadvantage. Generally, the duration of poor state of repair had an impact on the 'be healthy' and 'stay safe' aspects; while the effect of duration of overcrowding had more wide-ranging impacts – although not all statistically significant. The duration of 'inadequate heating' seemed to be less significant and more associated with economic indicators. It is also worth noting that families with at least one parent with a limiting, long-term illness were more likely to be living in an accommodation in poor state of repair, or inadequately heated. More broadly, there was a link between economic position of the family and the risk of experiencing bad housing.

'Poor quality' housing can not only affect a range of wellbeing outcomes in children, but also specific health behaviours. For example, a review of evidence on low cost housing and children's physical activities found that poor safety, crowding, inadequate facilities and poor neighbourhood relationship can be major contributors of reduced physical activities in children (Hanapi & Ahmad, 2016). The role of neighbourhood and other cross-cutting factors, confounders/ mediators, is discussed further in the next section.

Cross-Cutting and Confounding Factors

One of the notoriously difficult aspects of research on housing and health/wellbeing in general is the role that various other factors might play. In statistical terms, these factors can be distinguished broadly in 'confounders' (associated with both the exposure and the outcome), 'moderators' (affecting exposure) and 'mediators' (on the causal pathway between exposure and outcome). Much research in this field is cross-sectional in nature, partly because designing randomised controlled trials with a focus on the built environment is costly and logistically/ethically rather difficult. However, there is some data emerging from longitudinal and quasi-experimental studies that can also help tease out not only whether housing affects health/wellbeing, but also 'how'.

One of the most commonly discussed confounders in this field of research is the role of socio-economic status – household poverty, other indicators of disadvantage and the wider 'social determinants' of inequality often come in tandem with poor-quality housing. While a detailed discussion on the specific confounding role of these aspects is beyond the scope of this chapter, as previously discussed, poor housing does have an effect on children's wellbeing outcomes, independently of socio-economic status.

Data from the 2014 EHS also shows other inequalities aspects, for example, the prevalence of dampness is greater in ethnic minority households, those living in poverty and the lowest income groups. The proportion of dwellings with dampness also increases with local area deprivation (English Housing Survey, 2014). Figure 8.2 illustrates how even in the case of physical hazards such as moisture in buildings, the problem is of a socio-technical nature, whereby exposure is affected not only by building design and outdoor conditions, but also by behavioural aspects and socio-economic drivers.

The role of poor housing (and of other factors) on health inequalities is also discussed within the US context, for example, with disproportionately higher levels of asthma morbidity and mortality in African American and Latino children who live in low-socioeconomic-status urban environments. The research also highlights however that:

> It is clear that individual interventions will not work alone and that a comprehensive and multifaceted approach to reduce asthma disparities that incorporate interventions that address family, social, and behavioral factors, along with continued medical advances within a culturally competent health care system, is needed.
>
> *(Bryant-Stephens, 2009, p. 1205).*

An interesting study on housing and the wellbeing of low-income children highlights the complex web of effects and argues that the 'housing context may have direct as well as indirect associations with children's development' (Coley et al., 2013, p. 1778). In particular, they suggest that parental functioning

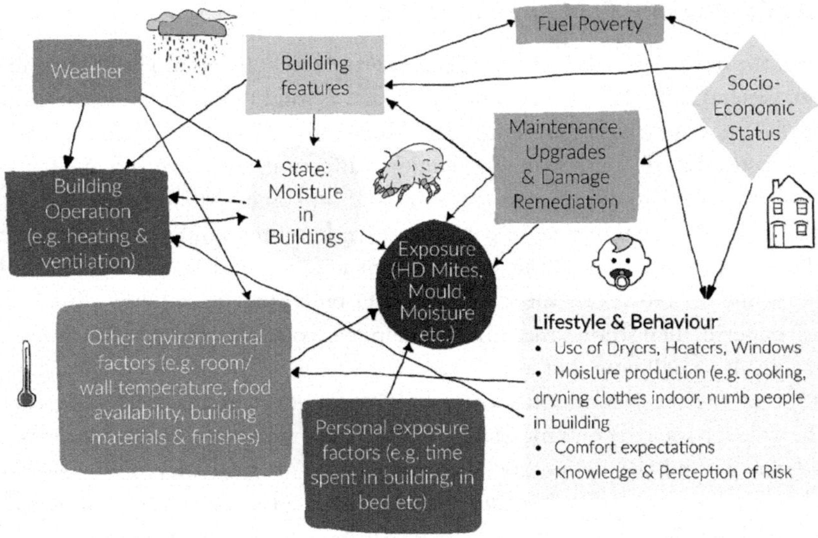

FIGURE 8.2 Exposure to physical hazards in housing as a socio-technical problem affected by engineering challenges, behavioural aspects and socio-economic drivers: example of moisture in buildings.

Source: Ramon Mendoza (graphic) and Marcella Ucci (idea).

and family processes can have a mediating role, and act as, 'a primary vehicle through which housing may influence children's functioning' (Coley et al., 2013, p. 1778), through an impact on parents themselves. The research is based on a longitudinal, multi-method study of the wellbeing of low-income children and families in Boston, Chicago and San Antonio. They considered four aspects of housing characteristics – housing quality, residential instability, housing type and housing cost burden – either reported by mothers or observed by interviewers. For outcomes, they considered a range of child functioning measures reported by mothers using the Child Behaviour Checklist, as well as interviewer-administered tests to evaluate children's reading and maths skills. Data on child and family characteristics were collected, as well as data on 'family processes', such as self-reported maternal psychological distress, and family stress. The results indicated that poor housing quality was the stronger predictor of child's behavioural and emotional problems, and was associated with lower average reading and math skills among adolescents more so than young children – contrary to the initial hypotheses. They also found that:

> …family processes related to both stress and stability were implicated such that low-quality housing may induce stress in parents, increase mental health problems, and limit their ability to regulate family activities, in turn affecting children's socioemotional functioning.
>
> *(Coley et al., 2013, p. 1778).*

Another powerful reminder of the indirect effect of housing on children through parents, and especially mothers, is the finding from Corman et al. (2016), based on US data, that maternal depression is a risk factor for children's inadequate housing conditions. In this case, there is a potential feedback loop where mothers with depression are at greater risk of living in poor-quality housing (which in itself can have a negative impact on children wellbeing), but this, in turn, can worsen even further parental stress and family functioning, and indirectly affecting children's wellbeing.

Besides the factors discussed so far, the effects of the wider neighbourhood's physical and social environments on exacerbating, or alleviating, the impact of housing on children's wellbeing should not be underestimated. A comprehensive overview of neighbourhood's effects on children's health is beyond the scope of this chapter. Villanueva et al. (2016) summarise some key aspects, highlighting evidence in support of associations between child development and neighbourhood destination, green spaces, interaction with nature, traffic exposure and housing density. Regarding the latter factor, the authors highlight that the evidence is mixed, and the pathways complex, at times contradictory. This is perhaps expected. For example, a greater urban density can facilitate walkability and access to facilities; however, dense inner-city environments are often associated with perceived fear of crime and poor environmental quality. Children living in high-rise buildings and densely built urban environments may be least likely to play outdoors.

Minh et al. (2017) outline a comprehensive discussion on neighbourhood's effects on early child development, arguing that there is still much to be learnt about the 'how', 'where' and for 'whom' neighbourhoods matter. Among other aspects, they emphasise that 'a lack of safety, increased neighbourhood social disorder, less belonging, less social cohesion and a lower potential for community involvement with children (or collective efficacy), was directly related to worse language, emotional and behavioural outcomes for children'.

Finally, it is important to note again the effect of duration of exposure, and their lifelong impacts: Barnes et al. (2010) found that duration of 'bad housing' had a range of negative effects on several wellbeing outcomes for children. Also, studies considering the effect of housing with a range of physical hazards have found that living with poor housing in the past can affect (adult) mental health in the present, regardless of current housing quality (Pevalin et al., 2017).

Figure 8.3 illustrates some of the factors discussed in this section, emphasising how children's wellbeing is deeply connected to their families' circumstances, life chances and wellbeing status. The home environment has wide-ranging and long-lasting impacts on a range of child wellbeing outcomes, including physical and mental health, child development, health behaviour and social wellbeing. Young children and pregnant mothers can be especially vulnerable to some risks, although the effect on older children's and adolescents' development and behaviour should not be underestimated. The effects are confounded, mediated or moderated by a number of other factors, illustrated in the outer circle

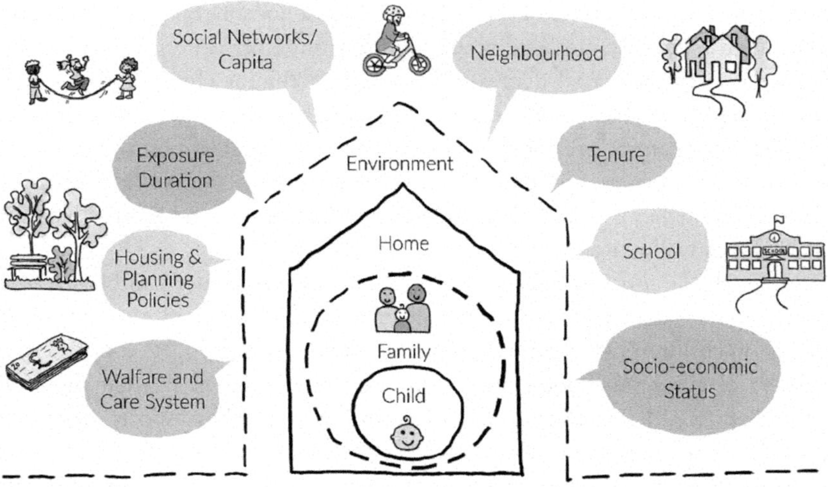

FIGURE 8.3 Role of the family, home and other environments on children's wellbeing, with key external drivers.
Source: Ramon Mendoza.

of the diagram. These can exacerbate or alleviate the problems, and should be considered when designing housing interventions.

Conclusions: What Works, Emerging Trends and Challenges

The earlier sections outlined the wellbeing (or rather the 'ill-being') effects of various housing dimensions on children. In this section, an overview of the effectiveness of various housing-related interventions is presented, and conclusions are drawn on design and research implications for future cities.

A systematic review on the health impacts of housing improvement studies from 1887 to 2007 identified 45 relevant studies (Thomson et al., 2009), concluding that housing improvements – and especially warmth improvements – can result in general health improvements with limited evidence of negative effects. Improvements touched general physical and respiratory health, as well as mental health. But the review also emphasised that the effectiveness of the interventions may depend on baseline housing conditions and on careful targeting of the intervention itself. While the review did not focus exclusively on children, its key findings are a good introductory overview – some more detailed examples are provided below.

Most studies demonstrate a positive effect of improved warmth on children's (and families') health and wellbeing outcomes – with some of the studies also combining greater energy efficiency for heating with adequate ventilation or reduced sources of pollution. The health co-benefits of energy efficiency interventions on housing have been discussed widely in the past decade (e.g. Wilkinson et al., 2009). The link with fuel poverty is also important: a review of evidence highlighted that while the effects on adult physical health of interventions to address fuel poverty is modest, the effects on perceived respiratory health, by caregivers and children, is significant (Liddel & Morris, 2010). The review suggested also a significant impact on the physical health of infants, in terms of weight gain.

The potential impact of improved warmth and air quality is exemplified in a randomised controlled trial in New Zealand, examining the impact of non-polluting, more effective home heating on 409 children (aged 6–12) with doctor-diagnosed asthma. It concluded that the intervention did not significantly improve lung function. However, it did reduce asthma symptoms, days off school, healthcare utilisation and visits to a pharmacist (Howden-Chapman et al., 2008). Another RCT study in Wales (UK) targeting 192 children with moderate or severe asthma aged 5–14 years aimed to evaluate the effectiveness of installing ventilation systems, and central heating where necessary, in their homes. The trial found some positive effects on parent-reported asthma-specific quality of life, and on physical problems included in the generic quality of life scale. The changes on psychosocial quality of life, and on parent-reported school attendance were both not significant (Woodfine et al., 2011). An economic evaluation of this study also concluded that the intervention is likely to be cost effective for the public healthcare system, and particularly so for children with severe asthma (Edwards et al., 2011).

Homelessness and housing instability can have significant and long-lasting impacts on children and their families. Availability of affordable (and decent) housing – which, in turn, is driven by market conditions, housing and welfare policies – all have an impact on homelessness and housing instability, but the phenomenon is also linked to other aspects including access to employment opportunities, the role of parental physical and mental health and so forth. Therefore, the scope for interventions aimed at ending homelessness and reducing housing instability is far wider than housing/cities design and planning approaches. In this sense, a detailed overview of effective interventions is beyond the scope of this chapter, but it is worth highlighting that research shows how the heterogeneity of potential interventions to end homelessness/instability and associated negative wellbeing outcomes makes the evaluation of interventions particularly difficult (Bassuk et al., 2014). This is compounded by different approaches to defining homelessness, for example, whether this is intended 'simply' as lack of a physical home, or also lack of access to supportive relationships, opportunity and participation in community life (ibid). A more recent systematic review of housing assistance and child health also emphasises similar problems with availability of suitably comparable studies, and concluded that the relationship remains unclear, with many studies showing no association. However, 'a sizeable proportion of observed relationships within the quasi-experimental and association studies were in favour of housing assistance (50.0% and 37.5%, respectively), and negative outcomes were less common and only present among association studies' (Slopen et al., 2018, p. 1).

Most of the intervention studies discussed so far address the most prevalent and significant causes of housing-related ill-health and ill-being in children and their families. However, we must also consider how emerging challenges and trends might affect these aspects in the future. In this respect, climate change and other types of environmental degradation at the macro and urban scale could have a profound effect on children wellbeing. For example, climate change can have a dramatic impact on indoor conditions in residential buildings and represents a challenge for public health. However, improved building design and passive measures can reduce the risk of overheating and overall climate change mitigation, and adaptation strategies in homes can benefit health (Vardoulakis et al., 2015).

Air pollution is also a significant challenge for public health and for children especially, in terms of both outdoor and indoor sources (RCP, 2016). There is still limited evidence on how housing may be an effect modifier of outdoor air pollution effects. There is also emerging evidence that a wider-than-considered range of pollutants may be dangerous to human health, and to children in particular, than previously known. Most housing-level design strategies addressing indoor air quality primarily rely on ventilation (i.e. diluting indoor sources with 'fresh air'). However, in heavily polluted urban areas, there is limited evidence to evaluate the trade-offs between ventilating with polluted, outdoor air, and letting indoor pollutant concentrations escalate. Of course, the real solution is the reduction of pollution sources, both from indoor and outdoor origins; however, this requires strong, political willingness and public opinion support. Besides ventilation, it is important to consider other, design-related factors affecting exposure to air pollution, including location of air-inlets and of rooms where residents spend most of their time when at home alongside the role of neighbourhood and city-scale factors, such as transport, location of green areas and location/distribution of building types across the city.

It is also imperative to consider how current trends and innovations, such as artificial intelligence, the Internet of Things, wearable technologies and the idea of 'smart cities', might deeply affect our experience of, and expectations from, the built environment in future, and how, in turn, these might impact on housing provisions and needs. It is plausible to expect that these technologies will allow for greater levels of customisation, adaptability and interactivity of the home environment, which might generate positive wellbeing outcomes but also unexpected negative ones (e.g. dependency on computer gaming), as well as a greater risk of inequalities. For children in particular, the role of gaming technologies and of virtual reality is likely to have a deep and profound effect on their perception of reality and of their surrounding environments, as well as on their social habits and broader lifestyle. In this sense, ensuring access to safe, good-quality green and playing areas is perhaps one of the important imperatives of urban design for the future. This is especially critical when considering that pressures on land are not likely to reduce, and that the current trend for smaller floor and volume sizes for homes is likely to continue.

Perhaps one of the most extraordinary aspects of this research area is the acknowledgement that the general housing design principles for good health and wellbeing have been known for some time:

- Sufficient space, and layout/details which meet the needs of residents;
- Good environmental quality (hygrothermal, lighting, sound, air quality, state of repairs);
- Housing stability;
- Access to safe and good-quality facilities (e.g. green areas, good schools), and to employment opportunities;
- Opportunities to form meaningful connections with the local community.

Yet it is sad to note that even in relatively wealthy countries, the majority of research studies still have to focus on how to remediate the effects of deep, societal inequalities and of wider pressures on the environment and the economy, as opposed to establishing the wellbeing gains that might be achieved with optimal housing design and operation. We know the 'essential ingredients' of good housing design and perhaps even a few 'good recipes', but we just do not know how societies should agree on finding the resources for these 'recipes'. As a result, most research to-date is focussed on how to guarantee a minimum level of housing conditions for all, instead of defining standards for 'optimal' housing that fully support wellbeing.

Academia, policy makers and communities should also more proactively debate and establish how the housing stock in future may be affected by, and need to be adapted for, the impact of:

- Future technologies, including artificial intelligence, virtual reality, wearables and the Internet of Things;
- Ageing populations and other demographic changes;
- Climate change and environmental degradation, such as pollution;
- Inequalities.

When considering the deep and long-lasting impacts of housing on children's wellbeing, there is compelling evidence of the need to consider the factors discussed earlier to future-proof our housing stock. In doing so, we are not only protecting but also enhancing the lives of many generations to come.

Acknowledgements

The contribution of Ramon Mendoza to the illustrations included in this chapter is gratefully acknowledged.

References

Akacem, L.D., Wright, K.P., Jr., LeBourgeois, M.K. (2016). Bedtime and evening light exposure influence circadian timing in preschool-age children: a field study. *Neurobiology of Sleep and Circadian Rhythms*. 1(2), 27–31.

Akacem, L.D., Wright, K.P. Jr., LeBourgeois, M.K. (2018). Sensitivity of the circadian system to evening bright light in preschool-age children. *Physiological Reports.* 6(5).

Babisch, W., Neuhauser, H., Thamm, M., Seiwert, M. (2009). Blood pressure of 8–14 year old children in relation to traffic noise at home—results of the German Environmental Survey for Children (GerES IV). *Science of the Total Environment.* 407(22), 5839–5843.

Barnes, M., Butt, S., Tomaszewski, W. (2010). The duration of bad housing and children's wellbeing in Britain. *Journal of Housing Studies.* 26(1), 155–176.

Barton, C., Kenny, C. (2018). *Health in private-rented housing. POSTnotes POST-PN-0573.* Parliamentary Office Science and Technology (POST). https://researchbriefings.parliament.uk/ResearchBriefing/Summary/POST-PN-0573

Bassuk, E., DeCandia, C., Tsertsvadze, A., Richard, M. (2014). The effectiveness of housing interventions and housing and service interventions on ending family homelessness: a systematic review. *American Journal of Orthopsychiatry.* 84(5), 457–474.

Belojevic, G., Jakovljevic, B., Stojanov, V., Paunovic, K., Ilic, J. (2008). Urban road-traffic noise and blood pressure and heart rate in preschool children. *Environment International.* 34(2), 226–231.

Braun, J.M., Sathyanarayana, S., Hauser, R. (2013). Phthalate exposure and children's health. *Current Opinion in Pediatrics.* 25(2), 247–254.

Brown, D., Benzeval, M., Gayle, V., Macintyr, e S., O'Reilly, D., Leyland, A.H. (2012). Childhood residential mobility and health in late adolescence and adulthood: findings from the West of Scotland Twenty-07 Study. *Journal of Epidemiological Community and Health.* 66, 942–950.

Bryant-Stephens, T. (2009). Asthma disparities in urban environments. *The Journal of Allergy and Clinical Immunology.* 123(6), 1199–1206.

Clark, C., Martin, C., van Kempen, E., Alfred, T., Head, J., Davies, H., Haines, M., Barrio, I., Matheson, M., Stansfield, S. (2006). Exposure-effect relations between aircraft and road traffic noise exposure at school and reading comprehension: the RANCH project. *American Journal of Epidemiology.* 163(1), 27–37.

Clark, M., Riben, P., Nowgesic, E. (2002). The association of housing density, isolation and tuberculosis in Canadian First Nations communities. *International Journal of Epidemiology.* 31(5), 940–945.

Coley, R.L., Leventhal, T., Lynch, A.D., Kull, M. (2013). Relations between housing characteristics and the wellbeing of low-income children and adolescents. *Developmental Psychology.* 49(9), 1775–1789.

Corman, H., Curtis, M.A., Noonan, K., Reichman, N.E. (2016). Maternal depression as a risk factor for children's inadequate housing conditions. *Social Science and Medicine.* 149, 76–83.

Edwards, R., Neil, R., Linck, P., Bruce, N., Mullock L., Nelhans, N., Pasterfield, D., Russell, D., Russell, I., Woodfine, L. (2011). Enhancing ventilation in homes of children with asthma: cost-effectiveness study alongside randomised controlled trial. *British Journal of General Practice.* 61(592), e733–e741.

English Housing Survey. (2014). *English housing survey. Table DA5103 damp and mould – households; Table 5102 damp and mould – areas.* https://www.gov.uk/government/statistical-data-sets/dwelling-condition-and-safety

Figueiro, M.G., Nagare, R., Price, L.L.A. (2018). Non-visual effects of light: how to use light to promote circadian entrainment and elicit alertness. *Lighting Research Technology.* 50, 38–52.

Fisk, W., Lei-Gomez, Q., Mendell, M.J. (2007). Meta-analyses of the associations of respiratory health effects with dampness and mold in homes. *Indoor Air.* 17(4), 284–96.

Hanapi, N., Ahmad, S. (2016). A review on environmental characteristic that influence children physical activities in low cost housing. *Procedia—Social and Behavioural Science.* 222(23), 19–27.

Howden-Chapman, P., Pierse, N., Nicholls, S., Gillespie-Bennett, J., Viggers, H., Cunningham, M., Phipps, R., Boulic, M., Fjällström, P., Free, S., Chapman, R., Lloyd, B., Wickens, K., Shields, D., Baker, M., Cunningham, C., Woodward, A., Bullen, C., Crane, J. (2008). Effects of improved home heating on asthma in community dwelling children: randomised controlled trial. *British Medical Journal*. 337.

Jevons, R., Carmichael, C., Crossley, A., Bone, A. (2016). Minimum indoor temperature threshold recommendations for English homes in winter—a systematic review. *Public Health*. 13, 4–12.

Leventhal, T., Newman, S. (2010). Housing and child development. *Children and Youth Services Review*. 32(9), 1165–1174.

Lomas, K., & Porritt, S. (2016). Overheating in buildings: lessons from research. *Building Research and Information*. 45(1–2), 1–18.

Minh, A., Muhajarine, N., Janus, M., Brownell, M., Guhn, M. (2017). A review of neighborhood effects and early child development: How, where, and for whom, do neighborhoods matter? *Health & Place*. 6, 155–174.

ODPM. (2004). *The impact of overcrowding on health and education*. London: Office of the Deputy Prime Minister (ODPM). http://dera.ioe.ac.uk/5073/1/138631.pdf

Pevalin, D.J., Reeves, A., Baker, E., Bentley, R. (2017). The impact of persistent poor housing conditions on mental health: A longitudinal population-based study. *Preventive Medicine*. 105, 304–310.

Public Health England. (2015). *Heatwave plan for England—making the case: the impact of heat on health – now and in future*. London: Public Health England. https://assets.publishing.service.gov.uk/government/uploads/system/uploads/attachment_data/file/429572/Heatwave_plan_-Making_the_case_-_2015.pdf

RCP. (2016). *Every breath we take: the lifelong impact of air pollution*. London: Royal College of Physicians (RCP). https://www.rcplondon.ac.uk/projects/outputs/every-breath-we-take-lifelong-impact-air-pollution

Schmeer, K., & Yoon, A.J. (2016). Home sweet home? Home physical environment and inflammation in children. *Social Science Research*. 60, 236–248.

Slopen, N., Fenelon, A., Newman, S., Boudreaux, M. (2018). Housing assistance and child health: a systematic review. *Pediatrics*. 141(6), pii: e20172742.

Solari, C.D, Mare, R.D. (2012). Housing crowding effects on children. *Social Science Research*. 41(2), 464–476.

Stansfeld, S., Clark, C. (2015). Health effects of noise exposure in children. *Current Environmental Health Reports*. 2(2), 171–178.

Thomson, H., Thomas, S., Sellstrom, E., Petticrew, M. (2009). The health impacts of housing improvement: a systematic review of intervention studies from 1887 to 2007. *American Journal of Public Health*. 9(S3), S681–S692.

Vardoulakis, S., Dimitroulopoulou, C., Thornes, J., Lai, K.M., Taylor, J., Myers, I., Heaviside, C., Mavrogianni, A., Shrubsole, C., Chalabi, Z., Davies, M., Wilkinson, P. (2015). Impact of climate change on the domestic indoor environment and associated health risks in the UK. *Environment International*. 85, 299–313.

Villanueva, K., Badland, H., Kvalsvig, A., O'Connor, M., Christian, H., Woolcock, G., Giles-Corti, B., Goldfeld, S. (2016). Can the neighborhood built environment make a difference in children's development? building the research agenda to create evidence for place-based children's policy. *Academic Pediatrics*. 16(1), 10–19

WHO. (2009). *WHO guidelines for indoor air quality: dampness and mould*. World Health Organisation. http://www.euro.who.int/__data/assets/pdf_file/0017/43325/E92645.pdf

9

FROM PRECARITY TO INTERDEPENDENCE

The Role of Age-Friendly Communities in Promoting Wellbeing in Excluded Communities

Mark Hammond, Stefan White and Christopher Phillipson

Wellbeing in an Age of Precarity

Promoting wellbeing in our future cities involves recognition of two key social trends. First, the impact of demographic changes associated with population ageing; second, the extent to which cohorts entering their 50s, 60s and beyond will have experienced a significantly higher level of social and economic instability in their working lives than previous generations. By 2050, there will be 2.1 billion people aged 60 and over, compared to 926 million people today (UN, 2017). While the majority of this growth will take place in the developing world, there will still be a significant, demographic shift in developed countries. In Europe, 34% of the population will be aged 60 and over by 2050, with greater numbers of older people living in urban areas (WHO, 2007).

The cohort of older people in 2050 will have had very different lives from those in 2020, reflecting the social and political changes affecting the late-twentieth and early twenty-first century. The chronic social and economic insecurity of modern capitalism has the potential to create an older cohort, defined by what has been termed 'precarity', a condition characterised by working lives increasingly shaped by casual labour contracts, unprotected tenancies, withdrawal of guaranteed pensions and reductions of public services (see Cooper & Whyte, 2017; O'Hara, 2015; Standing, 2012). While the current discourse around an emerging precariat has focussed on the challenges facing younger people (Dannefer & Huang, 2017), the cumulative disadvantage many will have experienced within their working lives will require us to re-examine the opportunities and support that society provides for people in later life.

We do not, however, need to wait until 2050 to see examples of precarity in our older population. The population of cities (notably in the Global North) are getting older and increasingly heterogeneous (Buffel & Phillipson, 2016). Growing inequality and austerity have created and exacerbated conditions of social isolation, spatial exclusion and multiple deprivation, leading to large divergences in wellbeing among different groups of older people. Older people, especially those affected by issues, such as migration, homelessness, dementia and gentrification, are already experiencing multi-dimensional insecurity, perpetuated by a social and political context that individualises both risk and responsibility. Experiences of precarity are negatively correlated with current understandings of wellbeing in later life, which rely on stability and predictability as the basis of ontological security (Grenier et al., 2017; Grenier & Phillipson, 2018; Lewis et al., 2015).

This chapter examines the role of what has been termed 'age-friendly cities and communities' in tackling issues faced by older people experiencing precarity in disadvantaged communities, using examples from the 'Manchester Age-Friendly Neighbourhoods' project in Manchester, UK. Building on this work, the chapter will demonstrate the importance of engaging in issues relating to precarity, spatial exclusion and social isolation within the Age-Friendly movement, and the opportunities to improve wellbeing by creating conditions that address and reduce the increasingly precarious experiences of people in later life.

From Precarity to Interdependence

The study of precarity is widely used to illustrate the vulnerabilities that many people face as a product of social, political and economic instability. Much of this work has focussed on structural inequalities derived from a global market system. Neoliberal politics which promote deregulation of labour markets, regulation of labour unions and global competition for attractive tax conditions (and thus lower social support), have resulted in the erosion of security for an increased number of people in the Global North (Standing, 2012). We can already see the ways this is affecting our current older population, through the rationing of social care, withdrawal of public amenities and repositioning of the social security system as a 'hostile environment' (Ryan, 26 April 2018; Streek, 2016).

While a structural understanding of precarity can help us to understand how current and future older people might experience a social or economic deficit as a result of precarity, our intention in this chapter is to explore how older people experiencing precarity can improve their lives through collective action. To do this, we turn to Butler's (2004) examination of the ontological condition of precariousness, which she suggests is a fundamental aspect of human life. She argues that this is the case because our lives can never be autonomous, and that we live contingent lives in which we are all '...physically dependent on one another, physically vulnerable to one another' (Butler, 2004, p. 27). Butler (2004) suggests that precarity and precariousness should be understood as discrete concepts: precariousness is a universal insecurity that results from our interdependence, whereas precarity is the unequal distribution of precariousness within different parts of society. Precarity is, therefore, an insecurity that goes beyond wealth distribution or labour market status, and additionally intersects with class, gender and ethnicity.

The transition to a precarious society has widespread effects on individual wellbeing. The ontological security that is offered through social and material stability may be replaced by a state of fear that basic human needs will not be met. By reinforcing individualist competition for a seemingly scarce range of resources, precarity produces mistrust and social conflict, which further undermine a sense of community and belonging that is central to our sense of wellbeing (Neilson, 2015). Butler's (2004) notion of precarity as a consequence of unequal relationships of dependence and interdependence also suggests an interpretation of social isolation as both a form of, and contributor to, precarity.

Butler (2015) also explores how the experience of precarity can be challenged through different forms of social action. She argues that, 'The opposite of precarity is not security, but, rather, the struggle for an egalitarian social and political order in which a liveable interdependence becomes possible' (p. 69). Central to this is the performative act of assembly, in labour movements, protest and civil society, in which people come together to assert power through collective acts of association. These new forms of collective engagement are predicated on coalitions that build on the difference between actors, rather than seeking homogeny based on prescriptive identity politics (Butler, 2015).

Age-Friendly Cities as a Response to Precarious Ageing

The call for active citizenship and the collective action that underpins Butler's response to precarity are mirrored in programmes aiming to improve the wellbeing of older people, a group who may experience marginalisation arising from the interaction between globalisation and urban change (Buffel & Phillipson, 2016). The World Health Organization's (WHO) 'Age-friendly Cities' approach is a global initiative that seeks to challenge societal perceptions of ageing as a process of medical decline and social disengagement. In response, Age-Friendly initiatives seek to promote the concept of 'active ageing' – opportunities for older people to participate in all areas of society in a way that values the diversity of capabilities older people might have (WHO, 2007).

Developing Age-Friendly communities requires both social and physical changes to communities, to ensure opportunities for meaningful participation of older people in civic society as part of providing opportunities for self-fulfilment (WHO, 2018). We argue that the Age-Friendly model should be understood as multi-factorial and place-based, engaging with the specific lived experience of actual older people existing in that location in order to address the barriers and opportunities of existing and potential relationships. It recognises the interconnections between aspects of the lived experience as vitally important, calling for coordinated action and partnership working around a shared goal of improving older people's quality of life (Doran & Buffel, 2018; Greenfield, 2018; Scharlach & Lehning, 2013; White & Hammond, 2018).

While the Age-Friendly movement seeks to address the exclusion of older people from decision-making processes, these forms of exclusion are best viewed as 'intersectional' (King et al., 2019). Risk factors such as poverty, health inequalities, intergenerational conflict or racial tensions all contribute to social exclusion and often are exacerbated in older cohorts. These experiences of social exclusion are personal but they are also spatially concentrated, often in disadvantaged urban communities where the issues facing older people are multiple and interrelated. As a result, the mechanisms for creating Age-Friendly cities and communities must seek to respond to local opportunities and barriers that prevent participation, acknowledging the heterogeneous needs of older people experiencing social exclusion (Buffel et al., 2013; Ogg, 2005).

The Global Network of Age-Friendly Cities and Communities (GNAFCC), launched by the WHO in 2010, had attracted over 1000 members by 2020, demonstrating its success in tapping into a growing interest in ageing within urban policy. There are, however, notable criticisms of the programme, and some have questioned how successful some Age-Friendly initiatives have been at activating those experiencing precarity, social isolation and spatial exclusion (Gonyea & Hudson, 2015; Greenfield, 2015; Phillipson, 2018). In response, a number of cities have adopted 'place-based' approaches to developing Age-Friendly cities, engaging with 'whole system' perspectives which promote increased interconnectedness between service institutions and local populations and which are in the process of being enacted on the ground. 'Place' is understood not as a purely material or geographical location, but as the embodied product of interrelations between a person and other bodies (friends, neighbours, institutions) enacted in space. Massey (2005) argues that 'Place' should be more than a representational 'place-holder' for more intense understandings of lived experience in a particular locale and location because space is '...always being made' through the coexistence of heterogeneous relations, which are embedded material practices (p. 9). The relationships of interdependence that determine experiences of precarity, therefore, include all multiply-determining aspects of our lived experience in a place; but moreover, they could usefully be seen to constitute the nature of the place where we live.

Consequently, place-based working seeks to develop collaborations within a specific locality to understand local issues, aspirations and opportunities informed by the lived experiences of those who, through their interactions with others, create places. These approaches attempt to transform the reciprocal relationship between people, society (social environment) and place (physical environment), each of which is subject to potential change over time. As space is relational, place is produced through the social interactions of those who inhabit or operate within a particular locale. In an Age-Friendly context, the potential of place-based working is to provide a means for personal, social and emotional fulfilment of older people rather than (just) provide a means of improving physical wellness (Greenfield et al., 2012).

The core feature of place-based working is the creation of a two-way, productive relationship of interdependence between citizens and institutions, where both parties are able to share decision-making and development powers as a means of addressing a common goal. These coalitions of difference that underpin place-based approaches, both within a community of people and between citizens and local institutions, provide the basis of interdependent relationships, which addresses the precarity faced by many older people who are normally excluded from influencing processes of change in their neighbourhood.

This chapter will draw upon three case studies derived from the 'Manchester Age-Friendly Neighbourhoods' programme, which elaborate on three key facets of interdependence and place that highlight the potential for Age-Friendly neighbourhoods to address experiences of precarity in urban communities. The first examines how interdependence can provide a means of overcoming structural issues that affect the production of place. The second demonstrates how interdependence can increase the capabilities of both actors within a relationship to realise spatial justice. The third shows how creating relationships of interdependence can be an inclusionary practice that addresses the complex, multifaceted forms of marginalisation.

Manchester Age-Friendly Neighbourhoods

The Manchester Age-Friendly Neighbourhoods (MAFN) programme utilises a place-based approach as a means of addressing social inequalities and precarity within four, deprived urban communities of Manchester, UK. The initiative was established by Manchester School of Architecture and Southway Housing Trust in 2016 and aims to work alongside communities of older people to develop four, Age-Friendly neighbourhoods over a four-year period. The programme was funded through the Big Lottery 'Ageing Better' fund, with additional financial support from Manchester City Council's 'Age-Friendly Manchester' team. The programme builds upon a previous pilot study, Age-Friendly Old Moat, developed with the University of Manchester in 2013 (Phillipson et al., 2013; White & Hammond, 2018).

The aim of the MAFN programme is to develop sustainable, resident-led partnerships in each neighbourhood in which older people and local institutions can work together to respond to challenges and opportunities within their neighbourhood. The programme is inspired by the Connected Communities (C2) approach (Durie & Whyatt, 2013), which starts from the critical position that traditional neighbourhood renewal policies have generally failed to address issues of social inclusion or poverty (and often made them worse).

Analysis of the C2 approach suggests that processes of cyclical decline in deprived neighbourhoods are the product of weak connectors that create disjointed relationships of interdependence between resident and agency worker, agency and agency, resident and resident. The negative effect of these situations is indicated by the emergence of shared, tacit beliefs that 'nothing can be done' to improve the quality of life of residents in deprived communities. This perpetually limits the possibility of change within agencies, or the development of robust, neighbourhood structures that tackle precarity and enable interdependence (Durie & Whyatt, 2007).[1]

The MAFN neighbourhood partnerships are underpinned by a series of activities: creating an action plan, supporting and funding small projects; and creating new relationships between organisations and older people.

Creating an Action Plan

Each partnership within the MAFN programme is centred around a co-produced neighbourhood action plan. Developed through a series of participatory methodologies in collaboration with local residents and institutional partners, the action plan is a spatial representation of older people's lived experiences, providing both robust evidence for action and a catalogue of ideas developed by the community. The plan consists of spatial census data, urban design analysis, neighbourhood survey data and findings from action planning workshops, with a focus on exploring the spatial manifestations of these data sources (Figure 9.1). As of January 2019, the MAFN research team have engaged in 4,800 interactions with local people and institutional partners in creating the four, neighbourhood action plans, sharing both experiences of living in those neighbourhoods and ideas about how to make it better for older people.[2]

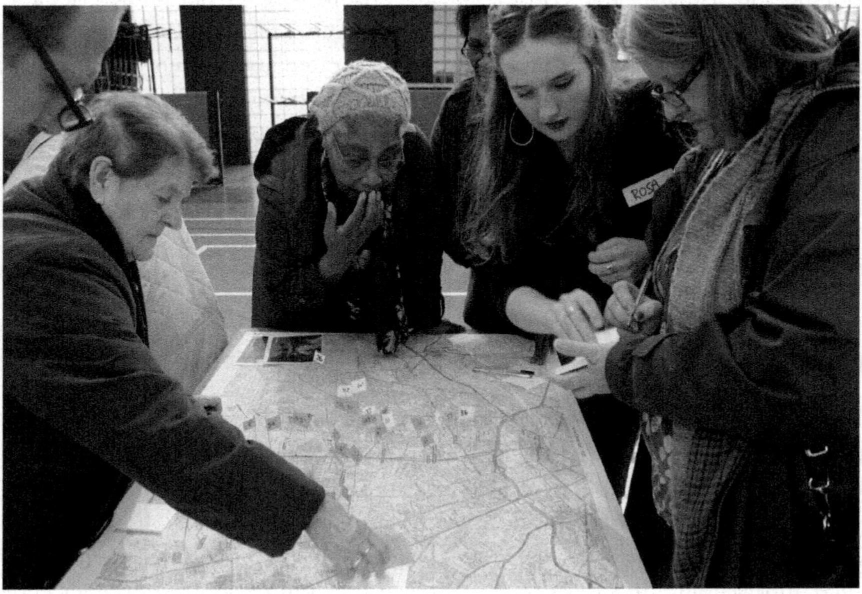

FIGURE 9.1 Older residents from Hulme and Moss Side taking part in an action planning workshop.

Source: Authors.

Developing and Funding Small Projects

Each partnership was provided with a resident investment fund to support the development of small projects (usually less than £2,000), which could be used to enact their vision of an Age-Friendly community. These projects were developed by local residents, with projects supported, reviewed and agreed by a resident-led board in each area. These boards consisted of older people and representatives of institutions and organisations that are active in the area.

Create New Relationships between Organisations and Older People

The purpose of a partnership approach is to enable new relationships and connections to occur, allowing individuals to affect each other in ways not currently possible. The aim is to generate systemic change, in which new relationships between actors are able to change how services are created and delivered. This offers a means of challenging models of dependency that are implicit in the labels that individuals have, such as those between volunteer and user, or provider and customer. This requires agencies and service providers to be open to develop new ways of working (both inter-agency, and with the community), and residents to be organised and engaged (usually through a commonly recognised issue that they want to respond to).

The programme was developed in five Manchester neighbourhoods: Burnage, Moston, Miles Platting, Hulme and Moss Side. Each has contrasting demographic and spatial characteristics, and by various metrics can be described as multiply deprived and precarious communities. Our focus in this chapter will be the Hulme and Moss Side neighbourhoods, located just south of Manchester's urban core. Both communities have a relatively young population of 34,189, of which only 12.4% are aged 50 and over (compared to 34.6% in England and Wales). The area has undergone significant change in recent years, with a new university campus and increasing affluent student population moving into the area. A number of demographic characteristics suggest risk factors for a precarity in the neighbourhood's older population (see Table 9.1).

Discussion: The Future, Age-Friendly City

The case studies presented in this chapter suggest how interventions that support interdependence can address the increased levels of precarity that might develop in urban environments in the future. While the challenges facing cohorts of older people will be significant, this needs to be seen as a call for action, rather than despair. Precarity raises the necessity to develop new models of interdependence: in the home, in the workplace, and in the community. From older people's cohousing to workers cooperatives, to Age-Friendly neighbourhoods and 'village' models, the focus on *relationships* becomes increasingly vital as a means of maintaining wellbeing in the face of an increasingly isolated, individualistic

TABLE 9.1 Data representing potential precarity risk factors in later life in Hulme and Moss Side, compared to the national average (England and Wales)

	Hulme and Moss Side (%)	*England and Wales (%)*
Proportion of retired population receiving pension credit support[a]	63.1	14.3
Economic activity: Inactive (50–64)[b]	50.8	33.6
Ethnic group: Black/African/Caribbean/Black British (50+)	35.4	1.6
Main language: Not English (50+)	16.1	4.1
Marital and civil partnership status: Single (never married), separated, divorce or widowed (50+)	69.0	38.7
Long-term health problems or disabilities: Day-to-day activities limited a lot/a little (50+)	52.5	36.8

Source: Authors.

a Note: Data from August 2018. Pension credits are a state-funded benefit for retired people on low incomes, available to older people whose normal pension is not enough to support basic living costs (which as of January 2019 is set at £163 per week for single people, and £248 per week for couples).

b Note: Data from 2011 Census.

Case Study 1: Creating an Age-Friendly 'partnership'

Using interdependence to address structural issues that limit how place is made. Following a series of initial engagement events, led by the research team, which involved hundreds of local residents and community representatives, 22 people agreed to become the founding board members of the Age-Friendly Hulme and Moss Side partnership. These were a broad mix of institutions (e.g. health professionals, council workers, police, university staff), established community 'champions' (e.g. community group volunteers, resident association chairs) and individual residents with no previous experience in civic participation or affiliation to existing groups. A number of situations experienced in the first year of the partnership board highlighted how institutions (including the University) were not engaging with the state of precarity that many older people faced, but demonstrate how actively addressing these conditions provides a means of greater engagement and collaboration. These reaffirm the notion that social exclusion is a systemic failure rather than an individual deficit, and thus is open to change through the concerted efforts of those within the system.

One of the key challenges faced within the early phases of the project was the conflict between a desire to support socially excluded people to do good in their community, yet still operating within the ethical and legal framework set by our external funders and University finance department. The role of the University in the programme had a fixed four-year time-frame, so the board recognised that a robust and sustainable set of structures and procedures would need to be developed.

In June 2016, the treasurer of the Age-Friendly Hulme and Moss Side partnership board investigated setting up a bank account, initially just for the £2,000 set aside to fund the management of the board. The board approached a number of banks to set up an account, but were turned down due to the poor credit history of some board members. This setback, both in terms of time and confidence, led the board to approach the South Manchester Credit Union, a not-for-profit cooperative that provides accounts and loans for local residents. While there were some inconveniences with this account, it also empowered the board to control their own budget and manage their own finances independently of the University.

Based on these experiences, the board set up mechanisms to support other groups and individuals who had no means of receiving funding. Institutions and voluntary groups on the board agreed to work in partnership with any applicant who needed support, removing a potential barrier that socially excluded people (such as those without bank accounts) from developing projects. Rather than a deficit, actively engaging with issues of precarity helped the board establish a more inclusive approach, which, in turn, enabled participation from individuals who are shut out of traditional funding mechanisms.

This case study shows how structural forces, such as the banking system, can influence the production of space. In previous community funding schemes in Hulme and Moss Side, the creation of spatial interventions was limited for those deemed worthy of credit by international banks, rather than those whose ideas and skills might address local needs or aspiration. Prior to the Age-Friendly partnerships in Hulme and Moss Side, these were not understood by many in the community as a component of place, and thus voluntary and community funding schemes were inaccessible to many in the community. By enabling a more diverse group of people to access financial support, the community are able to activate spaces in ways that were not previously possible. This, in turn, affects the spatial character of the neighbourhood by expanding where activities take place and who has access to these venues. The unequal distribution of insecurity, which undermines people's ability to enact change, is overcome when the barriers faced by people transition from being internal, individual insecurities to commonly understood conditions of precarity. For members of the Age-Friendly board, the first-hand experiences of financial precarity provided insights into how to achieve urban change, and greater understanding of the measures needed to address the inequalities faced by the most marginalised members of the community.

Case Study 2: New Hope Fellowship Church/Age-Friendly Bus

Relationships of interdependence increase the capabilities of both actors. One of the aims of an Age-Friendly community is to increase the capabilities of older people to enact change in the locale. In the case of Age-Friendly Hulme and Moss Side, one of the key concerns of residents was the relationship between older residents and a small number of larger institutions, including Manchester City Council. In response, the local Age-Friendly programme sought to engage in holistic processes that sought to address systemic issues of marginalisation, rather than specific interventions that might just provide a short-term 'fix' to the problem.

An example of a more holistic approach is provided by the St. Georges Estate located in the north-west corner of Hulme, which by many metrics can be seen as a community with multiple forms of deprivation. Through the development of the Age-Friendly Hulme and Moss Side action plan, we discovered that St. Georges was the part of Hulme with the highest number of older people reporting poor health, the worst access to public transport, the lowest levels of car ownership, and the highest number of older people living alone. The social exclusion experienced in St. Georges was exacerbated by a number of spatial qualities, with the estate located the furthest distance from shops and community facilities, other than a small and expensive corner shop.

The New Hope Fellowship Church is the only social infrastructure in St. Georges, but our research found that it was used infrequently. When we asked a council worker about why more events didn't occur there, they highlighted the lack of an accessible toilet. They noted that they did not want to exclude older people with disabilities, so felt the venue was not appropriate for them to use. Whilst this position is not illogical, the result was simply that an exclusionary position was transferred to another group: from the disabled people to the residents of St Georges. In responses, the research team worked with local St. Georges residents and the New Hope Fellowship church to convert their existing toilet to make it accessible for people with disabilities. The conversion cost £2,000 and was agreed by the Age-Friendly Hulme and Moss Side board in early 2017.

The project was successful in encouraging more activity located in St. Georges estate, including IT classes, a dinner club and a ten-week exercise programme, run by the city council. The existing lunch club also has noted increased numbers of older people in attendance, including two wheelchair users who didn't previously stay for the lunch club (which took place directly after the food bank) because they would be unable to use the facilities.

The marginalisation of St. Georges residents should be understood as the uneven distribution of precarity within space, a process that is informed by both physical environment (location, lack of facilities), and the social relationships which reaffirm these conditions. The physical solution was simple and low cost, but did not previously occur in St. Georges because the social environment perpetuated a series of norms which determined what kinds of spaces events should take place in and the Council services did not individually have the scope to act to address the underlying cause. This case study exposes not just how an altered set of relationships can enact transformative change for a spatially excluded group but how developing interdependence can increase the capabilities of both actors, in this case local residents and the local council. For the council, the relationship was not about handing over power to residents, but mutually increasing each other's power to address the spatial injustices. This is underpinned by reconceptualisation of relationships, from the perceived dependence of older 'service users' to a recognition that interdependence can both expand the field of possible actions for both parties.

Case Study 3: Ayeyyo Lunch

Relationships of interdependence can be an inclusionary practice. From the outset of the Age-Friendly Hulme and Moss Side programme, a central concern of the research team was undertaking intense forms of engagement as a mechanism of reaching socially isolated individuals and groups. The circumstances that cause social isolation are, by definition, a factor of the relationships external to the isolated individual. As a result, even targeted acts of inclusion by the research team (with whom genuinely isolated people have no relationship) are ineffective. Instead, our focus was on fostering a partnership network that was open to difference and actively seeking to expand itself. This process understands social isolation as a product of systemic marginalisation and thus seeks to address it through systemic change. While some communities might be hard to reach for the research team, they are imminently reachable for others within a partnership that is always looking to expand.

An example of this is the older Somali community, who had been identified anecdotally as a significant group at risk of social isolation. None of the members of the Age-Friendly partnership had any links to the Somali community, and there were no obvious gatekeepers to approach who could help facilitate connections.

In September 2016, the Age-Friendly Moss Side board were contacted by the 'Women's Support Group' (WSG). WSG was a small and informal group of younger Somali women who met at a local community centre to provide peer support for each other. The group were mostly first-generation migrants, but had grown up in the UK speaking fluent English. Members of the WSG first heard about the Age-Friendly programme after having a conversation with a community member who had previously designed and run a community project, funded by the Age-Friendly Hulme and Moss Side partnership. The WSG approached the Age-Friendly Hulme and Moss Side partnership to explore how they might be able to support their parents and grandparents, many of whom were isolated due to language and cultural barriers. Some of the older Somali community lacked documentation, which dissuaded them from seeking support or attending events. Two members of the Age-Friendly board agreed to meet with a group of older Somali women and the WSG to start developing a project that would address their specific social and cultural needs.

Rather than an accidental engagement reliant on chance encounters, this illustrates the success of the partnership, in which connections, advocacy and responsibility are devolved to all members, thus enabling the programme to engage 'exhaustively' or continually in a way unachievable by top-down processes of more targeted or representational engagement.[3]

The WSG decided to start a lunch club calling it 'Ayeeyo', which is Somali for 'Grandmother'. Ayeyyo was a weekly lunch club for 10–15 older Somali women, including food and informal socialisation. The sessions were organised by younger Somali women, who also cooked the lunch and drove older residents to the venue. In return, the older residents agreed to teach the younger generation songs and dances as a way of passing on Somali culture. Beyond just a chance to socialise, the Ayeyyo group were founded on a recognition of the unequal distribution of opportunities for older Somali women as a result of systemic barriers within society. One example of this was public health programmes, from which the older Somali women felt excluded. An explicit part of the project proposal was for the WSG to work with local community health professionals to provide an arena for public health initiatives to be communicated. The WSG invited various groups to attend their sessions, translating presentations from professionals from English to Somali. Once established, the group became embedded in the wider programme of work in the neighbourhood, as other members of the partnership had a means of reaching (physically, culturally, linguistically) a community that they would otherwise not have engaged with. For example, a local arts venue approached the group to talk about their programme of events and which might be interesting and appropriate for them, later provided free tickets for the group to attend a number of events.

Ayeyyo Lunch demonstrates the potential of devolved responsibility for engagement, in which the aim of creating social justice for the most socially isolated groups is shared by the local partnership as a whole. Like many projects, the initial participants in Age-Friendly Hulme and Moss Side were the already active citizens who were capable of attending public events. By promoting inclusion as a fundamental concept of an Age-Friendly community and the explicit methodological basis of the partnership, the programme was able to include people as active participants that were several degrees of separation removed from the previously empowered mainstream community institutions.

This case study demonstrates that relationships of interdependence provide a means of generating inclusionary practices that address complex and multifaceted forms of marginalisation. For the older Somali community, their language, gender, legal status and financial resources all influenced their capabilities to interact with others and therefore the capabilities to produce space. Through a systemic focus on inclusion within the project, the MAFN programme was able to identify and support the conditions for transformative interdependence – first between two generations of Somali women, and later between the Somali women and local institutions – which would not have been possible through engagements based on pre-determined interventions. Spatially, the impacts of this are small but significant. A community space that was not previously part of their experience of the neighbourhood is transformed into a space both of sociability and of comfort (for many, the only place where they can remove their hijabs outside of their home), and a space to generate wider forms of interdependence, including with people who could enable them to expand their territories to venues and facilities previously unavailable to them.

society (see further Monbiot, 2017). For the Age-Friendly city, precarity calls for place-based approaches, in which interdependence is fostered not just between the older cohort, but also with the myriad of institutions, agencies and groups who influence the lived experience of the neighbourhood.

The importance of the spatial dimension of precarity and precariousness can often be overlooked in both discourse and programmes seeking to address social inequality. Based on Butler's suggestion that precarity is the unequal distribution of precariousness, the case studies in this chapter demonstrate how this unequal distribution is also inherently and inextricably spatial. For those with bad credit ratings, or those without community facilities, or those whose language and culture exclude them, precarity has a clear impact on the relationships through which space is continually produced, and their capabilities to ensure that changes to their community address their needs and aspirations as older people.

The key aspect we seek to emphasise is that the relationships of interdependence required to enable 'active ageing', 'greater civic participation' or 'reduce social isolation' are not generic, but experiential. A recognition of spatiality is also a recognition of specificity and difference, as they '…force into the imagination a fuller recognition of the simultaneous coexistence of others with their own trajectories and their own stories to tell' (Massey, 2005, p. 11). The examples from the Manchester Age-Friendly Neighbourhoods project all demonstrate how the relationships between a heterogeneous array of actors can be the catalyst for social change, and that these relationships can be supported to flourish through coordinated, place-based initiatives.

This is not to discount the role of design and architectural construction in defining space. The numerous programmes of wholesale 'regeneration' in Hulme and Moss Side were highlighted by many older people as events that have both broken and strengthened relationships within the community. The benefit of a partnership approach, as taken in the MAFN programme, is that it enables the urban institutions that commission, influence or mediate urban development to do so without the need to adopt generic stereotypes about the older population. Rather than awaiting a process of community consultation, the development of enduring, two-way relationships between older people, community groups, institutions and local government should provide the basis for genuine forms of co-production of both the physical and social environment.

At this stage, it is important to recognise that precarity is a product of political decision-making; it should be viewed as a failure of policies that prevent the exploitation of labour and property, and marginalise the human rights of some groups (Berardi, 2016; Neilson & Rossiter, 2008). The contradictions between the adoption of the Age-Friendly concept, on the one hand, and the austerity-driven reduction in public services on the other, are glaring and ripe for critique (McGarry, 2018). In the face of these structural challenges, it is fair to question whether the Age-Friendly model will become a mere branding exercise for cities, or whether the movement is able to tackle issues such as '… widening inequalities, the impact of climate change, problems of homelessness, and the lack of affordable housing' (Philipson, 2018, p. 7). Herein lies the great potential of the Age-Friendly city movement: the opportunity to leverage interdependence and collective action is a route to challenging these wider structural systems. The collective act of assembly is not just a means of managing decline in the face of austerity, but a mechanism by which older people can show how an alternative way is possible, working together to demonstrate the transformative potential of collaborative, rather than competitive, approaches.

To conclude, precarity should not be understood as an individual deficit, but the consequence of systemic, multi-dimensional exclusion; a failure of the social, economic, political and spatial networks through which individuals generate agency. If an Age-Friendly city is to address the needs of an increasingly older population, interventions need to actively engage with the conditions of precarity, not just the symptoms. Each of the examples in this chapter demonstrates how the conditions of precarity are often hidden and individualised: the structural issues with financial services; experiences of spatial exclusion in certain locations; exclusion from some groups from the civic and voluntary offer of their neighbourhood. The Manchester Age-Friendly Neighbourhoods project shows that, through interaction, these conditions become explicit, and through interdependence, they can be overcome. This requires holistic processes in which residents and institutions are open to affect each other in meaningful ways, working towards common goals through shared practices. Through this, Age-Friendly programmes can create platforms for co-production based on genuine, two-way relationships between diverse actors, and in doing so create pathways for socially and spatially excluded older people to realise an equitable and just city.

Acknowledgements

Along with the hundreds of older people and institutional partners who have contributed to the MAFN programme, the authors would like to thank the team of researchers that have worked on the Manchester Age-Friendly Neighbourhood project over the last three years, and who contributed immensely to the field work documented in this chapter; Emily Crompton, Mark Hammond, April Manderson, Georgina Mitchell, Catherine Morris, Devon Poyser, Jude Wells, Stefan White, Katherine Wong and Matt Youngson.

Notes

1. Examples of the C2 approach, such as the 'Beacon Project' in Falmouth, UK, demonstrate how increasing the number of productive relationships of interdependence can reduce precarity in deprived communities. The Beacon project provided a mechanism for bringing together the various local agencies – police, housing, health, teachers, probation – and local residents to define shared problems, and thus work together for find new ways to enact positive change in their community. The initiative led to significant improvements in health, crime, education and employment outcomes (Fujiwara et al., 2016).
2. These interactions are noted because they are recorded by the MAFN team members. They do not represent unique individuals. Interactions between partners and residents in the area around age-friendly issues and projects have not been possible to track, but would involve much larger numbers of engagement actors (e.g. around 30–40 core members) with each contributing significant numbers of interactions.
3. It should be noted that the older Somali community also did not appear on the current census data.

References

Berardi, F. (2016). The impossibility of precarity. *Radical Philosophy*, 198 (July/August), 7–14.

Buffel, T., Phillipson, C., & Scharf, T. (2013). Experiences of neighbourhood exclusion and inclusion among older people living in deprived inner-city areas in Belgium and England. *Ageing & Society*, 33, 89–109.

Butler, J. (2004). *Precarious life: The powers of mourning and volence.* London: Verso.

Butler, J. (2015). *Notes towards a performative theory of assembly*. London: Harvard University Press.

Dannefer, D., & Huang, W. (2017). Precarity, inequality, and the problem of agency in the study of the life course. *Innovation in Aging*, 1 (3), 1–10.

Doran, P., & Buffel, T. (2018). Translating research into action: Involving older people in co-producing knowledge about age-friendly neighbourhood interventions. *Working with Older People*, 22 (1), 39-47.

Durie, R., & Wyatt, K. (2007). New communities, new relations: The impact of community organization on health outcomes. *Social Science and Medicine*, 65 (9), 1928–1941.

Durie, R., & Wyatt, K. (2013). Connecting communities and complexity: A case study in creating the conditions for transformational change. *Critical Public Health,* 23 (2), 174–187.

Fujiwara, D., Hotopp, U., & Lawton, R. (2016). *Lighting the way for C2 Connecting Communities: Social impact valuation of the Beacon Project 1995–2001.* Retrieved from https://www.c2connectingcommunities.co.uk/wp-content/uploads/2016/10/C2_LightingTheWay_FINAL.pdf

Gonyea, J. G., & Hudson, R. B. (2015). Emerging models of age-friendly communities: A framework for understanding inclusion. *Public Policy & Aging Report,* 25 (1), 9–14.

Greenfield, E. A. (2018). Age-friendly initiatives, social inequalities, and spatial justice. *Hastings Center Report,* 48, S41–45.

Greenfield, E. A., Scharlach, A., Lehning, J. K., & Davitt, J. K. (2012). A conceptual framework for examining the promise of the NORC program and village models to promote aging in place. *Journal of Aging Studies,* 26 (3), 273–284.

Grenier, A., & Phillipson, C. (2018). Precarious aging: Insecurity and risk in later life. *Hastings Center Report,* 48, S15–18.

Grenier, A., Phillipson, C., Rudman, D. L., Hatzifilalithis, S., Kobayashi, K., & Marier, P. (2017). Precarity in late life: Understanding new forms of risk and insecurity. *Journal of Aging Studies,* 43, 9–14.

Lewis, H., Dwyer, P., Hodkinson, S., & Waite, L. (2015). Hyper-precarious lives: Migrants, work and forced labour in the global north. *Progress in Human Geography,* 39 (5), 580–600.

Massey, D. (2005). *For space.* London: SAGE.

McGarry, P. (2018). Developing age-friendly policies for cities: Strategies, challenges and reflections. In T. Buffel, S. Handler, & C. Phillipson (Eds.), *Age-friendly cities and communities: A global perspective* (231–250). Bristol: Policy Press.

Monbiot, G. (2019). *Out of the wreckage: A new politics for an age of crisis*. London: Verso.

Neilson, B., & Rossiter, N. (2008). Precarity as a political concept, or, Fordism as exception. *Theory, Culture & Society,* 25 (8), 51–72.

Neilson, D. (2015). Class, precarity, and anxiety under neoliberal global capitalism: From denial to resistance. *Theory & Psychology,* 25 (2), 184–201.

Ogg, J. (2005). Social exclusion and insecurity among older Europeans: The influence of welfare regimes. *Ageing and Society,* 25 (1), 69–90.

Phillipson, C. (2018). Developing age-friendly work in the twenty-first century: New challenges and agendas. *Working with Older People* WWOP-12–2017–0037. Retrieved from http://www.emeraldinsight.com/doi/10.1108/WWOP-12-2017-0037

Phillipson, C., Stefan W., & Hammond, M. (2013). Age-friendly old moat. Retrieved December 6, 2013, from http://www.southwayhousing.co.uk/getattachment/Southway-in-Your-Community/Age-friendly-Neighbourhoods/Old-Moat-Age-friendly-Neighbourhood-Report.pdf.aspx

Ryan, F. (2018, April 26). The hostile environment? Britain's disabled people live there too. *The Guardian*. Retrieved January 8, 2019, from https://www.theguardian.com/commentisfree/2018/apr/26/hostile-environment-britain-disabled-people-windrush-benefits

Scharlach, A. E., & Lehning. A. J. (2013). Ageing-friendly communities and social inclusion in the United States of America. *Ageing & Society*, 33, 110–136.

Standing, G. (2012). The precariat: From denizens to citizens? *Polity*, 44 (4), 588–608.

UN (United Nations). (2017). *World Population Prospects-2017 Revision*. Retrieved from https://esa.un.org/unpd/wpp/Publications/Files/WPP2017_KeyFindings.pdf

White, S., & Hammond, M. (2018). From representation to active ageing in Manchester neighbourhood: Designing the age-friendly city. In T. Buffel, S. Handler, & C. Phillipson (Eds.), *Age-friendly cities and communities: A global perspective* (193–210). Bristol: Policy Press.

WHO (World Health Organisation). (2007). Global age-friendly cities: A Guide. Retrieved April 24, 2017, from www.who.int/ageing/publications/Global_age_friendly_cities_Guide_English.pdf

10

BUILDINGS FOR HEALTH, CITIES FOR WELLBEING

Ricardo Codinhoto, Christopher Boyko, Antony Darby and Margaret Watson

A Complex, Shifting Problem

By 2050, it is predicted that 70% of the world's 9.7 billion inhabitants will live in urban areas (UN, 2015). In the context of continuous global population growth and demographics showing a shift towards an ageing population, the value of planning and designing cities to support physical activity, sunlight, clean air, sustainable design and access to energy, access to healthy food and social inclusiveness will be paramount. This is a crucial time for understanding how cities influence healthy and unhealthy behaviours and for addressing the positive and negative impacts of cities' characteristics on moving the healthcare and wellbeing agenda further.

In this respect, the gradual transition from an agrarian to an industrial society has afforded unprecedented benefits as well as novel challenges to human health. Major causes of death changed from nutritional deficiency and infectious disease to non-communicable, degenerative chronic disease, an 'epidemiologic transition' that impacted on the way we live, evidencing the relationship between the physical environment (PE), health and wellbeing (Omran, 2005).

In the past and currently, various cases of epidemic disease outbreaks started within urban contexts that lead to pandemic events. Examples of epidemics that killed thousands include plague in Athens (Salway & Dell, 1955), measles in Boston (Melosi, 2008), cholera in London (Johnson, 2006), smallpox in Sidney (Mear, 2008), yellow fever in Philadelphia (Powell, 1993) malaria in Niamey (Keiser et al., 2004), influenza in Glasgow (Grist, 1979) and SARS-CoV-2 in Wuhan in 2019. In many cases, urban sanitation and infrastructure are key factors in the spreading of such diseases. Early literature mostly covers infectious diseases, but it is reasonable to argue that other problems related to mental health and wellbeing were also present in those societies.

Efforts to eradicate diseases followed different rationales. In the US, ideas shifted from zoning out harmful environments like industrial and residential areas to stimulate suburban economic developments that could promote healthier behaviours like diet and exercising. The governments also mandated the use of Environmental Impact Assessments (EIA) and Impact Statements (EIS) to increase urban compliance with health standards in place (Corburn, 2014).

In the UK and worldwide, EIAs are still used, generally for large projects that can impact on areas, such as pollutant emissions, traffic, noise and vibration, visual intrusion and surrounding ecology (MHCLG, 2018). Current EIAs are very extensive and include various dimensions that can impact on people's health and wellbeing, such as health, social, equality, transport, resilience, sustainability, ecology, cultural and life-cycle impact assessments (Glasson & Therivel, 2013; McCallum et al., 2018). The effectiveness of methodologies such as Health Impact Assessment (HIA) has been questioned (Wismar et al., 2004), but evidence shows that they can be effective, despite epistemological limitations (Wismar et al., 2007).

It is evident that interventions proposed in various areas are effective. As depicted in Roser (2018), the worldwide life expectancy range has improved from 30 to 55 years in 1918 to 55 to 85 in 2015. Europe, Canada, Japan, Australia and New Zealand lead the chart while African countries such as Central African Republic, Chad and Nigeria are among those with the shortest life expectancy. This is significant, considering a steady population increase from 1.65 to 7.4 billion in the same period and a continuous (slower) rise (Figures 10.1 and 10.2). For WHO (2018a), growth ratio is a direct outcome of health improvements (i.e. as the health of that population improves, the population growth ratio reduces).

Demographics is also changing as a consequence of better quality of life and increased life expectancy (Figure 10.3). Despite significant differences from bottom and top scoring countries, the increase in the total percentage of older people in the world is seen in all countries, as is the decreasing percentage of young people. While not all countries have the same demographic profile, all countries are experiencing a demographic shift, which puts current and future healthcare needs and strategies in a constant state of flux. Health and wellbeing needs will change as demographics change, thus requiring constant interventions to promote health and wellbeing.

Population ageing is a common, worldwide phenomenon. In the UK, 9.2 million residents are > 65 years 31% of whom live alone (the number of people aged 100 years or above reached 15,000 (ONS, 2016). The global, old-age dependency ratio (>65/(15–64)) was 12.6% in 2015 and is projected to double in advanced economies and to almost quadruple in developing economies over the next 85 years. As we age, we become more fragile and prone to diseases. Healing takes longer and our capacity to cope in unfamiliar and stressful environments diminishes. As a result, there has been a shift towards design for longevity which addresses all stages of our life. Countries like the UK and Japan, where the population is older and expected to age very rapidly, can experience an unprecedented quiet age humanitarian crisis if this is not looked closely.

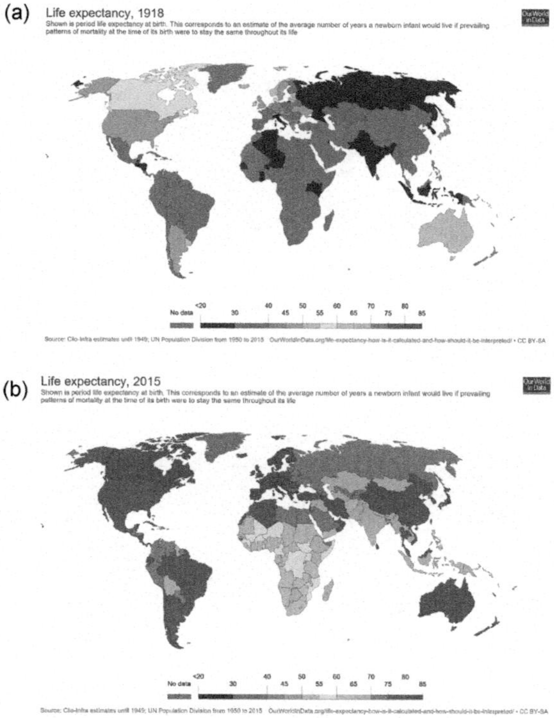

FIGURE 10.1 World life expectancy in 1918 (left) to 2015 (right).
Source: Roser (2018).

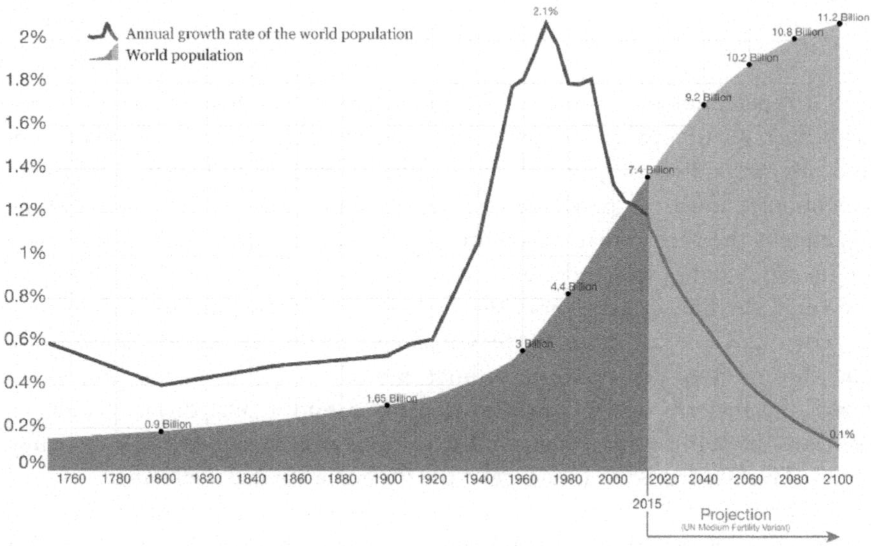

FIGURE 10.2 World population growth rate estimate.
Source: Roser (2018).

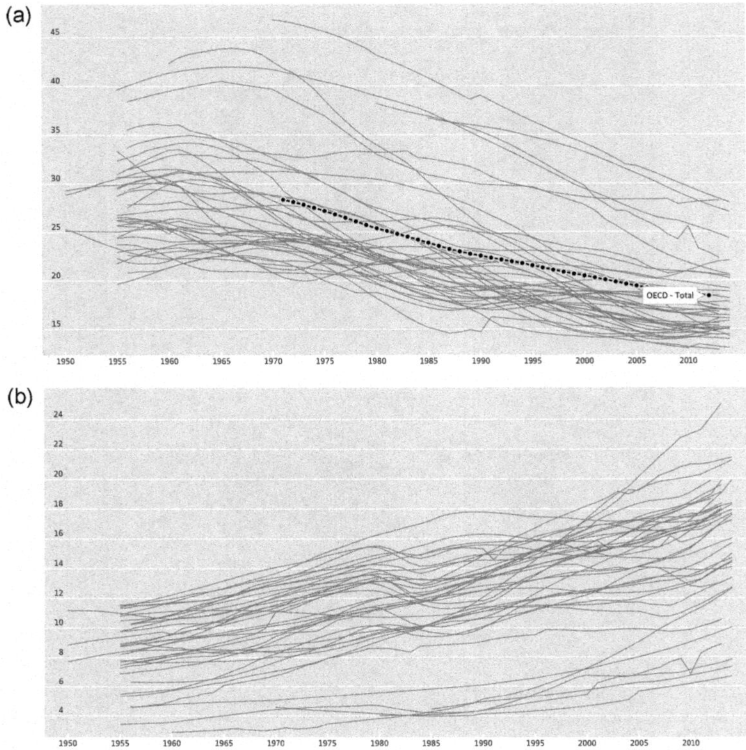

FIGURE 10.3 (a) Young and (b) elderly population: Total percentage of population, 1950–2014.

Source: OECD (2018a, b).

The epidemiologic transition (Omran, 2005) is another, ongoing, worldwide phenomenon. With economic development, problems such as malnutrition and infectious diseases give way to complex transitions in lifestyle and living conditions known to contribute to non-communicable diseases (NCDs). One example is the theory that urbanisation in developing economies is impacting on increased light exposure levels as regulated by day/night time, which impact circadian rhythm, causing onset sleep delays, thus decreasing total sleep time (Czeisler, 2013; Yetish et al., 2015). Circadian disturbances (Wang et al., 2011), and chronic sleep deprivation (Mullington et al., 2009), are associated with a significant increase in NCD risk, particularly cardiovascular disease (Rangaraj & Knutson, 2016), and accidents in the work environment (Powel & Copping, 2016). This illustrates the influence of the PE on health and wellbeing.

While the evidence is alarming, it only emphasises exposure to light and sleeplessness. However, other building and neighbourhood scale parameters that affect sleep include temperature (Okamoto-Mizuno et al., 1999), noise (Alessi et al., 2005), the presence of antisocial behaviour (Evans, 2014), time spent indoors (Morgan & Stewart, 1998a, b) and social parameters, such as cultural practices (Crawford, 1994). Thus, to further our understanding of how these PE parameters interact and altogether influence sleep is key (Cooper et al., 2011).

Obesity is another health condition impacted by urbanisation. Obesity is a worldwide rising NCD (WHO, 2000) related to cardiovascular disease and type 2 diabetes. It reduces individual's life expectancy and increases the complexity of healthcare and socio-economic provision at the neighbourhood, city and national levels (James et al., 2004). For GO-Science (2007), the PE plays an important role in the condition of obesity. In general, the physical dimension is the most commonly studied feature of obesogenic research with outdoor walkability receiving considerable research attention recently (Biddle & Mutrie, 2007; Boyko & Cooper, 2011; Kirk et al., 2010). Reduced urban mobility patterns and increased availability of energy-dense food and drink (Swinburn & Egger, 2002; Townshend & Lake, 2009) are other underlying issues impacting the susceptibility to obesity at city and neighbourhood (Black & Macinko, 2008). The current rise in obesity makes dwellings, hospitals and care homes unfit for the needs of bariatric patients and associated care workers.

Modern city and neighbourhood profiles tend not to support healthy lifestyles that are key to suppress the formation of obesogenic environments (Cooper et al., 2011; Swinburn et al., 1999). Poor urban design and form characteristics include areas dominated by commercial establishments offering unhealthy food and drink (Black & Macinko, 2008), with little or no places for physical exercise (Frank et al., 2007) and accessible green spaces (Gordon-Larsen et al., 2006), communities with unwalkable pavements and low-density homogeneous neighbourhoods (Frank et al., 2005), places perceived as unsafe and violent (Diez Roux, 2001) and the predominance of the private car and associated infrastructures (French et al., 2001).

Attempts to reduce the prevalence of obesogenic environments include guidelines focussed on 'active design' principles (Robbins, 2011), or policies that directly address obesity (Sallis & Glanz, 2009). Unfortunately, the evidence to suggest that PE factors have a correlation with the prevalence to obesity is still inconclusive (Townshend & Lake, 2009; WHO, 2000), and alternative strategies to prevent or reduce obesity, such as building levels of Non-Exercise Activity Thermogenesis (NEAT) remain largely unexplored (Marsh et al., 2020).

While it all sounds overwhelmingly negative, the challenges we face is the result of much improvement that led to the emergence of new problems. The vision is to transform the way in which health and wellbeing presented here are based on their consideration within and beyond the design of buildings and public spaces. Each building asset has the potential to contribute positively to health and wellbeing. For that to happen, a holistic, integrated view of health and wellbeing must be adopted to address the rapid increase in urbanisation coupled with a shift in demographics and increased awareness of physical and mental health conditions that have created unprecedented demands upon the world's health and social care systems.

PE Health Determinants

The health and wellbeing of individuals and communities are influenced by various environments. According to WHO (2018a), the key, impacting factors are those embedded within each individual profile, such as scholarly and income levels, living habits and genetics, and the surrounding environment, which, in turn, can influence behaviours. Even though less influential, remediative factors, such as access to healthcare, also have an impact on individuals.

Currently, most built environment interventions driven by increased urbanisation tend to focus on environmental efficiency, sustainability, lowering embodied carbon and cost with some consideration being also given to the occupiers and users of buildings and public spaces. There is an increasing pressure on social services and healthcare and a need to find ways of shaping the built environment to focus on improving the health and wellbeing of people from cradle to grave, whether at work, rest or play.

Improving inter-related areas, such as health and wellbeing, education and living conditions, is a priority in the UK and across the world. The United Nations predicts that, over the next 30 years, most of the world's population growth will occur in cities and towns. WHO, the UN and others identify the health of people in these growing, urban cityscapes as a key challenge (UN, 2014; WHO, 2009), so to ensure a healthy population, our cities need to be re-designed with people's health as a fundamental design objective. There are many sources that recognise this (Alker et al., 2014; Allen et al., 2016; USDoL, 2017), with key, contributing factors being indoor and outdoor air quality, thermal comfort and fuel poverty, access to natural and artificial light, biophilia and access to nature, noise, vibrations, building and city layout, look and feel, amenities and location.

This represents a siloed view, based on architecture and engineering alone, that leaves out wider social and psychological aspects. Related disciplines, such as sociology, psychology and physiology, must be considered together with enabling technologies supported by computer science and management disciplines, such as service design. Only a pan-disciplinary view can provide the ability to transcend traditional silos by considering wider health-related factors, such as connections between people, workforce resilience, human movement and mobility, active design, pollution, zoning, distinctions between public and private space, grief and bereavement, processes of social influence, behavioural economics, social demographics and inequality, disability, gender, race, religion, social isolation and overcrowding. As depicted in Figure 10.4, an individual's health and wellbeing baseline can be concomitantly impacted positively and negatively by the environments he/she is in throughout the different stages of his/her life.

Thus, to discuss health and wellbeing and healthy cities from a PE perspective means to discuss its relationship with the fabric and ambience of the environment while embracing a broader concept of healthcare provision that incorporates

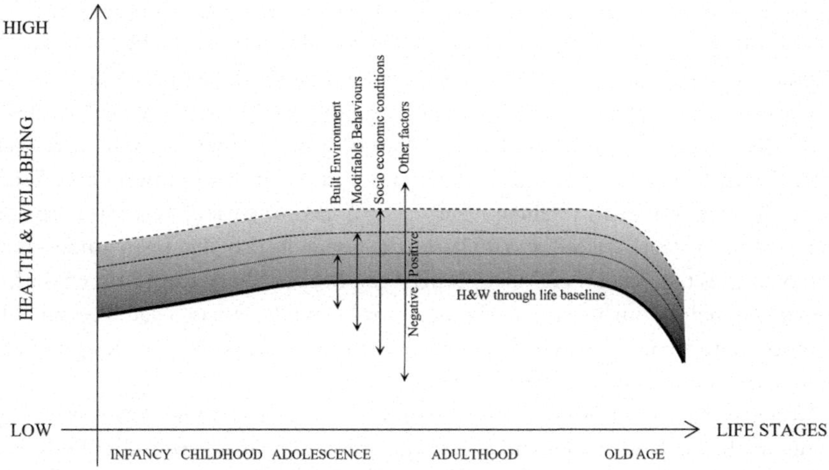

FIGURE 10.4 Hypothetical model of health determinants and its impacts on health and wellbeing.

Source: Ricardo Codnihoto.

prevention not only as part of a healthcare system, but also as part of education and work. This is what WHO (2018a) endorses by considering three, interconnected and interdependent determinants of health. The social and economic environments alongside with the PE entail the background characteristics that influence individuals' behaviours.

Arguably, there are side effects of socio-economic advancements. For instance, less economically developed economies tend to rely on adults to look after children and older members of the family. In Asia, for instance, approximately three quarters of older people still live with their adult children (Martin, 1989). In developed and developing economies, in general, all adult members of the family are actively working away from home. With reduced time to be with, and look after, their families, there is an increased dependency on the educational (nurseries and schools) and healthcare systems (hospital, care and nursing homes), which are two determinants of health. Staying at home may not always be appropriate or practical (Sulaiman et al., 2006a, b), with the expectation of institutional care for older people becoming the norm (Sulaiman, 2012). Increased obesity rates among older people add to the complexity. For instance, it becomes essential to take into account the emotional and physical needs of bariatric patients in care homes (Learner, 2014). In turn, the strain of providing extra space and resources (e.g. specialist mattresses, hoists, carers trained in manual handling of severely obese people, appropriate patient transport) often means increasing healthcare costs for patients, carers and providers (LGA, 2013; Yang & Hall, 2008).

Increasing obesity rates are putting care systems under great pressure. Evidence suggests that the provision of care for bariatric patients requires specific, ergonomic, PE designs and special services (Hahler, 2002; Hignett & Griffiths,

2009). However, these modifications can lead to increased costs and risks to patient and staff safety (Hignett et al., 2013; Xie & Carayon, 2015). From a PE perspective, inadequacy can hinder the provision of adequate care and living standards (Cooper et al., 2011), lead to undesirable health outcomes (Codinhoto et al., 2009), create stigma within care environments, increase staff turnover, foster dissatisfaction among staff and patients and result in spiralling costs. From a service perspective, an inefficient service can lead to patient and carer frustration and even death (Hahler, 2002). Little research also has been undertaken that examines the critical connection between hospitals' proximity to, or within obesogenic neighbourhoods and the need for hospitals and associated services to accommodate bariatric patients as well as consider changes to the design of the PE and services for the benefit of patients.

Nonetheless, the PE is not restricted to the built assets and infrastructures that enable (or hinder) the social and economic environment where individuals live. It also includes the space between buildings, roads and various other modes of transport, infrastructure for clean water, pure air and telecommunication. Psychological dimensions, directly related to physical envelope, such as the sense of density and crowding, and the sense of public private, security, safety and sacred are also part of what is considered the PE (Cooper et al., 2008).

The idea is that the mix of what is available (Figure 10.5) and how it is used influences a population's health positively and negatively. It is unlikely that the impact is linear or extensive as presented in those pictures; nonetheless any opportunity for improving people's wellbeing should be considered. For instance, individuals may live in an area where the physical and the socio-economic environments are prone to disease (e.g. fuel poverty, lack of clean water), but have opted for living a healthier life style through exercising and a healthy diet. Obviously (and unfortunately) many would not have that choice as they live in extremely poor areas where there is no access to basic sanitation and food, but still, some aspect of leaving can be healthier for those individuals who opted for a balanced diet or simply by avoiding smoking and binge drinking.

Adding to the problem is the fact that we deal with these complex relationships in a fragmented manner. The potential, non-medical interventions of achieving health through the PE are many and varied, encompassing technological, psychological and social factors; typically a mixture of all three. There is a need to examine the things we can do to the PE, through changing building usage, better design of new buildings, appropriate development of cities, community engagement, and housing and building support services, to improve health and wellbeing of people. Key, challenging areas where there is greatest potential impact are health in the work place, social housing and public spaces. These particular places can promote improvements to the health of older people, vulnerable and disadvantaged – typically those exposed to the poorest environments and those who rely on stretched health and care services. These core, envisaged 'places' are those where the responsibility for ensuring they are co-designed and maintained for the health of the users is shared collectively. Those places, which

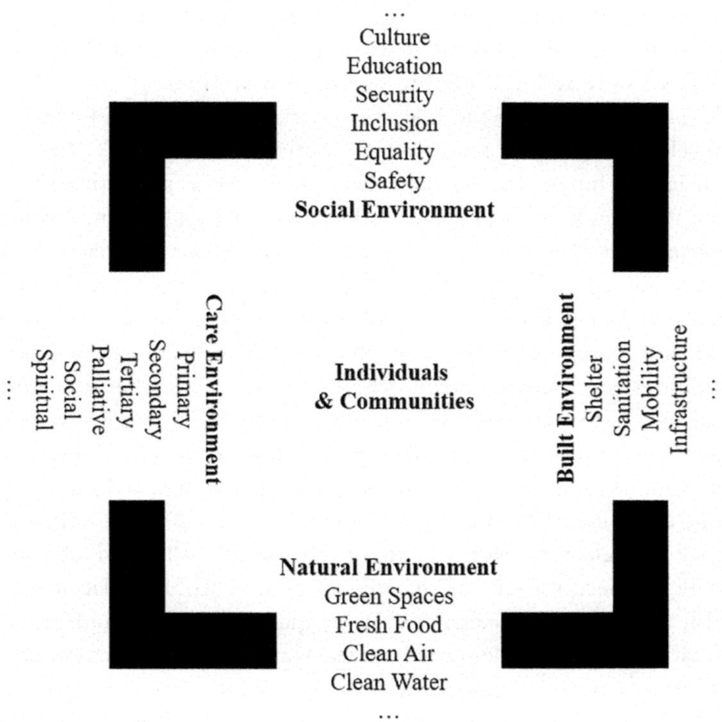

FIGURE 10.5 The determinants of health, adapted from WHO (2018a).
Source: Ricardo Codinhoto.

include key aspects of home, work and play, where the ability to design and manage buildings and spaces to be healthy will have greatest benefit are:

Health in the work place relates to the social, economic and PEs. Income can positively impact on wellbeing by enabling access to food, water, education; it can also enhance the feelings of fulfilment and social engagement. Negatively, if unbalanced, it can cause stress and be the source of physical and mental disorders. The WGBC report on Health, Wellbeing and Productivity in Offices presents a clear argument for building owners to consider employee health, stating that, 'there is overwhelming evidence which demonstrates that the design of an office impacts the health, wellbeing and productivity of its occupants'. With staff costs in a typical business accounting for 90% of the operating costs, anything that affects health, wellbeing and, hence, productivity, is of major concern (Alker et al., 2014). A US study puts the cost of absenteeism (at a typical rate of 3% per employee) amounting to approximately £1,500 per employee/annum (USDoL, 2017). Poor mental health costs UK employers £30bn a year (ACAS, 2018), and the cost of 'presenteeism' is estimated at a similar levels (DHS, 2017). Health in retail properties comes to similar figures (WGBC, 2016). However, there is still a need to further investigate the PE contributors to workplace health and develop widely applicable interventions to improve workforce health, resilience and, hence, productivity. **There is an urgent need to redesign jobs and workplaces to embed and enable health and wellbeing.**

Health in social housing in the UK, for instance, is seeing rapid urban growth and redevelopment, based on an ageing, existing building stock. The Building Research Establishment (BRE) carried out a study that states that the policies in the last 20 years have insufficiently addressed replacement, improvement and new housing (Nicol et al., 2015). As a result, problems associated with poor housing, including excessive cold, falls, overcrowding, fire, damp, mould, hygiene, noise, lighting, asbestos, radon and carbon monoxide, directly account for the substantial increase of NHS care costs (£1.4bn *per year*) (Nicol et al., 2015). Social housing is of particular concern, as it provides for the most vulnerable and disadvantaged in society (Lupton et al., 2009): older people, those on low incomes, those with physical or learning disabilities or mental health problems, those suffering from obesity or forms of Alzheimer disease, the socially isolated and ethnic minorities. The tragedy at Grenfell Tower in 2017 is a stark indication of the state of neglect for people living in UK social housing, which brings into sharp focus the need for safe and healthy environments. The National Institute for Health and Clinical Excellence (NICE) quality standards highlights design and adaptation of housing, leisure activities, planning and evaluation of services and involvement and contributions to the community, as an essential component of the pathway for supporting independent living and wellbeing. This is not just a question of bricks-and-mortar, but community, infrastructure and equality. In this area, **there is still a need to investigate integrated, cross-disciplinary solutions to meet the health demands of these occupiers**. Whilst many institutions, nationally and internationally, promote, fund and undertake research on ageing populations, none has a multidisciplinary approach based on socio-economic and environmental dimensions. A new, ecopsychosocial resilience model/philosophy is needed, prominent examples being the US National Institute of Ageing and the European Working Group on Ageing Populations and Sustainability.

Health in public spaces is a key subject addressed by reports from organizations, such as Project for Public Spaces (PPS, 2016), Healthy Spaces and Places (HSP, 2009) and Urban Green Spaces and Health (WHO, 2016). Public spaces, including parks, recreation grounds, museums, leisure centres, libraries and the space in-between buildings, all contribute to health. Parks, for example, can be beneficial by providing opportunities for social interaction and enhanced physical activity, but also noise buffering, absorption of air pollution, improved sleep, improved cognitive function and improved immune system. Equally, there are potential negative aspects, such as risk of allergies, exposure to UV radiation, pathogens and pollution, among others. Socially, the privatisation of public and semi-public spaces and gentrification is restricting access of people to public spaces. The ubiquitous digitalisation of life is also contributing to that. Therefore, urban planners, architects and managers face many conflicting demands, further complicated by the effect of the surrounding built environment and supporting infrastructure, which can have a huge influence on the quality of the public space (Cooper et al., 2008).

These three areas illustrate the various factors that influence population health, but also reveal the lack of understanding of what factors are important, how various, contributing factors are related, what changes are most effective and how improvements might be measured or quantified. While the issue itself is not a new one – health has after all been the rationale for swathes of reforms, and radical solutions have been implemented to housing crises, for example – a user-centred reform still needs to be coupled with advances in architectural engineering with the sole purpose of improving the health and wellbeing of communities who live, work and socialise in diverse (built) environments.

Truly Integrated Healthcare for Wellbeing

To continue to build our care system upon the same needs as 70 years ago to meet the encumbrance of accidents, emergencies and diseases is no longer appropriate (Ham et al., 2011). People are being failed by a fragmented care system that does not account for demographic changes, the epidemiologic transition and new health determinants. Only a truly integrated care system would address the problems that the current system has (Curry & Ham, 2010; Humphries & Curry, 2011; Lewis et al., 2010). An integration beyond the integration of care services.

Silent care inefficiencies are one of the key problems caused by fragmentation. A major example of this is the treatment of minor ailments at secondary care facilities (RPSGB, 2003). The Keogh report warned that 'urgent but non-life threatening' conditions can be treated in non-secondary care settings and identified community pharmacies as an 'under-utilised resource' that could substantially reduce the burden on other healthcare providers (Keogh, 2013). In the UK, Emergency Departments (EDs) and General Practices (GPs) receive substantial numbers of people with minor ailments (Fielding et al., 2015), which impact on waiting times while reducing the availability for more serious conditions and inflates the cost of service provision in both settings. Watson et al. (2015) demonstrated that, in the UK, 13% of GP and 5% of ED consultations could be efficiently and effectively treated in community pharmacies. Nationally, these estimates equate to approximately 18 million GP and 6.5 million ED consultations per year, costing approximately £1.1 billion (Fielding et al., 2015).

In the UK (and potentially worldwide) the majority of the population has access to community pharmacies (Todd et al., 2014) where no appointments are necessary, with relatively short waiting times and skilled personnel are available to advise and support people with minor ailments. Evidence in the UK shows that this idea is feasible (Paudyal et al., 2013), and increases satisfaction associated with higher rates of health and wellbeing (Watson et al., 2015). However, for a shift to happen, reassurance of safety and effectiveness of care at community pharmacies is needed. For that, over-the-counter (OTC) consultations still need to improve (Pearl, 2013; van Eikenhorst et al., 2017). For Watson et al. (2014), the main barriers to OTC are privacy, effective communication skills and perceived consumer knowledge regarding information provision. Privacy (visual, auditory, personal or spatial) is a dimension that can be enabled through building design, while communication and knowledge can be enabled through education. Thus, tackling building design without tackling education (or vice versa) would not be efficient.

For the above case, as well as for many other cases to work, it is necessary to have an integrated approach for health and wellbeing in cities. Here, integrated refers to:

> 'Working together across boundaries to deliver a successful and streamlined service to the end-user'. It is about putting people and communities at the centre of care delivery through a coherent process/set of processes between organisations, people and services that enable greater transparency between partners as well as enhanced benefits for service users. … creating an operational definition, shared values, goals and knowledge.
>
> *(Suter et al., 2009).*

Such a wide and open concept requires different types and levels of integration. It requires *real integration* as the merging of services and/or organisations by removing inter-departmental walls, and it requires trust to enable *virtual integration* (Ham et al., 2011). It requires *vertical integration* of care across distinctive levels within the same service organisation (such as the integration between social and health care) and *horizontal integration* for enabling the collaboration of care providers and multidisciplinary teams (Rumbold & Shaw, 2010). Also macro integration of policy where service providers seek to deliver integrated care across all available services to the whole population (Williams & Sullivan, 2010), *meso integration* of services for particular groups of people that have the same health problem and *micro integration* for supporting patient interaction through care approaches, such as coordination and care planning (Valentijn et al., 2013).

Freudenberg (2000) argued that the improvement of the health of urban populations can only be achieved by increasing access and the quality of healthcare, reducing risk behaviour, and improving social conditions. Similarly, the UK Department of Health and Social Care view is that healthcare and wellbeing is about more than providing care at a care facility. **There is an increasing need for further integration of different agencies and public bodies, such as education, transport and retail, to support the dissemination of preventive approaches** that are not yet part of any ministerial departments (DHSC, 2018). Frameworks that consider the contextual changes and health determinants discussed in this article have also been developed (Galea et al., 2005), but the issue of integration is not addressed to the necessary extent.

With regard to health indicators, WHO (2012) suggests that health is an important benchmark of sustainability of urban policies and as such, indicators should account for social equity, environment and development dimensions of sustainable cities linked to house improvement, pollution (sanitation), transport (in terms of safety and sustainable modes like walking and cycling), crime, equal access to health care services, green spaces, fresh food and waste. Like the WHO indicators, in Australia, the indicators of healthy liveable cities also converge on the idea of integration of other areas beyond healthcare, such as transport and education (Lowe et al., 2015). Integration is also embedded in views of person-centric healthcare design, which aims at designing out the problems and barriers that prevent health and wellbeing promoting behaviours (Tsekleves & Cooper, 2017).

However, for general health and wellbeing to happen through integration, it is necessary to move away from models of wellbeing that are focussed on provision of an uncountable, ever-increasing number of things. According to Sarah White (2017), 'The ubiquity of references to happiness and wellbeing indicates widespread anxiety that all may not be well…'. For her, '…individualist formulations of wellbeing in policy mimic or deepen the underlying pathology' (p. 121). Very much like the dopamine loop, these models are not designed for fulfilment, even if an individual has achieved what is essential for his/her own wellbeing. Other models have started to emerge, such as the relational wellbeing model (White, 2017) that integrates environmental, personal and societal dimensions and how we related to these dimensions that give us the sense of fulfilment sought and a downfall in an area can be compensated by upraising another.

Downfalls in health and wellbeing will continue to happen in future cities. Thus provision of (health and social) care is necessary. As shown in Figure 10.6

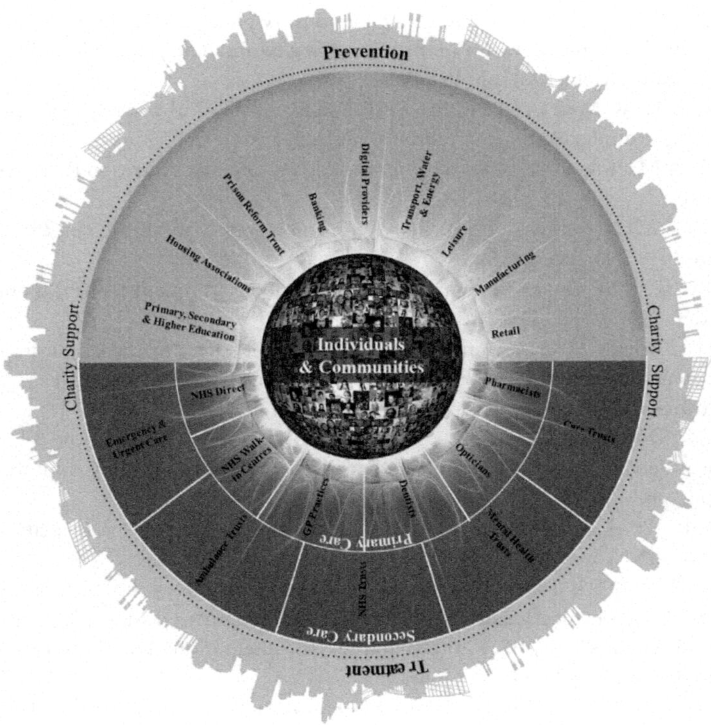

FIGURE 10.6 Integrated model of health and wellbeing in cities.
Source: Ricardo Codinhoto.

care provision forms the basis of a system that treats individuals from their physical or mental ailments. There is also a preventive layer that takes place everywhere, in every private or public building or space and is under the responsibility of individuals and communities living in those areas. Through integration, taboos will be dissolved through extensive public awareness, facilitated by the Internet and social media channels. This will be an important step in removing stigmas and stereotypes of health-related conditions, such as dementia, autism and many other physical and mental health conditions.

References

ACAS, (2018). Mental health in the workplace. [Online]. Available at: www.acas.org.uk/index.aspx?articleid=1900

Alessi, C. A. et al., (2005). Randomized, controlled trial of a nonpharmacological intervention to improve abnormal sleep/wake patterns in nursing home residents. Journal of the American Geriatrics Society, 53(5), pp. 803–810.

Alker, J., Malanca, M., Pottage, C. & O'Brien, R., (2014). Health, wellbeing & productivity in offices: the next chapter for green building. London: World Green Building Council.

Allen, J. G. et al., (2016). Building evidence for health: The 9 foundations of a healthy building. Boston: Harvard University Press.

Anderson, C., Blenkinsopp, A. & Armstrong, M., (2004). Feedback from community pharmacy users on the contribution of community pharmacy to improving the public's health: a systematic review of the peer reviewed and non-peer reviewed literature. Health Expectations, 7(3), pp. 191–202.

Biddle, S. J. H. & Mutrie, N., (2007). Psychology of physical activity: Determinants, wellbeing and interventions. London: Routledge.

Black, J. L. & Macinko, J., (2008). Neighborhoods and obesity. Nutrition Reviews, 66(1), pp. 2–20.

Boyko, C. T. & Cooper, R., (2011). Clarifying and re-conceptualising density. Progress in Planning, 76(1), pp. 1–61.

Codinhoto, R. et al., (2009). The impacts of the built environment on health outcomes. Facilities, 27(3/4), pp. 138–151.

Cooper, R., Boyko, C. & Codinhoto, R., (2008). The effect of the physical environment on mental wellbeing. Foresight: Mental capital and wellbeing project. London: Government Office for Science.

Cooper, R., Boyko, C. T. & Cooper, C. L., (2011). Design for health: the relationship between design and noncommunicable diseases. Journal of Health Communication, 16(sup2), pp. 134–157.

Corburn, J., (2014). Confronting the challenges in reconnecting urban planning and public health. American Journal of Public Health, 94(4), pp. 541–546.

Crawford, C. J., (1994). Parenting practices in the Basque country: implications of infant and childhood sleeping location for personality development. Ethos, 22(1), pp. 42–82.

Curry, N. & Ham, C., (2010). Clinical and service integration: The route to improved outcomes. London: The King's Fund.

Czeisler, C. A., (2013). Perspective: casting light on sleep deficiency. Nature, 497, p. S13.

DHS, (2017). Absence management & wellbeing: Survey results, s.l.: Direct Health Solutions.

DHSC, (2018). GOV.UK. [Online]. Available at: https://www.gov.uk/government/organisations/department-of-health-and-social-care

Diez Roux, A. V., (2001). Investigating neighborhood and area effects on health. American Journal of Public Health, 91(11), pp. 1783–1789.

Evans, G., (2014). Living in the city: Mixed use and quality of life. In: Wellbeing and the environment. Wellbeing: A complete reference guide, Volume II. s.l.:Wiley Blackwell, p. 702pp.

Fielding, S. et al., (2015). Estimating the burden of minor ailment consultations in general practices and emergency departments through retrospective review of routine data in North East Scotland. Family Practice, 32(2), pp. 165–172.

Folman, N. B. et al., (2006). Obesity, hospital services use and costs. Advances in Health Economics and Health Services Research, 17, pp. 319–332.

Francis, S., (2004). Making special places for health care. In: Designing better buildings: Quality and value in the built environment. Oxon: Taylor & Francis, p. 107.

Frank, L. D., Saelens, B. E., Powell, K. E. & Chapman, J. E., (2007). Stepping towards causation: do built environments or neighbourhood and travel preferences explain physical activity, driving, and obesity?. Social Science & Medicine, 65(9), pp. 1898–1914.

Frank, L. D. et al., (2005). Linking objectively measured physical activity with objectively measured urban form: Findings from SMARTRAQ. American Journal of Preventive Medicine, 28(2 suppl. 2), pp. 117–125.

French, S. A., Story, M. & Jeffrey, R. W., (2001). Environmental influences on eating and physical activity. Annual Review of Public Health, 22, pp. 309–335.

Freudenberg, N., (2000). Time for a national agenda to improve the health of urban populations. American Journal of Public Health, 90(6), pp. 837–840.

Galea, S., Freudenberg, N. & Vladhov, D., (2005). Cities and population health. Social Science & Medicine, 60(5), pp. 1017–1033.

Gates, B. & Gates, M., (2018). The ten toughest questions we get. [Online]. Available at: https://www.gatesnotes.com/2018-Annual-Letter

Glasson, J. & Therivel, R., (2013). Introduction to environmental impact assessment. Abingdon: Routledge.

Gordon-Larsen, P., Nelson, M. C., Page, P. & Popkin, B. M., (2006). Inequality in the built environment underlies key health disparities in physical activity and obesity. Pediatrics, 117, pp. 417–424.

GO-Science, (2007). Foresight. Tackling obesities: Future choices—obesity system atlas. London: Government Office for Science.

Green, S. M. & Gillet, A., (1998). Caring for patients with morbid obesity in hospital. British Journal of Nursing, 7(13), pp. 785–792.

Grist, N. R., (1979). Pandemic influenza 1918. British Medical Journal, 2(6205), p. 1632.

Hahler, B., (2002). Morbid obesity: A nursing care challenge. Medsurg Nursing, 11(2), p. 85.

Ham, C. et al., (2011). Where next for the NHS Reforms? The case for integrated care. London: The King's Fund.

Hignett, S., Carayon, P., Buckle, P. & Catchpole, K., (2013). State of science: human factors and ergonomics in healthcare. Ergonomics, 56(10), pp. 1491–1503.

Hignett, S. & Griffiths, P., (2009). Manual handling risks in the bariatric (obese) patient pathway in acute sector, community and ambulance care and treatment. Work, 33(2), pp. 175–180.

HSP (2009). Healthy spaces and places: A national guide to designing places for healthy living—An overview. Kingston: Planning Institute of Australia.

Humphries, R. & Curry, N., (2011). Integrating health and social care: Where next? London: The King's Fund.

Humphries, R. & Gregory, S., (2010). Place-based approaches and the NHS: Lessons from Total Places. London: The King's Fund.

James, W. P. T., Jackson-Leach, R. & Ni Mhurchu, C., (2004). Overweight and obesity (high body mass index). In: Comparative quantification of health risks: Global and regional burden of disease attributable to selected major risk factors. Geneva: WHO, pp. 497–596.

Jarrett, D., Stevenson, T., Huby, G. & Stewart, A., (2009). Developing and implementing research as a lever for integration: The impact of service context. Journal of Integrated Care, 17(5), pp. 38–48.

Johnson, S., (2006). The ghost map: The story of London's most terrifying epidemic—and how it changed science, cities, and the modern world. London: Penguin.

Keiser, J. et al., (2004). Urbanization in sub-saharan Africa and implication for malaria control. The American Journal of Tropical Medicine and Hygiene, 71(2_suppl), pp. 118–127.

Keogh, B., (2013). Transforming urgent and emergency care services in England. Leeds: DoH.

Kirk, S. F. L., Penney, T. L. & McHugh, T. F. L., (2010). Characterizing the obesogenic environment: The state of the evidence with directions for future research. Obesity Reviews, 11(2), pp. 109–117.

Learner, S., (2014). Growing number of care homes developing specialist bariatric rooms for obese people. [Online]. Available at: http://www.carehome.co.uk/news/article.cfm/id/1565071/ growing-number-care-homes-bariatric-rooms-obese

Lewis, R., Rosen, R. & Dixon, J., (2010). Where next for integrated care organisations in the English NHS? London: Nuffield Trust.

LGA, (2013). Social care and obesity: A discussion paper. London: Local Government Association.

LLSHAZ, (2002). A timely service: LSLSHAZ project on access to emergency hormonal contraception through accredited community pharmacies. London: Lamberth, Lewisham and South Health Action Zone.

Lupton, R. et al., (2009). Growing up in social housing in Britain: A profile of four generations, 1946 to the present day. London: Tenant Services Authority.

Marsh, A. T. M., Jahjab, N. A., Gleedb, F., Peacockc, O., Coley, D. & Codinhoto, R. (2020) Balancing supply and demand of non-exercise activity thermogenesis (NEAT) through building design. *Building Research & Information*. (In Print).

Martin, L. G., (1989). The graying of Japan. Population Bulletin, 44(2), pp. 1–42.

Martin-Hamblin GFK, (2002). Report of the osteoporosis pharmacy pilot study. London: Martin-Hamblin GFK.

McCallum, L. C., Ollson, C. A. & Stefanovic, I. L., (2018). An adaptable Health Impact Assessment (HIA) framework for assessing health within Environmental Assessment (EA): Canadian context, international application. Impact Assessment and Project Appraisal, 36(1), pp. 5–15.

Mear, C., (2008). The origin of the smallpox outbreak in Sydney in 1789. Journal of the Royal Australian Historical Society, 94(1), pp. 1–22.

Melosi, M. V., (2008). The sanitary city: Environmental services in urban America from colonial times to the present. Pittsburgh: University of Pittsburgh Press.

MHCLG, (2018). Environmental Impact Assessment. [Online]. Available at: https://www.gov.uk/guidance/environmental-impact-assessment#Preparing-an-Environmental-Statement1

Morgan, D. G. & Stewart, N. J., (1998a). High versus low density special care units: Impact on the behaviour of elderly residents with dementia. Canadian Journal on Ageing, 17(2), pp. 143–165.

Morgan, D. G. & Stewart, N. J., (1998b). Multiple occupancy versus private rooms on dementia care units. Environment and Behavior, 30(4), pp. 487–503.

Mullington, J. M. et al., (2009). Cardiovascular, inflammatory, and metabolic consequences of sleep deprivation. Progress in Cardiovascular Diseases, 51(4), pp. 294–302.

Nicol, S., Roys, M. & Garret, H., (2015). *The cost of poor housing to the NHS: BRE Briefing Paper.* Watford: Building Research Establishment.

OECD, (2018a). Young population. [Online]. Available at: https://data.oecd.org/pop/young-population.htm#indicator-chart

OECD, (2018b). Elderly population. [Online]. Available at: https://data.oecd.org/pop/elderly-population.htm

Okamoto-Mizuno, K. et al., (1999). Effects of humid heat exposure on human sleep stages and body temperature. Sleep, 22(6), pp. 767–773.

Omran, A. R., (2005). The epidemiologic transition: a theory of the epidemiology of population change. The Milbank Quartely, 83(4), pp. 731–757.

ONS, (2016). 2011 Census aggregate data. s.l.: Office fo National Statistics; National Records for Scotland; and Nothern Ireland Statistics and Research Agency.

Paudyal, V. et al., (2013). Are pharmacy-based Minor Ailment Schemes a substitute for other service providers? A systematic review. British Journal of General Practice, 63(612), pp. 359–362.

Pearl, J., (2013). Are some pharmacies failing? London: WHICH.

Pedersen, D. M., (1999). Model for types of privacy by privacy functions. Journal of Environmental Psycology, 19(4), pp. 397–405.

Pine II, J. B., (1993). Mass customization: The new frontier in business competition. Boston: Harvard Business School Press.

Powel, R. I. & Copping, A. G., (2016). Measuring fatigue-related impairment in the workplace. Journal of Engineering, Design and Technology, 14(3), pp. 507–525.

Powell, J. H., (1993). Bring out your dead: the great plague of yellow fever in Philadelphia in 1793. Philadelphia: University of Pennsylvania Press.

PPS, (2016). The case for healthy places: Improving health outcomes through placemaking. New York: Project for Public Places.

Pruitt, S. et al., (2002). Innovative care for chronic conditions. Geneva: World Health Organisation.

Ramsay, A., Fulop, N. & Edwards, (2009). The evidence base for integrated care. London: Department of Health.

Rangaraj, V. R. & Knutson, K. L., (2016). Association between sleep deficiency and cardiometabolic disease: implications for health disparities. Sleep Medicine, 18, pp. 18–35.

Roser, M., (2018). Life Expectancy. [Online]. Available at: https://ourworldindata.org/life-expectancy

RPSGB, (2003). Better management of minor ailments: using the pharmacist. London: RPSGB.

Rumbold, B. & Shaw, S. E., (2010). Horizontal and vertical integration in the UK: Lessons from history. Journal of Integrated Care, 18(6), pp. 45–52.

Sallis, J. F. & Glanz, K., (2009). Physical activity and food environments: Solutions to the obesity epidemic. The Milbank Quarterly, 87, pp. 123–154.

Salway, P. & Dell, W., (1955). Plague at Athens. Greece & Rome, 2(2), pp. 62–69.

Shaw, S., Rosen, R. & Rumbold, B., (2011). What is integrated care? London: Nuffield Trust.

Sulaiman, N., (2012). Opportunities for the transfer of UK best practices for the provision of residential care homes for the elderly in Malaysia to meet emerging and changing social needs. s.l.:The University of Salford.

Sulaiman, N., Baldry, D. & Ruddock, L., (2006a). Issues concerning housing for the elderly in Malaysia. Delft: Delft University of Technology.

Sulaiman, N., Baldry, D. & Ruddock, L., (2006b). Relationship between housing and social policy in Malaysia. Provision to the Elderly. Weimar: Bauhaus Universitat.

Suter, E., Scott, C. & Smith, L., (2009). All together now: A conceptual exploration of integrated care. Health Quartely, 12(Special Issue), pp. 6–15.

Swinburn, B. & Egger, G., (2002). Preventive strategies against weight gain and obesity. Obesity Reviews, 3, pp. 289–301.

Swinburn, B., Egger, G. & Raza, F., (1999). Dissecting obesogenic environments: The development and application of a framework for identifying and prioritizing environmental interventions for obesity. Preventive Medicine, 29, pp. 563–570.

Todd, A. et al., (2014). The positive pharmacy care law: An area-level analysis of the relationship between community pharmacy distribution, urbanity and social deprivation in England. BMJ Open, 4(8), p. e005764.

Townshend, T. & Lake, A. A., (2009). Obesogenic urban form: Theory, policy and practice. Health & Place, 15, pp. 909–916.

Tsekleves, E. & Cooper, R., (2017). Emerging trends and the way forward in design in healthcare: an expert's perspective. The Design Journal, 20(sup1), pp. 2258–2272.

UN, (2014). World urbanization prospects: The 2014 revision, highlights (ST/ESA/SER.A/352), s.l.: United Nations.

UN, (2015). World population prospects: The 2015 revision, key findings and advance tables. New York: United Nations.

USDoL, (2017). Labor force statistics from the current population survey: Household data annual average: 47. Absences from work of employed full-time wage and salary workers by occupation and industry. [Online]. Available at: https://www.bls.gov/cps/cpsaat47.htm

Valentijn, P. P., Schepman, S. M., Opheij, W. & Bruijnzeels, M. A., (2013). Understanding integrated care: a comprehensive conceptual framework based on the integrative functions of primary care. International Journal of Integrated Care, 13(10), p. e010.

van Eikenhorst, L., Salema, N. E. & Anderson, C., (2017). A systematic review in select countries of the role of the pharmacist in consultations and sales of non-prescription medicines in community pharmacy. Research in Social and Administrative Pharmacy, 13(1), pp. 17–38.

Wang, X. S. et al., (2011). Shift work and chronic disease: the epidemiological evidence. Occupational Medicine, 61(2), pp. 78–89.

Watson, M. C. et al., (2014). Using the theory of planned behaviour to develop targets for interventions to enhance patient communication during pharmacy consultations for non-prescription medicines. International Journal of Pharmacy Practice, 22(6), pp. 386–396.

Watson, M. C. et al., (2015). A cohort study of influences, health outcomes and costs of patients' health-seeking behaviour for minor ailments from primary and emergency care settings. BMJ Open, 5(2), pp. 1–14.

WGBC, (2016). Health, Wellbeing & Productivity in Retail: The impact of green buildings on people and profit. London: World Green Buildings Council.

White, S. C., (2017). Relational wellbeing: re-centring the politics of happiness, policy and the self. Policy & Politics, 45(2), pp. 121–136.

WHO, (2000). Obesity: Preventing and managing the global epidemic. Geneva: World Health Organization.

WHO, (2009). Global Health Risks: Mortality and burden of disease attributable to selected major risks. Geeva: WHO Press.

WHO, (2012). Health indicators of sustainable cities in the context of Rio+20: Initial findings from a WHO expert consultation. Geneva: s.n.

WHO, (2016). Urban green spaces and health: a review of evidence. Copenhagen: World Health Organization.

WHO, (2018a). Health Impact Assessment (HIA): The determinants of health. [Online]. Available at: http://www.who.int/hia/evidence/doh/en/

Williams, P. & Sullivan, H., (2010). Despite all we know about collaborative working, why do we still get it wrong? Journal of Integrated Care, 18(4), pp. 4–15.

Wismar, M., Blau, J., Ernest, K. & Figueras, J., (2004). The effectiveness of health impact assessment. Eurohealth, 10(3–4), pp. 41–43.

Wismar, M., Blau, J., Ernst, K. & Figueras, J., (2007). The effectiveness of health impact assessment: Scope and limitations of supporting decision-making in Europe. s.l.:Wold Heath Organisation.

Xie, A. & Carayon, P., (2015). A systematic review of human factors and ergonomics (HFE)-based healthcare system redesign for quality of care and patient safety. Ergonomics, 58(1), pp. 33–49.

Yang, Z. & Hall, A. G., (2008). The financial burden of overweight and obesity among elderly Americans: The dynamics of weight, longevity, and health care cost. Health Service Research, 43(3), pp. 849–868.

Yetish, G. et al., (2015). Natural sleep and its seasonal variations in three pre-industrial societies. Current Biology, 25(21), pp. 2862–2868.

11

HEALTH, WELLBEING AND URBAN DESIGN

Christopher T. Boyko, Rachel Cooper, Claire Coulton and James D. Hale

Introduction

Both high density and high deprivation in urban neighbourhoods have been connected with decrements in wellbeing, health and walkability (see Boyko & Cooper, 2014, 2017; Dempsey et al., 2012; Dunstan et al., 2014; Lee & Talen, 2014). While the combination of density and deprivation together and their impact on wellbeing and walkability have been *discussed* in the literature (see Guite et al., 2006), not enough is known *empirically* about the extent to which both density and deprivation impact wellbeing and the walkability of neighbourhoods. In particular, do high-density, high-deprivation neighbourhoods hinder wellbeing among its residents and discourage walkability through its design?

This chapter aims to investigate such a claim by exploring the relevant literature across three themes: density and wellbeing; deprivation and wellbeing; and walkability and health. Next, a quantitative study is presented that empirically tests the claim in different wards within three UK cities. The chapter ends with a critical discussion about the practical and policy implications from the study for urban design and health.

Literature Review[1]

Density and Wellbeing

Much of the literature exploring the impact of density on wellbeing suggests that higher densities are correlated with reductions in wellbeing.[2] People living in high-density neighbourhoods tend to suffer from lower quality of life (Cramer et al., 2004), more psychological stress (Gómez-Jacinto & Hombrados-Mendieta, 2002), greater chronic mental fatigue (Kuo, 1992) and less social interaction (Dempsey et al., 2012) compared with those living in lower-density neighbourhoods. Some residents also experience a greater share of mental health issues, including psychiatric illness (Duvall & Booth, 1978; Paulus et al., 1978) and higher admission rates to hospitals for schizophrenia (Faris & Dunham, 1939).

A few studies have demonstrated that high densities may improve wellbeing. Specifically, high-density neighbourhoods, comprising high residential, transport, park, intersection and other densities, may enhance social capital among residents through strengthening social contacts and ties (Bernard, 1939; Halpern, 1995; Moore, 1986), and facilitate social interaction (Talen, 1999; Young & Wilmott, 1957) and co-operation (Halpern, 1995). Living in high-density neighbourhoods may also improve physical activity (Sallis et al., 2016), may reduce behavioural and emotional problems in children (Silburn et al., 2006) and enhance the overall wellbeing of older people living in sheltered, social or retirement housing (Lawton & Nahemow, 1979; Lawton et al., 1980).

Deprivation and Wellbeing

Similar to the above literature, living in highly deprived neighbourhoods almost uniformly has been associated with decreased wellbeing.[3] Research has shown significant associations between neighbourhoods with a high presence of physical neglect (e.g. litter, graffiti) and residents' inability to form adequate social ties (Ross & Jang, 2000; Sampson et al., 1997) or receive social support (Hill et al., 2013). Wood and Giles-Corti (2008) also found a link between highly deprived neighbourhoods and residents' lack of sense of community.

Furthermore, perceptions of deprivation are linked with wellbeing deficits and ill health. Adult residents who perceive their neighbourhood to be of low, overall quality may suffer from depression (Burdette et al., 2011; Ellaway et al., 2009) and substance abuse (Burdette et al., 2011). This association may depend on the kind of environmental deprivation, however: street-scale incivilities, including graffiti or litter, explain more of the relationship than do other factors, such as infrastructural issues (Ellaway et al., 2009).

Walkability and Wellbeing

The relationship between neighbourhoods that are walkable – or perceived to be walkable – and wellbeing (and health) is strong.[4] In particular, walkable neighbourhoods tend to foster higher levels of general physical activity (Foster et al., 2011; Kaczynski & Glover, 2012; Saelens et al., 2003), higher levels of walking for leisure and transport, and higher levels of walking among children (Martin & Wood, 2014) and older adults (Li et al., 2005). Furthermore, when homes in walkable neighbourhoods are close to non-residential destinations, inhabitants are less prone to overweight or obesity compared with those living in neighbourhoods where private vehicles are needed more for travel (Ewing et al., 2003; Frank et al., 2004; Saelens et al., 2003). Finally, in neighbourhoods where there exists a strong sense of community, residents may walk more (Lund, 2003; Wood et al., 2010). This may be due to people feeling safer about walking around in the day and night, perceiving one's neighbourhood to be interesting (Lund, 2002), seeing other people in the area and feeling as though the place promotes social interaction (Leyden, 2003; Lund, 2002).

Conversely, neighbourhoods that are less walkable may encourage poor physical health and wellbeing. Areas low in density, high in air pollution and containing traffic congestion contribute to physical inactivity, overweight and obesity among residents and greater risks of hypertension (Frank et al., 2003; Frumkin et al., 2004; Sallis et al., 2009). Moreover, neighbourhoods with poor-quality public open spaces, pavements or no pavements, and those with low street intersection densities, are associated with reduced walking behaviour among residents, particularly older people (Badland et al., 2010; Gilbert & Galea, 2014; Li et al., 2005; Mullen, 2003).

Overall, the above literatures provide correlational evidence that socio-spatial characteristics of the urban environment may impact the wellbeing of residents. While there is robust evidence to suggest that people in high-deprivation, low-walkability places experience worse wellbeing, the connection with high density in particular remains somewhat tenuous. Even within deprived areas, residents may experience wellbeing through strong, social infrastructures that may or may not be fostered through the design of buildings and spaces. Due to these potential discrepancies, it becomes important to empirically test whether the combination of high-density and high-deprivation neighbourhoods affect wellbeing and walkability.

Methodology

As part of the *Liveable Cities* project,[5] research was undertaken in three UK cities to understand how density and deprivation affect walkability (all at the ward scale) and wellbeing (at the individual scale). The three cities are: Birmingham, a large, multicultural city in the Midlands (1,073,045 inhabitants); Lancaster and Morecambe, a connected market town and seaside town in the North West (138,375 inhabitants); and Southampton, a port city in the South (236,900 inhabitants) (ONS, 2011).

Population density data from the 2011 Census and deprivation scores from the 2010 estimated Index of Multiple Deprivation were used to rank all wards in each city from low to high density and low to high deprivation. Wards were then chosen based on the best combination of lowest and highest density and deprivation, forming a four-ward matrix: low-density, low-deprivation ward (Lo-den, lo-dep); low-density, high-deprivation ward (Lo-den, hi-dep); high-density, low-deprivation ward (Hi-den, lo-dep); and high-density, high-deprivation ward (Hi-den, hi-dep).

Participants

Research participants, all of whom were over 18 years old and lived within one of the 12 wards, were recruited using different methods. In Birmingham (N = 58), Ward Support Officers were asked to help suggest residents who would be willing to complete the wellbeing questionnaire. Residents were also recruited in specific locations, including a school fair or local library. In Lancaster (N = 104), questionnaires were hand-posted to dwellings. Finally, in Southampton (N = 117), the local authority provided 800 home addresses to which questionnaires were posted. In addition, an online version of the questionnaire was made available.

Wellbeing Questionnaire

The questionnaire helped to understand residents' perceptions of their wellbeing and the ward and city where they lived. Residents of each of the 12 wards received the 23-item questionnaire between 2013 and 2015 (see Boyko et al., 2015, for more details about the questionnaire). Questions were divided into five categories: (1) Your local neighbourhood; (2) Safety; (3) Your health and wellbeing; (4) Your environment and daily life and (5) Travel and public transport. A final question asked participants to write down their postcode, which would be used for the walkability audit. The questionnaire took between five and ten minutes to complete.

Walkability Audit

The audit helped understand the walkability of the wards where participants lived. An app-based version of the Irvine-Minnesota Inventory called State of Place (SoP) was utilised,[6] consisting of approximately 280 subjective and objective, closed-end questions that examine the built environment at the road segment scale.[7] The data from the questions were aggregated to create an overall SoP Index score; questions could be further sub-divided into ten urban design categories: form, density, proximity, connectivity, parks and public spaces, pedestrian amenities, personal safety, traffic safety, aesthetics and recreational facilities. For this study, road segments were aggregated to provide a ward-scale State of Place Index score.

Participants' postcodes were converted to an XY Ordnance Survey grid reference and displayed as points on a GIS map. Circular buffers of 300 m were generated around each point to indicate each individual's local spatial context. The 300 m buffer is viewed as one of the principal standards for the minimum distance that people should live from accessible, natural greenspace (see English Nature, 2003), and has been applied to other analyses (e.g. Barbosa et al., 2007). Once buffers were generated, a selection of road segments within the buffers was chosen for the audit.

Within each ward, 2,600 m of road segments were audited, representing approximately 10% of the total road length per ward. Segments of different road types were selected, so that their total lengths were proportional to the road composition of each ward.[8] In total, 484 road segments were audited (approximately 40 per ward) using the State of Place app. Each audit began at the junction of a selected road segment and the intersecting road, and ended at the next junction, taking between 10 and 30 minutes per road segment, depending on the complexity of the segment (e.g. many mixed-use buildings).

Results

Wellbeing Questionnaire

MANOVA uncovered a statistically significant difference in wellbeing based on ward type across the three cities, F (69, 619) = 2.305, $p < 0.0005$; Wilk's $\Lambda = 0.505$, partial $\eta^2 = 0.204$ (see Table 11.1).
Post-hoc analyses using Tukey's tests revealed further nuance:

Low-density, low-deprivation wards. People living here:

- Were more satisfied with the beauty or physical setting of their neighbourhood compared with people living in Hi-den, hi-dep and Lo-den, hi-dep wards;
- Felt they had better access to parks and play areas in their neighbourhoods compared with people living in Lo-den, hi-dep wards;
- Felt safer when walking around during the day and at night compared with people living in Hi-den, hi-dep and Lo-den, hi-dep wards;
- Felt safer when their children were playing outside compared with people living in Hi-den, hi-dep and Lo-den, hi-dep wards;
- Were less anxious compared with people living in Lo-den, hi-dep wards;
- Had more pride in their city compared with people living in Hi-den, hi-dep and Lo-den, hi-dep wards.

High-density, low-deprivation wards. People living in here:

- Were more satisfied with the beauty or physical setting of their neighbourhood compared with people living in Lo-den, hi-dep wards;
- Felt that they lived closer to green and blue spaces compared with people living in Lo-den, hi-dep wards;
- Had more face-to-face conversations with close relatives or friends compared with people living in Hi-den, hi-dep wards.

Low-density, low-deprivation and high-density, low-deprivation wards. People living in here:

- Felt more satisfied with their lives 12 months ago compared with people living in Lo-den, hi-dep wards.

TABLE 11.1 Wellbeing questionnaire significant results based on ward type (N = 233)

Question	*Mean scores*				
	Lo-den Lo-dep (N= 85)	*Lo-den Hi-dep (N= 32)*	*Hi-den Lo-dep (N= 70)*	*Hi-den Hi-dep (N=46)*	*Significance*
1 In the neighbourhood where you live, are you satisfied or dissatisfied with the beauty or physical setting?	2.20	3.00	2.46	2.93	$p < .0005$
2 Do you live within a 5-minute walk of a natural "blue space" or "green space"?	1.12	1.28	1.01	1.13	$p = .001$
3 What do you think of the parks and play areas in your neighbourhood in terms of quality?	2.12	3.34	2.14	2.61	$p < .0005$
4 What do you think of the parks and play areas in your neighbourhood in terms of access?	1.91	2.63	1.97	2.13	$p = .006$
5 How safe do you feel walking alone in your neighbourhood at night?	3.83	2.59	3.40	2.93	$p < .0005$
6 How safe do you feel walking alone in your neighbourhood during the day?	4.59	3.75	4.51	3.98	$p < .0005$
7 My neighbourhood is safe for children to play outside.	3.52	2.84	2.94	2.87	$p = .001$
8 Overall, how anxious did you feel yesterday?	2.05	2.69	2.30	2.54	$p = .009$
9 Overall, how satisfied were you with your life 12 months ago?	3.66	2.94	3.51	3.30	$p = .008$
10 I feel a sense of pride in the way my city looks and feels.	3.35	2.63	3.10	2.67	$p < .0005$
11 Roughly how often do you have a face-to-face conversation with a close friend, relative or someone else close to you about how you're feeling or just to catch up?	3.46	3.81	3.91	2.78	$p = .022$

Low-density, low-deprivation; high-density, low-deprivation and high-density, high-deprivation wards. People living here:

- Felt the parks and play areas in their neighbourhoods were of better quality compared with people living in Lo-den, hi-dep wards.

Walkability Audit

Table 11.2 reveals the outcome of the walkability audit across the four ward types. High percentages in the ten urban design categories suggest that a ward type has performed well on the component parts of walkability, and a high percentage on the SoP Index suggests that a ward type has performed well as a composite of walkability.

Across the three cities, the Hi-den, lo-dep wards had the best SoP Index percentage (56.5%), followed by Hi-den, Hi-dep (55.6%); Lo-den, low-dep (53.6%); and Lo-den, Hi-dep wards (47.1%). Additional findings, divided into the ten urban design categories by ward type, include:

- Lo-den, lo-dep wards were perceived to have the best personal safety and were perceived to be the most aesthetically pleasing;
- Lo-den, hi-dep wards had the best connectivity to other places and had the most parks and public spaces;
- Hi-den, lo-dep wards had the best urban form and pedestrian amenities;
- Hi-den, hi-dep wards had the best densities, best proximity to a mix of uses, were perceived to be the safest from a traffic perspective and had the most public and private recreational facilities.

TABLE 11.2 Walkability audit percentages by aggregated ward

Categories / *Wards*	*Lo-den, lo-dep (%)*	*Lo-den, hi-dep (%)*	*Hi-den, lo-dep (%)*	*Hi-den, hi-dep (%)*
Form	69.7	66.1	75.4	72.9
Density	60.2	65.1	71.1	74.9
Proximity	5.1	4.8	10.2	16.8
Connectivity	89.7	92.1	89.1	91.5
Parks and public spaces	25.8	33.8	21.9	25.2
Pedestrian amenities	36.2	42.6	47.8	45.5
Personal safety	91.1	80.5	84.1	72.5
Traffic safety	33.2	32.8	40.0	45.2
Aesthetics	78.0	57.8	68.6	62.8
Recreational facilities	0.0	0.0	1.8	5.6
State of place index	**53.6**	**47.1**	**56.5**	**55.6**

Source: Authors.

Discussion

This chapter began by asking whether living in high-density, high-deprivation neighbourhoods were bad for residents' wellbeing and for walkability. The results suggest a different story: although there was only one significant finding for this ward type from the wellbeing questionnaire, it managed to achieve the second best score from the walkability audit. In particular, this ward type had the highest densities conducive to walking, the closest proximity to amenities and services, the best sense of traffic safety and the most recreational facilities. While these results do not indicate that high-density, high-deprivation neighbourhoods are great places to live, they begin to dispel ideas that residents living here receive little health and wellbeing benefits.

Examining the remaining ward types, additional patterns emerged. Residents living in low-density, low-deprivation wards exhibited the highest wellbeing scores, perceived their neighbourhoods to be aesthetically pleasing, accessible and safe, had the most pride in their city and felt the least anxiety and most satisfaction with their past lives. This might be expected, as people who are better off tend to have better access to resources, and more control over their lives (Beaverstock et al., 2004). In terms of walkability, these wards were shown to be less walkable than the two high-density wards. One reason for the lower walkability score may be due to the predominantly residential land use and the lack of local amenities and services in the area. Given that high-walkability neighbourhoods are perceived to encompass characteristics such as higher density, street connectivity and land use mix (Saelens et al., 2003), the finding makes sense. Furthermore, while this ward type scored relatively low on the amount of parks and public spaces category, anecdotally, the areas were plentiful with *private* greenspaces.

Another pattern was that the high-density, low-deprivation ward type and the residents inhabiting these areas performed best in terms of the combined wellbeing and walkability results. Residents living in this ward type perceived their area to be more beautiful, closer to green and blue spaces and were closer to better-quality greenspaces. Residents also believed they had more face-to-face conversations and felt more satisfied with their past lives. In terms of walkability, this ward type had the highest SoP Index percentage alongside the best form and pedestrian amenities. These findings confirm that high-density neighbourhoods with a good mix of amenities and uses have the capacity to be both walkable and beneficial for health and wellbeing (Halpern, 1995; Leyden, 2003; Southworth, 2005; Talen, 1999; Vine et al., 2012).

Finally, the poorest performing ward type was the low-density, high-deprivation ward. There were no significant results implying that residents living here were better off with respect to wellbeing compared with others. Likewise, the low-density, high-deprivation ward type had the lowest SoP Index score, only rating highly on connectivity to other areas and amount of parks and public spaces. While this latter finding corroborates other research (i.e. those with greatest access to greenspace appear to be those most in need, Barbosa et al.,

2007), the overall results suggest that the combination of low densities and high deprivation in neighbourhoods is not working for inhabitants.

Limitations

The above results need to be considered in light of three limitations, related to our sample for the wellbeing questionnaire:

- Small sample size: 233 participants may not represent the population living in our ward types within these cities;
- Uneven sample size: the four ward types were quite different in sample size, which could lead to confounding of the data (Martin & Bridgmon, 2012);
- Sampling strategy: the different recruitment methods used for each city make it unclear if results could be generalised to other people and places.

Conclusions

Despite these limitations, there are two important considerations from this research that are applicable for the design of future cities. First, the research has highlighted that high-density, high-deprivation neighbourhoods need not be associated with poor wellbeing and walkability. Rather, they possess walkable characteristics that architects, urban designers and planners should exploit, enhance and possibly transfer to other ward types.

Second, concentrated efforts are needed to understand the social, environmental and economic value of increasing the walkability of lower-density, more-deprived neighbourhoods through a variety of means. Co-designing and co-managing public spaces should be considered, particularly given the amount of greenspaces and parks found in lower-density, more-deprived neighbourhoods. This should be done with local people to improve the location, availability, access and quality of public and greenspaces (Colding & Barthel, 2013; Franz et al., 2008), which have been linked to enhancements in wellbeing.

Both of these considerations point to the idea that there is a definite relationship between wellbeing, walkability, density and deprivation within neighbourhoods. While some of these relationships are stronger than others, there likely are many more intervening variables that play a moderating or mediating role. Additionally, such research needs to be translated into interventions and tested *in situ* with stakeholders who would most benefit from these interventions. Doing so is a positive step in designing future cities for wellbeing.

Notes

1 Much of the literature in this section may be found in Boyko and Cooper (2014).
2 Density can be defined spatially as the number of units in a given area (e.g. number of dwellings per hectare, Boyko & Cooper, 2011). Wellbeing may be defined as "a dynamic state in which the individuals is able to develop their potential, work

productively and creatively, built strong and positive relationships with others, and contribute to their community" (Government Office for Science, 2011, p. 10).

3 Deprivation concerns deficits in income; employment; and education, skills and training; poor health and disability; presence of crime; barriers to housing and services; and problems with one's living environment (ONS, 2015).
4 Walkability refers to the capacity of an area to be suitable for pedestrians (Lee & Talen, 2014; see also Southworth, 2005).
5 Information about the project may be found here: www.liveablecities.org.uk
6 The Irvine-Minnesota Inventory questions have been psychometrically tested for inter-rater reliability (Boarnet et al., 2006; Day et al., 2006). For more information about State of Place, please see www.stateofplace.co
7 Road segments refer to a portion of a total road between junctions.
8 A roads and B roads are public roads that connect areas of regional and local importance, respectively; minor roads are public roads that connect to A or B roads and may be unclassified; local streets are public roads that provide access to land and/or dwellings with limited through-traffic (DfT, 2012).

References

Badland, H. M., Kearn, R., Witten, K., & Kearns, R. (2010). Examining public open spaces by neighbourhood-level walkability and deprivation. *Journal of Physical Activity and Health, 7* (6), p.818–824.

Barbosa, O., Tratalos, J. A., Armsworth, P. R., Davies, R. G., Fuller, R. A., Johnson, P., & Gaston, K. J. (2007). Who benefits from access to green space? A case study from Sheffield, UK. *Landscape and Urban Planning, 83* (2–3), p.187–195.

Beaverstock, J. L., Hubbard, P., & Short, J. R. (2004). Getting away with it? Exposing the geographies of the super-rich. *Geoforum, 35* (4), p.401–407.

Bernard, J. (1939). The neighborhood behavior of school children in relation to age and socioeconomic status. *American Sociological Review, 4* (5), p.652–662.

Boarnet, M., Day, K., Alfonzo, M., Forsyth, A., & Oakes, J. M. (2006). The Irvine-Minnesota Inventory to measure built environments: Reliability tests. *American Journal of Preventive Medicine, 30* (2), p.153–159.

Boyko, C. T., & Cooper, R. (2014). Density and mental wellbeing. In E. Burton & R. Davies-Cooper (Vol. Eds.), *Wellbeing: A complete reference guide: Wellbeing and the environment* (pp. 69–90). London: Wiley-Blackwell.

Boyko, C. T., & Cooper, R. (2017). Wellbeing in neighbourhoods: Current research and future practice. In C. L. Cooper & J. C. Quick (Eds.), *The handbook of stress and health* (pp. 555–569). London: John Wiley & Sons.

Boyko, C. T., Cooper, R., & Cooper, C. (2015). Measures to assess wellbeing in low-carbon-dioxide cities. *Urban Design and Planning, 168* (4), p.185–195.

Burdette, A. M., Hill, T. D., & Hale, L. (2011). Household disrepair and the mental health of low-income urban women. *Journal of Urban Health, 88* (1), p.142–153.

Colding, J., & Barthel, S. (2013). The potential of 'urban green commons' in the resilience building of cities. *Ecological Economics, 86,* p.156–166.

Cramer, V., Torgersen, S., & Kringlen, E. (2004). Quality of life in a city: The effect of population density. *Social Indicators Research, 69* (1), p.103–116.

Day, K., Boarnet, M., Alfonzo, M., & Forsyth, A. (2006). The Irvine-Minnesota Inventory to measure built environments: Development. *American Journal of Preventive Medicine, 30* (2), p.144–152.

Dempsey, N., Brown, C., & Bramley, G. (2012). The key to sustainable urban development in UK cities? The influence of density on social sustainability. *Progress in Planning, 77,* p.89–141.

Department for Transport (DfT). (2012). *Guidance on road classification and the primary route network*. London: DfT.

Dunstan, F., Fone, D. L., Glickman, M., & Palmer, S. (2014). Objectively measured residential environment and self-reported health: A multilevel analysis of UK Census data. *PLOS ONE, 8* (7), e69045.

Duvall, D., & Booth, A. (1978). The housing environment and women's health. *Journal of Health and Social Behavior, 19* (4), p.410–417.

Ellaway, A., & Macintyre, S. (2009). Are perceived neighbourhood problems associated with the likelihood of smoking? *Journal of Epidemiology and Community Health, 63* (1), p.78–80.

English Nature. (2003). *Providing accessible natural greenspace in towns and cities. A practical guide to assessing the resource and implementing local standards for provision*. Worcester: English Nature.

Ewing, R., Schmid, T., Killingsworth, R. E., Zlot, A., & Raudenbush, S. (2003). Relationship between urban sprawl and physical activity, obesity, and morbidity. *American Journal of Health Promotion, 18* (1), p.47–57.

Faris, R. E. L., & Dunham, H. W. (1939). *Mental disorders in urban areas: An ecological study of schizophrenia and other psychoses*. Chicago, IL: University Press.

Foster, S., Giles-Corti, B., & Knuiman, M. (2011). Creating safe walkable streetscapes: Does house design and upkeep discourage incivilities in suburban neighbourhoods. *Journal of Environmental Psychology, 31* (1), p.79–88.

Frank, L. D., Andresen, M. A., & Schmid, T. L. (2004). Obesity relationships with community design, physical activity, and time spent in cars. *American Journal of Preventive Medicine, 27* (2), p.87–96.

Frank, L. D., Engelke, P. O., & Schmid, T. L. (2003). *Health and community design: The impact of the built environment on physical activity*. Washington, DC: Island Press.

Franz, M., Gules, O., & Prey, G. (2008). Place-making and 'green' reuses of brownfields in the Ruhr. *Journal of Economic and Social Geography, 99* (3), p.316–328.

Frumkin, H., Frank, L., & Jackson, R. (2004). *Urban sprawl and public health: Designing, planning and building for healthy communities*. Washington, DC: Island Press.

Gilbert, E., & Galea, S. (2014). Urban neighborhoods and mental health across the life course. In E. Burton & R. Davies-Cooper (Eds.), *Wellbeing: A complete reference guide: Wellbeing and the environment* (pp. 23–50) Chichester: Wiley Blackwell.

Gómez-Jacinto, L., & Hombrados-Mendieta, I. (2002). Multiple effects of community and household crowding. *Journal of Environmental Psychology, 22* (3), p.233–246.

Government Office for Science (2008). *Mental capital and wellbeing: Making the most of ourselves in the 21st century*. London: Government Office for Science.

Guite, H. F., Clark, C., & Ackrill, G. (2006). The impact of the physical and urban environment on mental wellbeing. *Public Health, 120* (12), p.1117–1126.

Halpern, D. (1995). *Mental health and the environment: More than bricks and mortar?* Oxford: Taylor & Francis.

Hill, T. D., Burdette, A. M., Jokinen-Gordon, H. M., & Brailsford, J. M. (2013). Neighborhood disorder, social support, and self-esteem: Evidence from a sample of low-income women living in three cities. *Cities and Community, 12* (4), p.380–395.

Kaczynski, A., & Glover, T. (2012). Talking the talk, walking the walk: Examining the effect of neighbourhood walkability and social connectedness on physical activity. *Journal of Public Health, 34* (3), p.382–389.

Kuo, F. E. (1992). Inner cities and chronic mental fatigue. In E. Arias & M. Gross (Eds.), *EDRA 23/1992: Equitable and sustainable habitats*. Paper presented at the environmental design research association. Boulder, CO: EDRA.

Lawton, M. P., & Nahemow, L. (1979). Social areas and the wellbeing of tenants in housing for the elderly. *Multivariate Behavioral Research, 14* (4), p.463–484.

Lawton, M. P., Nahemow, L., & Yeh, T.-M. (1980). Neighborhood environment and the wellbeing of older tenants in planned housing. *International Journal of Aging and Human Development, 11* (3), p.221–227.

Lee, S., & Talen, E. (2014). Measuring walkability: A note on auditing methods. *Journal of Urban Design, 19* (3), p.368–388.

Leyden, K. M. (2003). Social capital and the built environment: The importance of walkable neighborhoods. *American Journal of Public Health, 93* (9), p.1546–1551.

Li, F., Fisher, K. J., Brownson, R., & Bosworth, M. (2005). Multilevel modelling of built environment characteristics related to neighbourhood walking activity in older adults. *Journal of Epidemiology and Public Health, 59* (7), p.558–564.

Lund, H. (2002). Pedestrian environments and sense of community. *Journal of Planning Education and Research, 21* (3), p.301–312.

Lund, H. (2003). Testing the claims of New Urbanism: Local access, pedestrian travel, and neighboring behaviors. *Journal of the American Planning Association, 69* (4), p.414–429.

Martin, K. E., & Wood, L. J. (2014). "We live here too"...What makes a child-friendly neighborhood? In E. Burton & R. Davies-Cooper (Eds.), *Wellbeing: A complete reference guide: Wellbeing and the environment* (pp. 147–184). Chichester: Wiley Blackwell.

Martin, W. E., & Bridgmon, K. D. (2012). *Quantitative and statistical research methods: From hypothesis to results*. San Francisco, CA: Jossey-Bass.

Moore, R. C. (1986). *Childhood's domain: Play and place in child development*. London: Croon Helm.

Mullen, E. (2003). Do you think that your local area is a good place for young people to grow up? The effects of traffic and car parking on young people's views. *Health and Place, 9* (4). p.351–360.

Office of National Statistics (ONS). (2011). *2011 Census: Population and household estimates fact file, unrounded estimates, local authorities in England and Wales (Excel spreadsheet)*. London: ONS.

Office of National Statistics (ONS). (2015). *Measuring what matters. National statistician's reflections on the national debate on measuring national wellbeing*. London: ONS.

Paulus, P. B., McCain, G., & Cox, V. C. (1978). Death rates, psychiatric commitments, blood pressure and perceived crowding as a function of institutional crowding. *Environmental Psychology and Nonverbal Behavior, 3*, p.107–116.

Ross, C. E., & Jang, S. J. (2000). Neighborhood disorder, fear, and mistrust: The buffering role of social ties and neighbors. *American Journal of Community Psychology, 28* (4), p.401–420.

Saelens, B. E., Sallis, J. F., Black, J. B., & Chen, D. (2003). Neighborhood-based differences in physical activity: An environment scale evaluation. *American Journal of Public Health, 93* (9), p.1552–1558.

Sallis, J. F., Cerin, E., Conway, T. L., Adams, M. A., Frank, L. D. et al. (2016). Physical activity in relation to urban environments in 14 cities worldwide: A cross-sectional study. *The Lancet, 387*, p.2207–2217.

Sallis, J. F., Saelens, B. E., Frank, L. D., Conway, T. L., Slymen, D. J. et al. (2009). Neighborhood built environment and income: Examining multiple health outcomes. *Social Science and Medicine, 68* (7), p.1285–1293.

Sampson, R. J., Raudenbush, S. W., & Earls, F. (1997). Neighborhoods and violent crime: A multilevel study of collective efficacy. *Science, 277* (5328), p.918–924.

Silburn, S. R., Zubrick, S. R., De Maio, J. A., Shepherd, C., Griffin, J. A. et al. (2006). *The Western Australian aboriginal child health survey: Strengthening the capacity of aboriginal children, families and communities.* Perth: Curtin University of Technology and Telethon Institute for Child Health Research.

Southworth, M. (2005). Designing the walkable city. *Journal of Urban Planning and Development, 131* (4), p.246–257.

Talen, E. (1999). Sense of community and neighborhood form: An assessment of the social doctrine of New Urbanism. *Urban Studies, 36* (8), p.1361–1379.

Vine, D., Buys, L., & Aird, R. (2012). Experiences of neighbourhood walkability among older Australians living in high density inner-city areas. *Planning Theory and Practice, 1* (3), p.421–444.

Wilson, N., Syme, S. L., Boyce, W. T., Battistitch, V. A., & Selvin, S. (2005). Adolescent alcohol, tobacco, and marijuana use: The influence of neighborhood disorder and hope. *American Journal of Health Promotion, 20* (1), p.11–19.

Wood, L., Frank, L., & Giles-Corti, B. (2010). Sense of community and its relationship with walking and neighborhood design. *Social Science and Medicine, 70* (9), p.1381–1390.

Wood, L., & Giles-Corti, B. (2008). Is there a place for social capital in the psychology of health and place? *Journal of Environmental Psychology, 28* (2), p.154–163.

Wood, L., Giles-Corti, B., & Bulsara, M. (2012). Streets apart: Does social capital vary with neighbourhood design? *Urban Studies Research, 2012,* p.1–11.

Wood, L., Giles-Corti, B., Zubrick, S., & Bulsara, M. (2011). "Through the kids…we connected with our community": Children as catalysts of social capital. *Environment and Behaviour, 45* (3), p.344–368.

Young, M., & Willmott, P. (1957). *Family and kinship in East London.* London: Routledge and Kegan Paul.

12

MAKING SPACE FOR CULTURE AND WELLBEING IN THE CITY

Andy C. Pratt

Introduction

The focus of this chapter is an exploration of the conditions that favour or undermine culture and wellbeing in the city. Like other chapters in this collection, I take a particular interpretation of wellbeing. I resist the dominant individualistic and subjectivist approaches to happiness and wellbeing (Frey, 2008), or liveability and wellbeing (Morrison, 2007; Okulicz-Kozaryn, 2013). Instead, I am concerned with the framing of the possibilities for wellbeing. These framing processes are constituted through the design, planning and governance of the City. Simply, the interpretation of wellbeing discussed in this chapter has two dimensions of inclusion: within a diverse culture (that is reflective of a host society); and, within a fair society (economic, social and political).[1]

A well-documented phenomenon of our societies, in particular our biggest cities, is inequality of income and opportunity; moreover, it is getting worse (Castells, 1996; Mollenkopf & Castells, 1991; Sassen, 2001). The normal processes of growth and development of our cities (which now account for more than half the world's population) have clearly gone wrong. Instead of cities being the highest achievement of humanity, they too often are the bearers of immiseration and produce the very opposite of wellbeing.

It is not only social and economic inequality, but environmental problems as well that the contemporary city generates. Striving for sustainable cities whilst carrying on 'business as usual', but with superficial changes like low-pollution vehicles, is short term and ineffective (Urban Task Force, 1999). More radical approaches have advocated a reverse of urbanisation, smaller cities which would, their advocates argue, be less damaging to the planet, and better for our way of life (Rogers, 2008). Size and scale are hoped for coordination aids; other commentators have pointed out the need to begin by addressing the coordination of cities (Jarvis et al., 2001; Pratt, 1996).

This chapter brings together the challenges of urbanisation and those of inequality. Whilst Wilkinson and Picket (2010), Albor et al. (2014), Dorling (2012) and others have pointed out the health dis-benefits of inequality and cities, the argument has not been extended previously to include fully a more general notion of wellbeing associated with culture.

The chapter takes as its focus the UK, by examining the last 100 years or so, in a long sweep of the co-development of cities and culture to discern both the drivers of change, and the tensions that open up between them. It uses this as a perspective from which to evaluate the current and future challenges to cities in relation to culture. The chapter is not concerned with the detail of policy and actions, but of the understanding the nature of the problems that we face, and where we need to focus our efforts to mitigate them.

Accordingly, the way in which the planning and governance of culture can lead to wellbeing is not a 'smart bullet' fix, but one that is complex and multifaceted: an ecosystem rather than a linear, mono-causal process(-es). Any analysis of urban change must confront the dynamism and complexity of the processes involved; moreover the dynamics are also subject to recalibration. We are more familiar with accounting for changes in technology and by extension economic growth, and with shifts in governance between the public and private sectors, but less so with the 'dark horse' of culture.

I will show that culture has underdone dramatic changes as other fields; most notably developing from a form of moral improvement and idealism, to a transformative process of economy and society. Above and beyond the complexities and details of any individual component of the city: the built environment is the container, or the platform on/in which these processes play out. Each one of these components has their own dynamics; what I want to highlight in this chapter is the meshing of the processes that generate a city which affords a particular space for culture at any particular moment.

The built environment with its life span, and lagged building cycles,[2] is but one example of how the intersection (or meshing) of processes generates huge challenges even if individual systems are well governed. The theme of the chapter is to examine the 'space' open for culture in the city. I interpret this cultural space in two interrelated ways: the physical spaces afforded cultural activities, and the organisation space or opportunity given to culture. The lessons from this chapter are two-fold: that we need to develop a more robust understanding of the dynamics of culture; and, that positive wellbeing results from the development of transversal modes of governance, and negative results from siloed forms of governance (Tett, 2015). The chapter primarily views the cultural as interactive and relational: meanings and actions, positive and negative are only defined in situ. Such a perspective sets the chapter against more functionalist insights that often result in urban life being reduced to economic rationalities, or basic needs (culture is not usually recognised as being a basic need: incorrectly).[3]

Four Historical Snapshots

In this section I summarise the ways in which governance has framed, and used, wellbeing and culture in the context of the City in the UK in the last hundred or so years. Broadly, this helps us to see the cultural dimension of the city through the lens of a four-phase schema of the renewal of the built environment, each which acts first as an enabler and then becomes a constraint (in the form of an everyday condition that can generate ill-being). I provide snapshots highlighting the balance of economic, cultural and state forces and the resultant legacy of the Civic movement (from the turn of the twentieth century), the Modern age of post-war rebuilding in the 1960s, the Post-industrial destruction and reconstruction of the 1970s onward, and the Current Austerity period (2010–).[4]

Civic Spaces (Late nineteenth century-1945)

The period from the turn of the twentieth century until the Second World War in many senses provides a foundation for the built environment and its presumed usage today. However, most inner-city street patterns were established in mediaeval times, and supplemented by the establishment of large-scale manufacturing and warehousing activities, which led in turn to a remaking (diminishing) of the public realm.

Many UK city centres were reconstructed in the late Victorian period delivering a civic centre, that is, a group of buildings associated with government and the public support of the arts. Either adorned in a gothic, or neo-classical style, these buildings, and the public spaces that accompanied them in the form of squares and parks, reveal a set of assumptions about the role of the (local) state in a paternalistic advocacy of respect for a social order, and a right to leisure. A key part of this vision was culture, viewed by many thought leaders of the time as a 'civilising' force. The local municipalism that characterised this period also demanded a softening of the mercantilism of large manufacturers, who sought to legitimate and establish their position in the social order, by supporting galleries, museums and concert halls. The output of state broadcaster, the BBC, echoed this cultural order. The spirit of self-help was also evident in the community-organised groups of cultural and educational provision. In between was the private sector provision of music halls, working men's clubs and public houses.

The population decline in the post-First World War period, and recession, did not stress the urban model; when growth took off again it was in the form of suburbanisation. This growth bore the mark of the garden city movement (which was a private sector initiative), which had a rather puritanical ethic with respect to culture and entertainment, as exemplified by the lack of provision of pubs in many of these developments. The development of the suburbs was stimulated by economic growth and fed by links to the British Empire. Port cities were a case in point; many key cultural institutions were initiated based on the profits of such trade, the traces can still be found in the naming of major buildings.

The Second World War, with the extensive urban bombing, inevitably changed cities, potentially creating an opportunity for a recalibration; however, as we will see, rebuilding took place for the most in the pattern of the old.

Modernisation (1945–1975)

The mark of urbanisation in this period was modernisation. Large sections of the built fabric of cities had been damaged, and there were many attempts to rebuild modern facilities for a growing population, often in place of the old. Many cities were rebuilt entirely, and the state-initiated 'new towns' movement sought to counter the 'sprawl' of suburbanisation, facilitated by the increasing domination of the motor car. Cities increasingly were rebuilt with the motor car not just 'in mind', but as a first priority. The inevitable contradiction of most cities was the congestion of old street patterns, and consequentially a disincentive to their use for both shopping and entertainment.

The massive changes in the nature of the (nation) state and its functions in the post-war period was characterised by the establishment of a welfare state providing universal social support, and the Town and Country Planning Act, which sought to rationalise land use. The support of culture by the state was developed as a function that was funded like the welfare state, on the principle of addressing market failure in the provision of public goods. Culture is a problematic notion as a cultural good, not in principle, but in particular: what sort of culture should be supported? The paternalistic view was to support 'high culture'; continuing the legacy of the pre-war period, and leave the dramatic growth of popular culture to the market.

The shaping of the cultural landscape of cities followed these patterns. It was one that had obvious continuities with the Victorian foundations, and whilst the new build, and new towns, adopted different architectural styles, and had different ideas about the separation of traffic, the notion of the civic centre remained: public (high) cultural facilities. However, the growth of popular music and the increase of youth consumption of all products increasingly challenged the position of high culture. Furthermore, the development of nightclubs and alternative music venues challenged the cultural provision of cities. The social changes also gave rise to a crisis of the paternalistic cultural system to one that was more democratic; this was further leveraged by significant (urban) immigration that led to particular city centres becoming ethnically and culturally diverse, which was in many respects a significant provocation to the existing cultural social order. Youth cultural forms were seldom state-supported, but they began to mark inner-city cores as 'scenes', which created a new identity for some cities.

Finally, television played an increasing role in its impact on the cultural life of cities, providing an individualised form of entertainment (of course with limited channels, the product was collective, but the experience of consumption was in the home). One of the key aspects of the cultural built environment that saw a visible change was the cinema. Cinema had been a mass urban presence at the start of this period, but television made significant inroads to its audience, and inevitably cinemas, that were often iconic structures in cities, closed down, finding a limited life as bingo halls, or churches serving new immigrant communities, before being demolished.

The growth in personal disposable income, and consumption, drove retailing to expand and helped to modernise the city. The innovations of the interwar period meant the Department Store still represented the 'anchor' tenants of the city centre, but they were increasingly challenged by mass fashion retailers, and a range of retailers focussed on youth trends. Food retailing was transformed by the emergence of the supermarket. The problem with transportation was resolved (temporarily) by the establishment of, first, pedestrianised streets, and, then, enclosed shopping centres. Shopping centres had a significant impact of removing 'the street' from the public realm; indoor shopping centres were private spaces that did not grant the same rights of use and assembly as the old street.

De-industrialisation (1975–2010)

The mid-1970s was a period of traumatic economic and social change in the UK, with labour unrest-, inflation- and recession-marked cities in terms of much physical dereliction of the building stock. Most cities had been built on a manufacturing base that provided employment and growth. De-industrialisation (from closure, or relocation abroad) was obviously significant in job losses and unemployment, but it marked the built environment by leaving a huge amount of vacant buildings for which there was seldom an alternative use. Moreover, many of these buildings constituted substantial parts of the urban built environment. The closure of massive sites, such as dockyards, and regions, such as coalfields, had an impact that went beyond job losses.

At the same time the logic of government began to shift towards a distrust of the state and public funding, in favour of private enterprise, and de-regulation. Accordingly, rebuilding was weakly planned, and had to await an upturn in the market (instead of the state engaging in regeneration to kick-start growth). Although the state continued to take the risk of remediating 'brown-field sites', the developments were usually private initiatives. As such, the provision of public spaces, and public goods, that is the everyday cultural environment, was seldom supported (as it did not make money). Cash-strapped local authorities tried, mostly unsuccessfully, to pick up the slack.

Aside from a number of key exceptions, private developers were less keen to deal with the challenges of brown field development, and preferred to build on green field sites. The logic of transportation planning (that favoured the car), and mostly unregulated sprawl and suburbanisation, created an obvious logic in favour of the 'out of town' retail centre. First, it was individual mega stores (based on food or DIY), then whole shopping centres moved out of town. On the one hand, this ripped the retail core out of cities; on the other hand, it created somewhat soulless shopping centres that were dead (and closed) when the shops closed, offering little, if any, cultural sustenance, and generally required a car to access them. An early addition to the new shopping centres (and further loss of the city) was the cinema multiplex (enabled by digital distribution of film).

As a consequence, the inner city became a neglected and declining space; often, the only remaining markers were the Department Stores (that were now out of fashion), and convenience stores. Once a mainstay of urban culture, the public house became an endangered institution. People dependent on the city centre faced poorer choices, and more expensive purchases. The decaying property did create an opportunity for those seeking to make a career out of (new) culture-making commercial premises relatively cheap, and available for short lets. The growth of cultural production, which had been promoted by the economic wealth and the demographic changes of the 1960s, began to reach a critical mass, yielding jobs, income and cultural influence, by the turn of the twentieth century.

However, short-life accommodation and cheap rents soon ended. As regeneration schemes advanced, cities sought to remake themselves. One way was to provide office-based activities, which replaced many jobs, and put a little breath back into urban retail (at least in the day time). Another way was to encourage cities to 're-brand' and 'sell' themselves to attract mobile investors and jobs. A common pattern was to promote quality of life, particularly cultural life, of the city as an attractor for mobile firms, and their staff. Cities thus embarked on 'place management', and 'supporting the experience economy'. Bound up in this struggle to lure visitors and employees to a city were the reverberations of the Internet, and online shopping. If people were to continue to use cities, the experience had to offer something better than online. Aside from street animation, and experience retailing, cities also sought to develop new cultural institutions: galleries, museums and concert halls (often part funded by the lottery). Sadly, many were built as promotional tools, and they failed to attract visitors, or generate local support.

Austerity and Beyond (2010–)

An emblematic moment of austerity was when Newcastle City Council set a zero budget for culture in 2013. This was a signal of the dire straits of local government funding by central government, as well as how low culture is in our priorities (returning to Maslow). Ironically, cities are investing in policies for 'place making' whilst places are being 'un-made', or neglected. A less obvious impact of the decline in public funding for culture has been the social and physical infrastructure of culture. There is evidence of (cultural) building closures due to lack of funds and maintenance, and the increased practice of offering experienced staff fractional contracts, or replacing them altogether with volunteers (Pratt & Hutton, 2013).

Underlying Themes

Nothing is constant like change; in terms of cities and culture, this is equally true. However, what we can learn from our snapshots of roughly 30-year periods is that, as a society, we have changing ideas of what and how culture should be provided. Moreover, this provision cannot be isolated from more general shifts in economic cycles, and related technologies, as well as the shifting role of the state. An increasingly commercial dimension to culture has seen the state relatively, and absolutely, withdrawing from the field: whether in direct investment, or in terms of governance. The danger is that culture, so often imagined as the 'glue' that holds together a city, let alone generates its distinctiveness, is increasingly falling between the cracks of traditional policy silos (such as transport, economic development, housing, etc.).

Why does this matter? What has not been stressed in the review of the last century is that culture was initially seen as the right of everybody, and the state sought to ensure that (its choice of culture) was made available. Culture (albeit limited) had a place in the city, as symbolised by the built environment, and the everyday activities of its population. In the complex cycles of economic and technological changes, and of the waxing and waning of state control, culture has lost its guarantor. It is true that (consumer and experience) culture is now deployed, instrumentally, to animate cities. The wave of 'place making' strategies characteristic of the current period are well-meaning, but deal with symptoms not causes. First, the notion that 'places' can be re-made from the top-down by dictate or plan, or by a marketing team, is contradictory as it will most likely alienate those who are already embedded and have their own 'sense of place'. Second, such place making is like trying to lock the stable door after the horse has gone: the long period of de-industrialisation the UK suffered has disinherited populations, and stripped them of a sustainable heritage; or, for some, the recent wave of gentrification has necessitated their relocation.

Cultural production, and cultural employment, commonly fails to find resonance with this view of the city. In fact, one of the dilemmas that has recently been recognised is that cultural producers can no longer afford to remain in the city. This gives us pause to take a close look at the space we allot to culture in our cities, and perhaps take on board a reconceptualisation of culture. Certainly, many of the debates about creative cities and the cultural economy have begun to raise these issues, namely that cultural production is more sustainable and resilient than cultural consumption. Moreover, it is the source of innovation and new ideas that can contribute to wider growth and change (Pratt, 2010, 2015). But, capping all of this, culture provides a means of re-forging and developing identity and community; something that we often hear is missing from our cities.

The dangers of adopting a superficial consumer experience of culture to underpin the city are several. First, it is prone to the theme park problem: it is always necessary to build a new ride to keep the visitors coming back each season. This is another way of saying that they are high maintenance. Second, that the audience, those who you attract to the city, are limited. If an adequate return on investment in cultural consumption is to be attained, then a focus on high net worth individuals makes sense. Tailoring the experience to 'cultural tourists', or to 'high spending shoppers', or, selling the image of a city to investors targets a small proportion of the population, and a narrow (and necessarily) conservative notion of culture. This can generate a somewhat ironic view of the 'creative/cultural' innovativeness of a city. Third, the consequences are that the cultural offer is for outsiders, and not residents (whose taxes may be paying for it). Far from bolstering a local cultural identity, locals may feel alienated from the cultural provision. This has led to some commentators asking the pertinent question: 'whose city, whose culture?' (Zukin, 1995).

One of the advantages of cities, like all 'off-line' activity, is that it is difficult to ignore 'difference'. In an online community you can easily be protected by an echo-chamber of your own views, and if challenged, you have the option to 'log off'. The city has always been the fora for dealing with diverse people, and viewpoints. Indeed, the very word, fora, has its roots in a tightly braided political-built environment structure. The governance of culture that makes it easy to exclude a proportion of the population has the potential to engineer the material world to resemble the online world.

This is the reason that we need to look closely at the particular cultures we are promoting, and those we are undermining, in our cities. A partial perspective, supporting an elite, may sound economically attractive, but socially and culturally (and therefore economically), it will be a disaster. We need to recognise that cultural as well as social diversity are a strength; they are one of the wellsprings of urban growth. Diversity of ideas, opinions and outlooks matched by an urban order (or governance) that supports and legitimates this range has been the hallmark of cities (whether they are called creative cities or not). Promotion of a diversity of ideas is inclusive of the whole population: it makes no sense to exclude, when the diversity is the resource that drives a successful city.

It is for these reasons that we need to interrogate our cultural policies for cities, and the notions of culture that we hold as a society, and the ways that they are governed. As noted above, there is a trend that has seen culture lose its 'place' in the city, and the spaces, both public spaces and policy spaces, have been neglected. We risk the danger of seeding division and stagnation, as well as a return to the utilitarianism that writers such as Charles Dickens reacted against in the first blush of industrialisation, which paid little heed to people, their cultures and wellbeing and the city.

What Have We Learnt?

The long view of the relationship between culture and wellbeing, and governance, sketched out in this chapter has trained our focus on the ways that cultural wellbeing has been conceived of, and the shifting mode and the imagined engagement of citizens with culture (consumption and production). This underlines the point that culture is as much about setting a frame of reference, or a way of being, rather than the delivery of a service.

With the benefit of the historical narrative, we can discern the changing patterns of the field of tensions within culture are located: between the state, economy and civil society. At various points in time we can see culture drawn closer, or pushed further, from particular elements. This is an important point: culture does not exist separately, outside of, or beyond, the city (and its internal tensions within and between civil society, economy and the state); rather, culture is practised and situated. Thus, interventions, policies and practices, are situated and cannot be simply mapped from one place or time to another.

Moreover, we can note that each of the components of the city have their own cycles that fail to mesh with the others. The most significant 'mis-match' is the built environment. Critically, the built environment as the platform, or stage, upon which action is played out, its good or ill-adaptation to the players and processes, has an enabling or constraining effect on any actions. The conventional core city functions and their associated planning activities quickly get out of sync, and need to be modified to bring them back closer to the intended arrangement. Transversal activities such as culture and wellbeing that cut across the matrix of other functions will fail to mesh. Furthermore, they will not be recognised as 'failing', as they are not the primary focus of policy.

This chapter has sought to recognise that the often-hidden or obscured, positive relationship between culture and wellbeing is contingent on situational change; consequentially, it points to the challenge that cities present if we seek to align culture and wellbeing and to reap the benefits: this chapter has highlighted three 'challenge complexes'.

The first challenge concerns culture itself. City authorities, citizens and economic actors have vied for control of the physical spaces of the city, and the organisational spaces (the organisational configurations to affect policy: marginal or dominating). The initial understanding, one that coincided with a particular hey-day of city planning, was that of the provision of open space and recreational activities: culture and relaxation from the labours of work; green 'lungs' for the city and its citizens. These spaces were conceived of as being balanced with economic and state land uses. For example, we can see the civic centre as a blending of 'public culture' and the state. Cultural organisation was perceived to assist in the delivery of a well-ordered city, and hence was not given an autonomous role.[5] However, in the contemporary period, these patterns and processes have been more or less reversed, as public spaces are removed in favour of private spaces and economic productivity, and with culture being viewed as a support for consumption and marketing of the city (Ward & Gold, 1994).

The second challenge follows on from this: for much of the period, surveyed culture has generally been viewed as residual, something to be added in when other issues have been solved, or, as instrumental, as a tool to ease some identifiable problem. Cultural land uses are invariably demoted or valued as secondary, and the contribution of culture is reduced to one of passive or ornamental support: the intrinsic value of culture being discounted. This seems to be a case of both culture 'falling between the cracks' between the economic state (the first challenge) and that culture's instrumental values being accounted for, but not its intrinsic values. It is this intrinsic value that can engage the senses and demonstrate care and attention to both the city, and its citizens. We can highlight that a continuing problem has been that the organisational field of capability (planning and governance) has not been expanded to reflect the extended use of culture by the citizenry and its contribution to wellbeing.

The third challenge is the increasingly individualised interpretation of urban change as legitimated by policy making and politics. Despite the celebration of the public realm of Victorian cities, and the dreams of the Garden City pioneers, such spaces are now interpreted as wasted, or non-profitable. It is emblematic that, currently, much privately promoted development supports the virtues of 'co-working spaces', and interaction zones, but that these all take place within a bounded (private) realm; the actual real (public) spaces between the buildings are neglected, or erased (Pratt, 2017). This process has been aided and abetted by the immiseration of local authorities who can no longer 'service' public spaces, and even when they can, they are forced to contract out such public tasks (Pratt & Hutton, 2013).

What Is To Be Done?

The three challenge complexes indicate the need for a networked and holistic solution, one that runs against the current tide of 'smart solutions'. A new way of addressing the problem is required, based on a new conception of culture and wellbeing as relational and situated. It also follows that narrowly defined functional governance, or land use regulation, are unlikely to be effective, and more likely to generate further problems. We can take our lead from debates about environmental sustainability and cities that point to the necessity of understanding the city in a more interconnected and interdependent manner (Jarvis et al., 2001; Pratt, 2008, 2009).

Returning to our starting point, it does seem to make sense to see increases in urban inequalities being related to poorer health and quality of life, as well as wellbeing. This is a conundrum as cities also seem to offer the possibility of a diverse and positive sense of wellbeing. The barrier is inequality, part of which is structural, and part of which is coordination (which can be manifest as lack of jobs, transport, homes and culture). Taking inspiration from environmental perspectives on the city, we can perhaps look for a more holistic solution. The physical and organisational 'space' accorded for culture in the city is seldom right or appropriate; what is needed is a more systematic and cross-cutting approach. In the same way that we now conceive of the potential mitigation of environmental issues being addressed at both the local and the global scales, perhaps we can see culture in the same way.

In order to achieve this, we will need to move away from single-purpose solutions: a way of putting sticking plasters over far greater issues. We need to recognise the intrinsic values of culture and the ways in which they contribute to wellbeing, not all of them being amendable to quantification, or singular equivalence (Crossick & Kaszynska, 2014; Oman & Taylor, 2018). This, in turn, suggests that we need to look at culture as a transversal aspect of the city, one that needs to be delivered as part of every activity. By simply thinking of culture and…, not culture or…, we might begin to recognise the values of culture, and the ways that those values may enhance particular activities, such as work, home or transport; and in so doing contribute to a more general wellbeing. However, as Wilkinson and Pickett (2010) have reminded us, we need to begin with addressing inequalities (or income, access and opportunity). In short, we need to start with a principle and ethic of inclusion in our cities: there would seem to be no better place to begin than with culture.

Notes

1 I am using the notion of inclusion, not participation or access, on purpose; I reference wider debates on social exclusion which recognises that people can self-exclude, but that the systemic focus is on inclusion, but not forcing, or requiring action. In short, it is about opportunity (See Byrne, 2005; Healey, 1998; Levitas, 2005; Sen, 2000; Silver, 1994).
2 Building cycles are invariably out of sync with demand due to the time that it takes to construct a structure.
3 The problem is rooted in the outdated basic needs framework developed by Maslow (1943).
4 The detail of this long history of culture and the city is only summarised here; it is based on a comprehensive account, found in Pratt (2014).
5 An example is the Garden City movement, and the idealised plans of their progenitors (Hall, 1988).

References

Albor, C., Uphoff, E., Stafford, M., Ballas, D., Wilkinson, R., & Pickett, K. (2014). The effects of socioeconomic incongruity in the neighbourhood on social support, self-esteem and mental health in England. *Social Science & Medicine, 111*, p1–9.

Byrne, D. S. (2005). *Social exclusion* (2nd ed.). New York: Open University Press.

Castells, M. (1996). *The rise of the network society.* Cambridge, MA: Blackwell Publishers.

Crossick, G., & Kaszynska, P. (2014). Under construction: Towards a framework for cultural value. *Cultural Trends, 23*(2), p120–131.

Dorling, D. (2012). Inequality and Injustice: some news from Britain. *Urban Geography, 33*(5), p621–629.

Frey, B. S. (2008). *Happiness: A revolution in economics*: Cambridge, MA: MIT press.

Hall, P. (1988). *Cities of tomorrow: an intellectual history of urban planning and design in the twentieth century.* Oxford: Basil Blackwell.

Healey, P. (1998). Institutionalist theory, social exclusion and governance. *Social exclusion in European cities*, p53–73. London: Jessica Kingsley.

Jarvis, H., Pratt, A. C., & Wu, P. C.-C. (2001). *The secret life of cities: the social reproduction of everyday life.* New York: Pearson Education.

Levitas, R. (2005). *The inclusive society?: social exclusion and New Labour* (2nd ed.). Basingstoke: Macmillan.

Maslow, A. (1943). A theory of human motivation. *Psychological Review, 50*, p370–396.

Mollenkopf, J. H., & Castells, M. (1991). *Dual city: restructuring New York.* New York: Russell Sage Foundation.

Morrison, P. S. (2007). Subjective wellbeing and the city. *Social Policy Journal of New Zealand, 31*, p74.

Okulicz-Kozaryn, A. (2013). City life: rankings (livability) versus perceptions (satisfaction). *Social Indicators Research, 110*(2), p433–451.

Oman, S., & Taylor, M. (2018). Subjective wellbeing in cultural advocacy: a politics of research between the market and the academy. *Journal of Cultural Economy*, p1–19. doi: 10.1080/17530350.2018.1435422

Pratt, A. C. (1996). Coordinating employment, transport and housing in cities: An institutional perspective. *Urban Studies, 33*(8), p1357–1375.

Pratt, A. C. (2008). What are the factors that could influence the future of work with regard to energy systems and the built environment? *Energy Policy, 36*, p4646–4651. doi:10.1016/j.enpol.2008.09.068

Pratt, A. C. (2009). Social and economic drivers of land use change in the British space economy. *Land Use Policy, 26*(S1), S109–S114. doi:10.1016/j.landusepol.2009.09.006

Pratt, A. C. (2010). Creative cities: Tensions within and between social, cultural and economic development. A critical reading of the UK experience. *City, Culture and Society, 1*(1), 13–20. doi:doi:10.1016/j.ccs.2010.04.001

Pratt, A. C. (2015). Resilience, locality and the cultural economy. *City, Culture and Society, 6*(3), p61–67.

Pratt, A. (2017). The rise of the quasi-public space and its consequences for cities and culture. *Palgrave Communications, 3*(1), 36. doi:10.1057/s41599-017-0048-6

Pratt, A. C., & Hutton, T. A. (2013). Reconceptualising the relationship between the creative economy and the city: Learning from the financial crisis. *Cities, 33*(0), p86–95. doi:http://dx.doi.org/10.1016/j.cities.2012.05.008

Rogers, R. (2008). *Cities for a small planet.* New York: Basic Books.

Sassen, S. (2001). *The global city: New York, London, Tokyo* (2nd ed.). Princeton, NJ: Princeton University Press.

Sen, A. (2000). *Social exclusion: concept, application, and scrutiny.* Manila: Asian Development Bank.

Silver, H. (1994). Social exclusion and social solidarity: three paradigms. *International Labour Review, 133*(5, 6), p531.

Tett, G. (2015). *The silo effect: why putting everything in its place isn't such a bright idea.* London: Little, Brown.

Urban Task Force. (1999). *Towards an urban renaisance.* London: Spon

Ward, S. V., & Gold, J. R. (1994). *Place promotion: use of publicity and public relations to sell places.* London: Belhaven Press.

Wilkinson, R. G., & Pickett, K. (2010). *The spirit level: why equality is better for everyone* (New ed.). London: Penguin.

Zukin, S. (1995). *The cultures of cities.* Cambridge, MA: Blackwell.

13

DIRECTIONS FOR CHANGE IN TECHNOLOGY AND WELLBEING IN THE CITY

Andrew Laing

Reclaiming the Promise of Technology

The chapter explores how information technology has transformed the way we work and live and, in so doing, is also transforming the contribution that cities make to wellbeing. Technology has the potential to add value to the purpose and meaning of cities, and to enrich citizens' wellbeing. This promise of technology is at risk from the ways in which the ideas of 'smart cities' have evolved and been practised. The technocratic and exclusive character of smart city technologies can be challenged by alternative views of how technology can be used and accessed to contribute to wellbeing in cities.

In exploring the ideas of wellbeing and place in relation to technology, I propose a view of wellbeing that enables self-fulfilment, meaning and purpose through a collective dynamic of action, sometimes referred to as a eudaimonic concept of wellbeing.[1] This perspective contrasts with the hedonic view of wellbeing that has emphasised an individualistic view of a 'good life' by enabling happiness, pleasure or utility for the greatest number of individuals (Atkinson et al., 2012). I argue that the dominant concepts of the smart city have so far emphasised a utilitarian and efficiency-driven model of wellbeing that has restricted the ability and participation of users and citizens in the making of their collective wellbeing in the urban environment. In this sense, the smart city has ironically perpetuated the Modernist functionalist view of the city as a centrally planned, ordered and highly segregated environment in which the use of space and the city is highly controlled and regulated, and in which the use of space is monolithic, hierarchical and homogeneous.

Within the history of ideas about technology and the city, and within the concepts of the smart city, it is possible to identify both a pessimistic and an optimistic vision of how technology can contribute to wellbeing in cities. These divergent perspectives allow us to imagine an alternative view of how technology is evolving to enable citizen users to engage with the city. In so doing, it is possible to imagine different futures, futures in which technology will enrich and enchant our experience of the city and open possibilities for wide participation in the design, planning and use of urban environments. In this alternative view, the smart city could be reclaimed and reinvented, requiring the creation of a new kind of 'civics' that empowers citizens. While these arguments are exploratory and speculative, there is enough evidence to indicate what might be possible, and the directions of change.

To develop an alternative view of the possibilities for technology to contribute to wellbeing in cities, it is valuable to re-examine the history of ideas of technology and the city in relation to the body, machines and our experiences of the city.

From the Industrial Machine City to the Post-modern Computer City

The Challenge to the Modernist City

The Modernist industrial city of the twentieth century was designed and planned to functionally and efficiently segregate and distribute activities in space and time (Banham, 1960; Evenson, 1969; Gideon, 1980; Le Corbusier, 1973, 1987; Mumford, 2000, 2009; Wiebenson, 1969). This was codified most thoroughly by Le Corbusier in 1934 for CIAM in *The Athens Charter* (Le Corbusier, 1973), in which healthy and productive 'machines' for living, working, healthy recreation and the enjoyment of nature were distributed across the city, connected by fast highways and rail transportation. The ordered layout of the city would enable recovery from the damaging impacts of the older manufacturing city with its chaotic congestion, pollution and disease (see Figure 13.1).

The Modernists drew on the engineering logic of the nineteenth century in thinking of the city as a circulation system for a social body that needed to be sanitised (Swyngedouw, 2006). Gandy (2005), following Vidler (1990), notes that the Modernist home was considered an exoskeleton, a prosthesis or prophylactic for the body, providing warmth, water, light and other essentials. Beyond the home was the network infrastructure of the industrial city, the hidden but essential pipes and wires that enabled the 'body machine' city to function along with the arteries of new transportation systems and highways that allowed citizens to speed efficiently from one functional zone or activity to another.

Information technology challenges the functionalist modernist programme for cities that dominated the architecture and planning of the twentieth century. It raises the promise of what Boyer called a 'nonlinear vision' in which computational connectivity enables non-hierarchical, multi-centred, open forms of community (Boyer, 1996, p. 19). Her formulation that 'the machine is to modernism what the computer is to postmodernism' (Ibid, p. 10) is a fertile starting point to explore the evolving relationships between technology, the city and wellbeing. Boyer highlights that in the shift from the 'machinist'

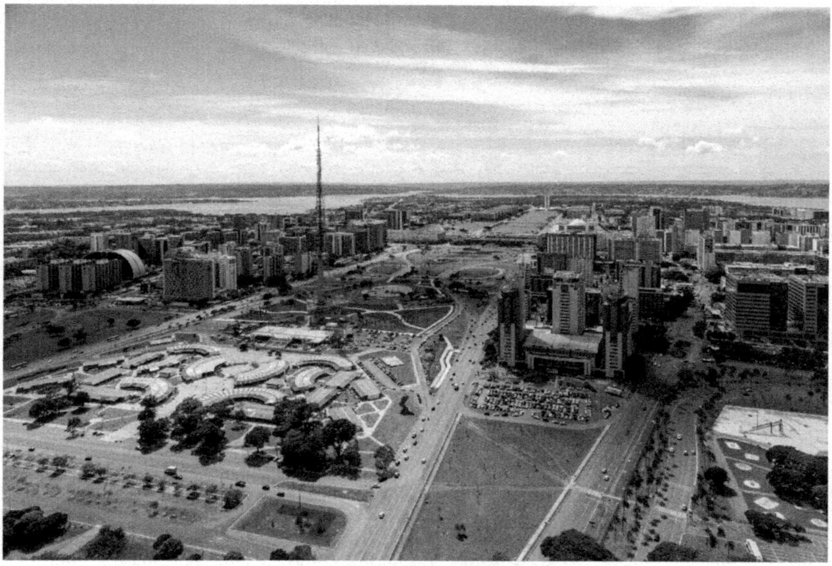

FIGURE 13.1 The Modernist city of Brasilia, an example of the functionalist segregation and distribution of functions and activities in city planning.

modernism to a 'computerist' postmodernism, the computer begins to drive our idea of what the city is or what it might become (Boyer, 1996). The question becomes: what kind of computer city, for whose benefit, and how might it serve wellbeing?

The Cyborg City in the Computer Age

The origins of ideas about the computer-driven, post-modern city derive from early-twentieth-century views of the body itself as a machine, a body that could be increasingly industrialised and technicised (see Figure 13.2).

If the body was a kind of industrial process, it could be augmented, replicated and partially, if not wholly, replaced by machines that would evolve to have intelligence. The body as machine could be adapted and morphed into robots or cyborgs.[2] Mitchell (1995, 2003) foresaw the cyborg as a post-human liberated from the body, a spatially networked urban citizen. The body could be externalised to the city, through the spatial extension of computerised intelligence in networked spaces, buildings and the city. Then, the city itself begins to be thought of as having intelligence, 'the brain or "thinking space" of the city…. is dispersed through innumerable nodes and networks' (Gandy, 2005, p. 31). The idea of the body-machine hybrid (the cyborg) was extended such that even buildings and cities could be thought of as extensions of bodies, as metabolic machines, having sentience, intelligence and eventually the 'smartness' of what became known as the smart city (see Figure 13.3).

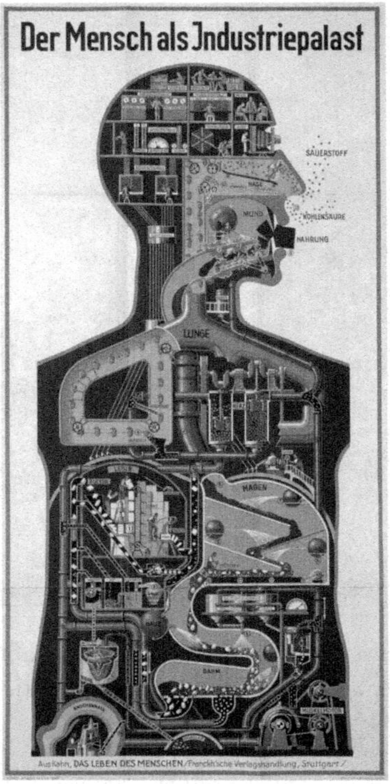

FIGURE 13.2 The body as machine: Der Mensch als Industriepalast (Man as Industrial Palace), Fritz Kahn, 1926.

The role of architecture and planning would then increasingly be one of programming, designing and providing systems and tools for cities that could themselves be active agents or collaborators in intelligently and systematically programming for their citizens' needs. The computer is therefore the critical device of transition from the idea of the human cyborg to the concept of city intelligence. The networked computer became the means of mediating the spatial distribution of intelligence that could be embodied in the city at-large.

Cyborg Foragers in Networked Post-sedentary Space

The computer and information technology are enabling a new understanding and experience of space (Castells, 2004; Duffy, 2008; Sassen, 2001; Varnelis & Freidberg, 2008), associated with networked global cities in what has been called a 'space of flows', an electronically connected, interactive network in which 'the global city is not a place, but a process' (Castells, 2000, p. 417; see also Batty, 2013; Mitchell, 1995; Picon, 2015; Sennett, 2012). Gandy (2005) describes this as a post-metabolic city in which the exchange of information supplants the role of material exchange as the dynamic shaping urban space.

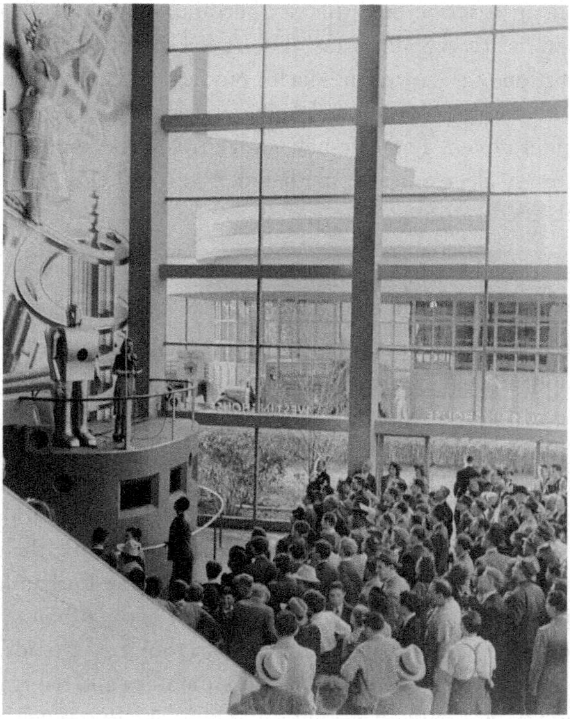

FIGURE 13.3 The body replaced or augmented by intelligent machines – the robot or cyborg. Lucy Ashjian, 'World's Fair 1939, Interior of Westinghouse Pavilion with Robot and Visitors'.

This technologically enabled space re-orders the logic of the nineteenth- and twentieth-century city. The industrial city segregated living and working areas, and with the use of the telegraph and telephone, separated management and administration from the factory, leading to the creation of central business districts and their associated mass commutation patterns (Mitchell, 2003). In its place, Mitchell argued, the nomadic 'information worker' appropriates multiple, diverse sites as workplaces and breaks down the former, specialised spatial programmes of home/office, café/office, hotel/workplace with more dynamic and complex patterns of use. Buildings and urban environments in the future city would need fewer specialised spaces. Space could be appropriated in more *ad hoc* ways.

Information technology is changing our understanding of patterns of space use. Ambient virtual information is augmenting the material world in communicating the meaning of places (Shepard, 2011). Shepard suggests that, as the 'data clouds of the twenty-first century descend on the streets, sidewalks and public spaces of the city', they may be becoming more important than the formal organisation of space and matter in shaping our experience of the city (Ibid, p. 18).

Crang and Graham describe how the city becomes a 'haze of software as much as a constellation of bricks and mortar' (Crang & Graham, 2007, p. 790). Rather than the substitution of electronic media for physical encounter, the environment is permeated with communication technologies, forming a hybrid space in which the digital is interwoven. For Mitchell, citizen users become 'cyborg foragers navigating through electronically mediated resource fields' in post-sedentary space (Mitchell, 2003, p. 159).

From Body as Cyborg to City as Computer

For the potential of the computer to distribute intelligence in the city, a series of mutations and mutual transformations of the body as cyborg and the city as computer had to occur. Not only did the network infrastructure to support distributed computing need to be created, the computer had to escape from the computer room to the desktop and then, in another mutation, become untethered via laptops, tablets and smart phones with their GIS geolocation capabilities. These devices and networks are instrumental in transforming the body into the twenty-first-century cyborg and the city into a networked urban landscape.

The smart phone especially fulfils the realisation of the urban cyborg idea enabled by wireless networks and geolocation. It is a tool that extends the mind and the body (Ratti & Claudel, 2016), outsourcing memory and navigation to create a converged digital 'post-human' condition: 'Digital technologies have become a dynamic extension of our bodies and minds, demanding a constant and two-way cybernetic exchange' (Ratti & Claudel, 2016, p. 60).

Yet paradoxically and ironically, the smart phone and other digital assistants, with their unprecedented ability to converge and blend the digital and physical domains, have radically re-focussed the human relationship to space and the city. They allow for 'a radical pivot back to physical space', transforming our 'corporeal inhabitation of cities', as the 'city unfolds inside every pocket' (Ibid, p. 63). Graham (2004) argues that, rather than replacing place, information technology tools act as prostheses extending human actions, identities and communities in time and space. They are embedded in urban life, surprisingly re-engaging our relationship to the physical world (see Figure 13.4).

Emergence of the Smart City

From Military Cybernetics to the Smart City

Halpern (2017) identified the emergence of the idea of the smart city as a hybrid in which the physical environment is an organism supported by machines. She traces the history of the idea of 'responsive environments' in which computation is integrated into the design of built environments, notably by Nicholas Negroponte in the Architecture Machine Group at MIT (later the Media Lab), which had itself drawn on earlier experiments in the 1960s and 1970s on cognitive

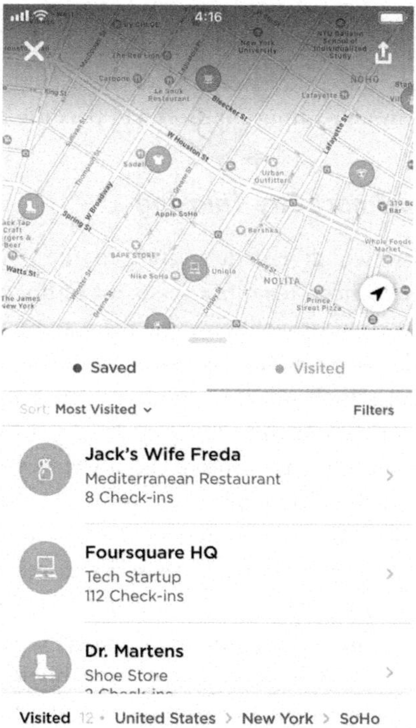

FIGURE 13.4 The map-based interface of the smartphone application Foursquare, a pioneer of location-based social media services.

science, urban computation and simulation. Picon (2015) also locates the beginning of the smart city ideas with the Cold War desires of administrators to pose urban problems as questions of cybernetic management, originating with military industrial research (see Norbert Wiener's book *Cybernetics* published in 1948). Then the city was viewed as a cybernetic problem of regulating human behaviour within a technical environment of information processing and feedback loops.

The emerging idea was that the subject of design was systems rather than discrete buildings, replacing architecture with media (Halpern, 2017). Central to the emerging idea of designing urban intelligence was that humans were not good pattern seekers, could not solve systematic problems and would be better supported by machines that could scale between the urban or planetary environment (Ibid.). The machine knows better.

Intelligent machines could be distributed and embedded into the city. Halpern notes that Negroponte's argument supporting CAD was that it responded to the need for a new kind of intelligence that is 'no longer beholden to the individual', a machine intelligence with decentralised urban sensors, effectors and processors. The goal of computing would be to make the built environment of the city responsive to the needs of the individual; the computerised city as a cybernetic machine (Ibid, p. 137). By 1975, with his publication of Soft Architecture Machines, Negroponte described the computer disappearing into the environment as an omnipresent machine; computing itself had become an 'environment'.

Diverging Strands of Smart City Thinking

Picon (2015) identifies two divergent strands in the evolution of smart city thinking that have implications for our assessment of how the smart city can be conceptualised to better support wellbeing: (1) the ways in which smart cities can provide artificial intelligence for the management of the city and its infrastructure and; (2) the way in which smart technology can couple human stakeholders with urban government and infrastructure through forms of hybridisation. Regarding the first strand, the aspiration of the smart city in this sense is to provide a better quality of urban life based on improved environmental efficiency, as the city is increasingly designed and managed as a system of information. The relationships between physical infrastructure, services and users are reconfigured to provide higher levels of reactivity and flexibility. The driver of the smart city in this first sense is 'the desire to anticipate and master everything' (Picon, 2015, p. 67), and can be tied into the hedonic model of wellbeing, that is, government in the smart city is designed to maximise individual and collective actions to provide for the greatest happiness or utility for all.[3]

The risk with this approach is that the city cannot be reduced to 'a system founded on a feedback loop between parameters that are finite in number' (Ibid, p. 50). Picon argues that this view of the smart city is narrowly, technologically determinist in the way in which commercial stakeholders define a new urban ideal and impose a top down view of what the city should be and how it can be used. He argues that this technocratic view is most evident in 'smart' urban developments, such as Songdo International Business District in South Korea, Masdar near Abu Dhabi, and in the PlanIt Valley planned city near Porto in Portugal.

Yet, as Picon (2015) notes, the 'smart city' can provide valuable monitoring of city functions, mitigate risks of disaster and reveal new dimensions of urban functionality. Townsend (2013) illustrates this benign aspect of the smart city, with examples of how the city of Chicago cross-referenced the data on meals-on-wheels with tax records to generate a map of elderly people living alone who may need to be checked on during heat and cold emergencies (Townsend, 2013, p. 209). Singapore's Smart Nation (2018) programme also has introduced many kinds of Apps to help citizens navigate the city, learn more about their health and access other services of many kinds.

Picon's second strand is a neo-cybernetic approach that can support high levels of citizen participation in urban administration, with citizens engaged in co-developing applications to drive the functionality of the city. As such, it has a much greater potential to activate citizens in urban decisions that will influence their wellbeing in both the short and longer term. The hypothesis he explores is that 'smart city' technology can enable the city in a sense to become 'conscious', provided with intelligence. In this more optimistic view, digital tools allow for: 'the optimization of its functioning and sustainability, as well as of its inhabitants' quality of life and the types of relationships they can maintain with one another' (Picon, 2015, p. 29).

Hill provides the example of how the city of Chicago predicts rat infestations (Hill, 2014a) and the example of the former Bridj bus service in Boston where 'the bus stop comes to you', enabled by data on patterns of transport use and social media analytics. Projects such as those of MIT's SENSEable City Lab indicate ways in which citizens can become actively engaged through technology in learning and acting on information about their lives in the city, the power structures in which they are embedded, and choices they have (or do not have) to make change. One example project tracked and analysed the microbiota of sewage. In another project, trash was tagged and tracked globally: 'The fact that we know where our trash ends up should make us more aware of the problem we create by throwing things away' (de Waal, 2011, p. 194). MIT Media Lab has collaborated with Deloitte on a project called DataUSA, an open-source government data visualisation website that features datasets from cities displayed in a way that is easy to access for non-tech savvy users.

In these examples, we see a further shift from the dominant emphasis on individualised wellbeing to longer-term, collective responsibility for planetary wellbeing in terms of resilience and environmental sustainability. This is a shift that Atkinson et al. (2012) note is characteristic of eudaimonic concepts of wellbeing, which 'consider not just the sustainability of wellbeing within an individual life-span, but equally, if not more importantly, beyond and into future lives' (p. 3).

The important question that Picon (2015) asks is: who controls or directs this form of the smart city? Is it through a politics as we have known it or through a set of algorithms that are out of reach of the citizen? Is there an alternative in which a new kind of technological empowerment mobilises collective action, demonstration and the invention of new forms of community? Can this alternative view of the smart city enable a new kind of 'right to the city', following Lefebvre (Picon, 2015).

Critique of the Smart City

The mechanistic and functionalist character of the new, ground-up, 'smart cities' has been critiqued by Picon (2015) and others such as Greenfield (2013), Koolhaas (2014), Sennett (2012), and de Waal (2011). Greenfield and Sennett both contrast the richness and complexity of existing historic cities with the inadequacy of the modernist architecture and urbanism that has been repeated within the technologically determinist urban plans of the new smart cities. The creative spontaneity of great, old cities is compared with the sterility of the new, smart cities. The irony is that, although technology allows for a post-functionalist programme of the city and how its spaces might be managed and controlled, the new 'smart' cities are remarkably conventional in their twentieth century, modernist layout and planning, with rigidly defined and segregated zones of activity, and highly centralised forms of management and control (see Figure 13.5).

Anderson and Rainie (2018) note that, while the broader expansion of technology in people's lives is still thought to be valuable, there are growing concerns about a digital dystopia creating higher levels of stress and information overload. There are concerns that the smart city movement has suffered from a lack of systematic critical thinking, dominated as it has been by corporate interests (Kitchin, 2015) and lack of clarity on how to define the smart city as such (Cavada et al., 2014). It is an unusual feature of the smart city movement, as Greenfield (2013) notes, that the concepts originated within technology businesses rather than from urban planning theory. As such, this dominant view of the smart city failed to account for broader trends in the social use of technology, notably the adoption of the smart phone and other more decentralised and participatory technologies and software, such as social media. The result was an over-specification and centralisation of the technological framework of the smart city and a 'willed blindness' to the complexity of real urban places (Greenfield, 2013).

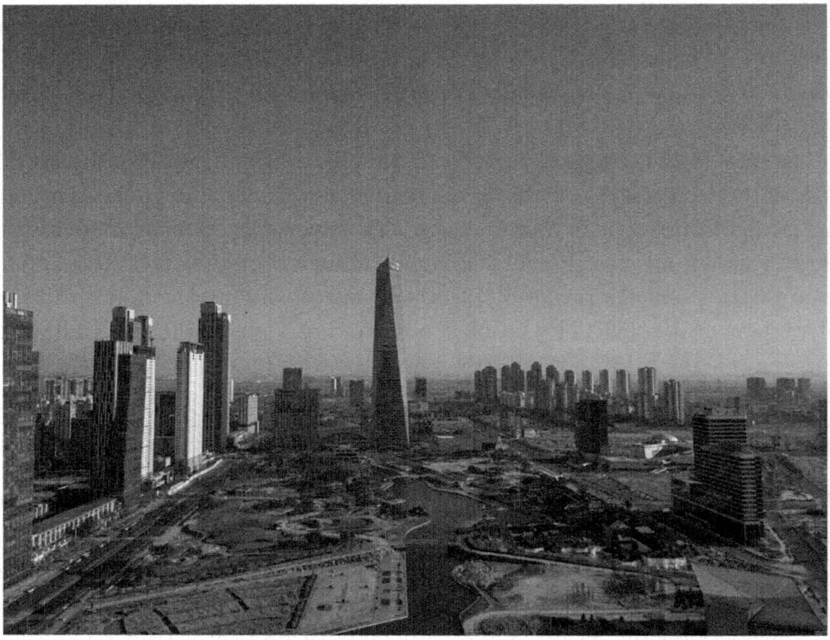

FIGURE 13.5 The smart city of Songdo, South Korea, from the 29th floor observation deck of G-Tower.

The typical smart city model, Greenfield argues, is incapable of replicating or enriching the true vitality of complex and chaotic, large-scale urban areas with their *ad hoc* and serendipitous behaviours, thereby reducing the purpose of the city to a model of streamlined, efficient convenience (Greenfield, 2013). This same critique of smart city concepts was made by Boyer back in 1983, when she noted that the elements of uncertainty, complexity and surprise that rule the city render urban command and control techniques ineffective (Boyer, 2015). The attempts to impose cybernetic rationality on the city require expert systems that side-step citizen democracy and rely on post-political, technocratic management (Boyer, 2015). These algorithmic models of urban governance cannot solve structural urban problems of inequality or weigh ethical concerns. They limit the potential of the smart city to contribute to wellbeing.

Technology Erodes the Public Realm but May also Shape It Anew

A further critique about the smart city model is how it might weaken the urban public realm. De Waal (2011) notes that new technologies may contribute to the demise of traditional public spaces such as town squares, multi-functional streets and public parks. These spaces have been the cornerstones of democratic assembly and engagement in cities for centuries. However, they also have the potential to contribute to new forms of public life and exchange. They have the capability to shape our urban experience in new ways (de Waal, 2011, p. 191).

The promise of technology in the smart city is thus a contested terrain requiring political engagement to design appropriate solutions. However, the smart city goals of improving urban efficiency and functional urban management have largely avoided the politics of technology in the city. In this sense, as Greenfield (2013) argues, the smart city movement has not been ambitious enough. It has aimed low in its focus on convenience and efficient optimisation, rather than recognising that cities are so much more than machines with workflows. Smart city concepts have ignored the complex pleasures and delights of the city that can be augmented and enriched by a technology that amplifies citizen and user engagement in its design and use. Indeed, many of the same technologies that have evolved to support the top down view of the smart city could be re-designed, re-purposed or re-imagined to be responsive and to enrich the wellbeing of citizens.

Re-enchanting the Smart City for Wellbeing

Re-imagining the City for Wellbeing

Our uses of spaces, buildings and the city are being re-designed and re-purposed in ways that allow us to re-imagine how the city enables or contributes to wellbeing. The categories of functional spaces and their patterns of use that formed the standard typologies of buildings in the Modernist architecture and city planning of the twentieth century are being decomposed and eroded by the mobility, autonomy and flexibility that technology provides. Work no longer happens exclusively in buildings called offices or factories. Our ways of living increasingly take place in blended, multi-functional environments across the city at-large. Technology has transformed how all kinds of spaces are programmed, designed and used.

As information technology disrupts the conventional programmes for spaces and buildings, it is also disrupting how such environments are briefed and programmed. The city augmented by technology, collaborative design tools and open-source architecture allows for new kinds of participatory architectural programming and design by citizens (Fok & Picon, 2016; Picon, 2010; Ratti & Claudel, 2016). The opportunity is for citizen users to be increasingly empowered to dynamically control how they use spaces and how such spaces are programmed and designed through new sharing applications and services (Laing, 2014). Users could become activist consumers of space, as space becomes a service (Hill 2014b; Laing, 2013; Waber et al., 2014). In this sense, the city becomes a resource to be more intensively used and shared over time, providing both individual user benefits and collective gains in longer-term environmental and sustainability performance.

Yet, this potential for technology to enrich lives and further wellbeing has been largely obscured by the technocratic ideology of the 'smart city' in its focus on providing infrastructural and operational systems driven by narrow views of efficiency. The fulfilment of the opportunities for a participatory, technologically enabled urbanism that can enrich wellbeing will require a new 'civics' (Townsend, 2013). It will require vigilance against the risks to privacy that are inherent in a smart city that relies on citizens sharing information. The optimistic view of this potential is that it represents a genuine revolution, 'comparable in significance to the birth of the major industrial cities in the nineteenth century and the emergence of the networked city as both an urban ideal and a physical process of city transformation' (Picon, 2015, p. 154).

The Purpose of the City Is Augmented by Technology

The purpose of cities as places in which connections between people can be accelerated and multiplied to provide valuable social, economic and cultural benefits is massively augmented and qualitatively transformed with technology (Duffy, 2008). Batty (2013) argues that cities have always been where people come to interact. Technology is enabling people to interact in systems of cities in new and different ways, 'cities are devices enabling us to communicate' (Ibid, p. xvii).

The mobility and choice enabled by technology provides for a more nomadic, exploratory, serendipitous way of living and working in which users optimise the density and proximity of cities to enrich their experience and promote their wellbeing. As such, the city can be a condenser of sustainable, healthy, pleasurable activity in which users empowered with technology are agents of its programme and design. Technology has the potential to enrich the purpose, meaning and pleasure of the city and to thereby contribute to citizen's wellbeing.

This opportunity given by technology is to augment the city and 'recoup the "right to the city", which Henri Lefebvre powerfully characterised in terms of heterogeneity rather than monoculture, encounter rather than separation, and simultaneity instead of sequence' (Mitchell, 2003, p. 165). We might also recall what Mitchell (2005) described as the new great challenge for architects, designers and planners: to 'create fusion spaces that satisfy important human needs in effective new ways, and that surprise and delight us through digitally enabled combinations of the unexpected' (Ibid, p. 23).

New Urban Typologies and Patterns of Use Contribute to Wellbeing

Technology that allows for a 'post sedentary' way of using space enables more mixed and overlapping uses of buildings and neighbourhoods. Duffy, following Mitchell, points to how knowledge work takes place in wider and more complex spatial and temporal landscapes, allowing for the use of space to be intensified (Duffy, 2008). The office building is no longer an isolated container for work. Technology is, as he describes it, 'dissolving the two iron laws that have shaped the buildings and cities in which we accommodate work': synchrony and colocation (Duffy, 2008, p. 16). Dan Hill has explored this shift from the industrial rhythms of the 'clockwork city', structured by rush hours and the spokes and hubs of transportation serving central business districts to a post-digital, mixed-use urban environment in which patterns or work and living are more diverse and fragmented (Hill, 2014a).

Duffy (2008) lists the kinds of benefits that should result from this paradigm shift in how the city works, highlighting: more mixed-use building, more opportunities for intensive and interconnected uses of spaces, and more differentiated and interactive spaces. But beyond the diversification and intensification of space use, he also highlights 'the rediscovery of how to drive harder the intellectual potential of cities, given that the city itself is such a powerful networking and communications device', and 'the rediscovery of serendipity – the creation of the overlapping and interstitial spaces that are immensely inherently valuable in the more loosely programmed knowledge economy' (Ibid, p. 19).

Re-spatialising the City

Technology is 're-spatialising' the city, creating new urban typologies (Ratti & Claudel, 2016) that break down the rigid zoning and segregation of activities in the city characteristic of Modernist planning and design. Ratti and Claudel note that innovations in digital fabrication may allow for restructuring of how and where things are produced. 3D printing challenges the laws of mass production and economies of scale. Computer-controlled machines enable new kinds of fast

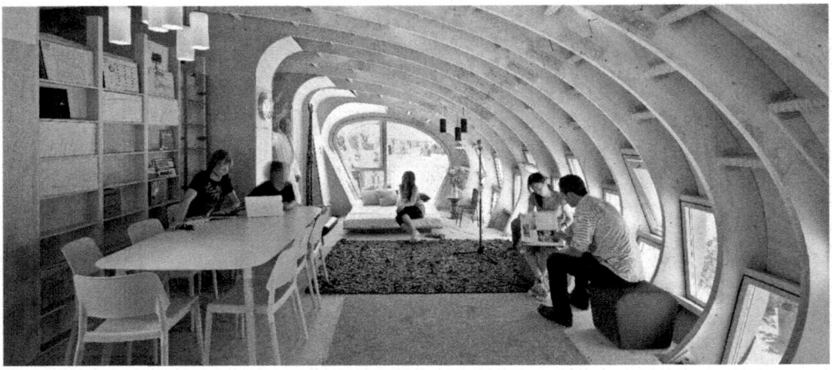

FIGURE 13.6 Fab Lab House, Barcelona.

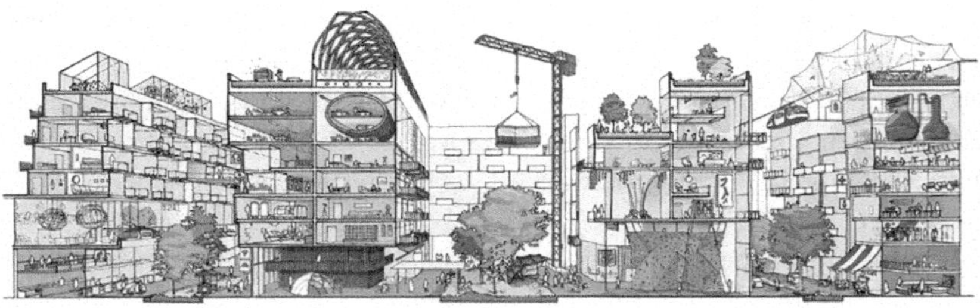

FIGURE 13.7 Sidewalk Labs' proposal for new kinds of mixed-use neighbourhoods in Toronto.

customisation. With intuitive, open-source software, a much wider socialisation of design is possible with new forms of participation and collaboration. Fabrication can take place at smaller scales and even domestic settings. New types of spaces for production and learning are emerging, such as FabLabs (see Figure 13.6).

Production may be realigned with domestic life and no longer take place in factories. At the Sidewalk Labs proposed new neighbourhood in Toronto (Badger, 18 October 2017); the development intended to demonstrate a flexible loft building typology with a simple shell and minimalistic interior that is easy to convert to other building uses. The new neighbourhood loft buildings would have enabled enable 'radical mixed uses' of residential, commercial and 'other', with co-housing and microunits (Sidewalk Labs, 2017, p. 123) (see Figure 13.7).

Technology Re-enchanting the City

More than the re-design of urban building typologies and patterns of use, technology can be used to reactivate the urban public sphere. Digital geotagging and annotation provides new narratives and meanings in urban space. Picon describes how, in the 'sentient and sensual city, augmented reality and geolocation enhance every square meter of urban space, investing it with new and unexpected functionalities and meanings' (Picon, 2015, p. 113). Varnelis and Friedberg (2008) describe how the geospatial web and ubiquitous computing can enable people, objects and places to tell their stories.

Thrift (2014) sees technology forming a 'new skin' of data across all the surfaces of the city, 'a skin which can have it owns life at least in part arising from the way it can be so easily integrated with so many activities' (Ibid, p. 1264). Dana Cuff foresaw this as an 'enacted space' in which computing is spatially embodied in all things around us as well as in our skin and bodies (Cuff, 2003). Thrift argues that the ubiquity of data in our environment will change our notion of place as cities take on a 'sense of themselves' (Thrift, 2014) (see Figure 13.8).

McCullough (2015) has described this as a new kind of 'information commons', unlike the earlier expectations of the disembodiment of cyberspace (Boyer, 1996). The city as information commons can be tagged with situated technologies, revealing the city as a collective public work. In re-enchanting and re-animating the city (Crang & Graham, 2007), technology may encourage new forms of public activism that make visible and knowable the workings of the city and its power structures. Users may be able to see previously invisible digital

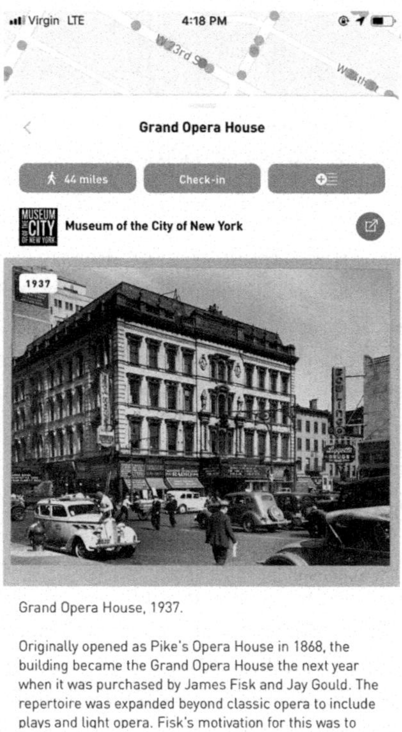
Virgin LTE
4:18 PM
Grand Opera House
44 miles
Check-in
Museum of the City of New York
1937
Grand Opera House, 1937.
Originally opened as Pike's Opera House in 1868, the building became the Grand Opera House the next year when it was purchased by James Fisk and Jay Gould. The repertoire was expanded beyond classic opera to include plays and light opera. Fisk's motivation for this was to

FIGURE 13.8 Non-commercial instances of geotagging technology, such as the Urban Archive app, can situate users in the history and geography of their urban environments.

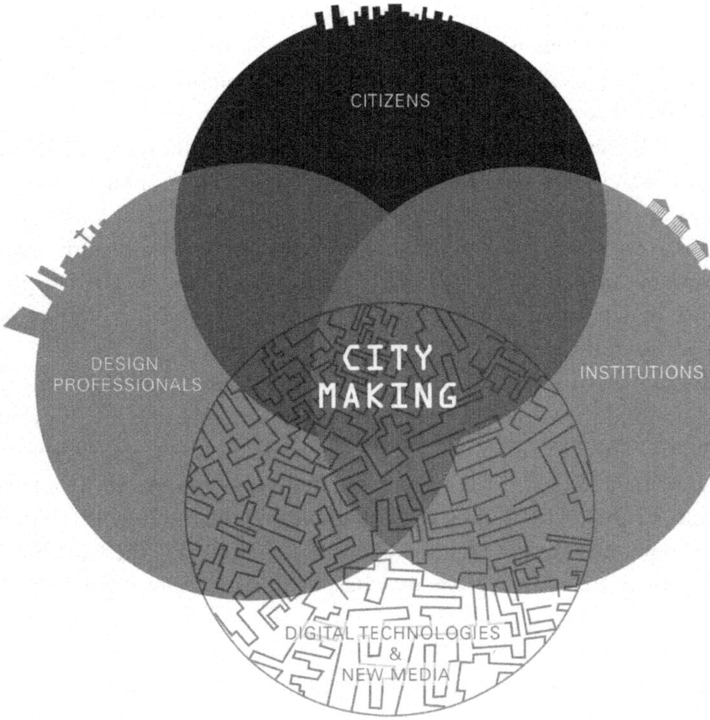

FIGURE 13.9 The Hackable City, with kind permission of Professor Martijn de Waal, Amsterdam University of Applied Sciences (AUAS).

structures and appropriate their technology for alternative uses to challenge and subvert conventional narratives. Crang and Graham suggest the possibility of a kind of collaborative authoring of the city to make it transparent or aesthetically problematic, 're-enchanting' the environment through overcoding it, 'taking virtual community out of the wires and onto the streets' (Crang & Graham, 2007, p. 806) (see Figure 13.9).

A New Civics for Wellbeing in the Smart City

Greenfield (2013) argues that the same technologies already being used in the smart city can be turned into ways that extend the abilities of citizens and communities to determine their conditions of existence. The enabler of this potential is the smart phone and similar mobile devices, given that they are already part of most people's daily experiences in every city. But it is not only a question of the distribution of smart phones but also a question of how so-called smart city big data can be harnessed by citizens for their own use, to 'post questions rather than deliver sterile solutions' (Greenfield, 2013, p. 95). This would require replacing the corporate proprietary control of data with free and open use by citizens.

Townsend (2013) emphasises the need to put citizens first in the approach to the smart city, to create a 'new civics' for the smart city. This would include enabling the public ownership of big data and an acknowledgement that participation in civic life would need to proactively ameliorate the conditions of uneven access and participation that currently exist. He notes that it is very likely there will be unintended consequences of the most at-risk communities being the least likely to access smart city resources. He suggests the development of new roles for data intermediaries who might provide skills and training for those excluded from access. Yet the engagement of citizens or users with the smart city requires investment by them to do so. In the evolution of the Web 2.0, Picon (2015) notes that the distinction between operators and users is blurred, and that being 'smart' requires users to co-manage the services such as energy and waste water treatment that are offered to them. Glasmeier & Nebiolo (2016) conclude that the focus should not be on strengthening the outcomes of a smart city for better urban living, but on collecting data on what better urban living is thought to be via its citizens, requiring more democratic forms of government that seek to achieve these as measurable outcomes.

Boyer (2015) asks, can the smart city overcome the 'digital divide', given that the United Nations has declared that the Internet is a fundamental human right, or will citizens remain mere 'unpaid data tabulators, voluntarily contributing information to an urban database that is monetized by private companies' (Ibid, p. 401). Dan Hill notes that the shift to digital processes represents a change in how government interacts with people, with the potential for planning based on averages to be replaced by citizens being provided with responsive services on-demand, using data to predict citizen needs (Hill, 2014b). It is then a political challenge for city government to provide services that are 'responsive, location-aware, personalized, well-designed and reflexive', and a design challenge 'to better understand and shape the ideologies underpinning network urbanism, to combine a sophisticated understanding of the rich urban data with a holistic collaborative approach to design and governance' (Ibid.).

Greenfield (2013) argues that smart city data could be used to empower networked citizens with tools to innovate, share and learn, strengthening the resilience of communities, and improving their understanding of challenges, risks and opportunities (Ibid, p. 97). The technology of the smart city can be used to assert Lefebvre's 'right to the city', enhancing personal mobility, citizen engagement and self-determination (Ibid, p. 96). This is a fundamentally different idea of the networked smart city, one in which wellbeing is politically enabled through technological empowerment.

The contribution that technology can make to wellbeing in the city is at risk of being compromised by top down utilitarian and efficiency-driven models of the smart city. In its place, alternative ways of harnessing technology to enrich and enchant citizen's urban experiences should be actively planned and designed for. This will require efforts to reframe the roles of architects, designers and planners to encourage participation in design, as well as efforts by city governments and corporations to open up participative technologies to empower citizens to be active users in making their wellbeing in the city. The potential is for technology to augment and enrich how citizens experience the city.

Notes

1 Atkinson et al. (2012) explore the differences between eudaimonic and hedonic views of wellbeing and place.
2 'Cyborg' short for cybernetic organism, a being with both organic and biomechatronic body parts. The term was coined in 1950 by Manfred Clynes and Nathan S. Kline.
3 As in Atkinson et al.'s (2012) discussion of the distinction between hedonic and eudaimonic concepts of wellbeing and place.

References

Ampatzidou, C., Bouw, M., van de Klundert, F., de Lange, M., & de Waal, M. (2016). *The hackable city: A research manifesto and design toolkit.* Retrieved from http://thehackablecity.nl/2018/03/17/new-publication-the-hackable-city-a-research-manifesto-and-design-toolkit/

Anderson, J., & Rainie, L. (2018). *The future of wellbeing in a tech-saturated world.* Retrieved from http://www.pewinternet.org/2018/04/17/the-future-of-wellbeing-in-a-tech-saturated-world/

Atkinson, S., Fuller, S., & Painter, J. (Eds.) (2012). *Wellbeing and place.* London: Routledge.

Badger, E. (18 October, 2017). *Google's founders wanted to shape a city. Toronto is their chance.* Retrieved at https://www.nytimes.com/2017/10/18/upshot/taxibots-sensors-and-self-driving-shuttles-a-glimpse-at-an-internet-city-in-toronto.html

Banham, R. (1960). *Theory and design in the first machine age.* New York: Praeger.

Batty, M., (2013). *The new science of cities.* Cambridge, MA: MIT Press.

Boyer, M. C. (1996). *Cybercities: Visual perception in the age of electronic communication.* New York: Princeton Architectural Press.

Boyer, M. C. (2015). The 'smart city' in the twenty-first century. In W. Ding, A. Graafland, & A. Lu (Eds.), *Cities in transition: Power, environment, society* (pp. 382–405). Rotterdam, NL: NAI Publishers.

Castells, M. (2000). *The rise of the network society, the information age: Economy, society, and culture.* Oxford: Wiley Blackwell.

Castells, M. (2004). Spaces of flows, space of places: Materials for a theory of urbanism in the information age. In S. Graham (Ed.), *The cybercities reader* (pp. 82–93). London: Routledge.

Cavada, M., Hunt, D., & Rogers, C. (2014). Smart cities: Contradicting definitions and unclear measures. *The 4th World Sustainability Forum.* Conference proceedings paper. www.sciforum.net/conference/wsf-4

Clynes, M., & Kline, N. S. (1960). Cyborgs and space. *Astronautics,* (September), 26–76.

Crang, M., & Graham, S., (2007). Sentient cities, ambient intelligence and the politics of urban space. *Information Communication and Society, 10,* 789–817.

Cuff, D. (2003). Immanent domain: Pervasive computing and the public realm. *Journal of Architectural Education, 57* (1), 43–49.

de Waal, M. (2011). The urban culture of sentient cities: From an Internet of Things to a public sphere of things. In M. Shepard (Ed.), *The sentient city* (pp. 190–195). Cambridge, MA: MIT Press.

Duffy, F. (2008). *Work and the city*. London: Black Dog Publications.

Evenson, N. (1969). *Le Corbusier: The machine and the grand design*. New York: George Braziller.

Fok, W., & Picon, A. (2016). The ownership revolution. *Architectural Design, 86* (September/October), 6–15.

Gandy, M. (March 2005). Cyborg urbanization: Complexity and monstrosity in the contemporary city. *International Journal of Urban and Regional Research, 29*, 26–49.

Gideon, S. (1980). *Space, time and architecture*. Cambridge, MA: Harvard University Press.

Glasmeier A, & Nebiolo, M. (2016). Thinking about smart cities: The travels of a policy idea that promises a great deal but so far has delivered modest results. *Sustainability, 8* (11), 1122.

Graham, S. (Ed.) (2004). Introduction to the cybercities reader. In *Cybercities reader* (pp. 1–29). London: Routledge.

Greenfield, A. (2013). *Against the smart city*. New York, NY: Do Projects.

Halpern, O. (2017). Architecture as machine: The smart city deconstructed. In A. Goodhouse (Ed.), *When is the digital in architecture?* (pp. 122–175). Berlin: Sternberg Press.

Hill, D. (2014a). *Clockwork city, responsive city, predictive city and adjacent incumbents*. Retrieved from https://medium.com/butwhatwasthequestion/clockwork-city-responsive-city-predictive-city-and-adjacent-incumbents-684b96df3417

Hill, D. (2014b). Urban parasites, data-driven urbanism, and the case for architecture. *Architecture + Urbanism, 11*, 6–10.

Kitchin, R. (2015). Making sense of smart cities: Addressing present shortcomings. *Cambridge Journal of Regions, Economy and Society, 8 (1)*, 131–136.

Koolhaas, R. (2014). *Rem Koolhaas asks are smart cities condemned to be stupid*. Retrieved from https://www.archdaily.com/576480/rem-koolhaas-asks-are-smart-cities-condemned-to-be-stupid

Laing, A. (2013). *Work and workplaces in the digital city*. New York: Center for Urban Research, Columbia University. Retrieved from https://www.aecom.com/What+We+Do/Design+and+Planning/Practice+Areas/Strategy+Plus/_thoughtLeadership/Work+and+workplaces+in+the+Digital+City

Laing, A. (2014). The implications of a networked urban landscape for architectural programming. *Volume, 42*, 68–75.

Le Corbusier. (1973). *The Athens charter*. New York, NY: Grossman Publishers.

Le Corbusier. (1987). *The city of tomorrow and its planning*. New York: Dover Publications.

McCullough, M. (2015). *Ambient commons, attention in the age of embodied information*. Cambridge, MA: MIT Press.

Mitchell, W. J. (1995). *City of bits, space, place and the infobahn*. Cambridge, MA: MIT Press.

Mitchell, W. J. (2003). *Me ++: The cyborg self and the networked city*. Cambridge, MA: MIT Press.

Mitchell, W. J. (2005). After the revolution instruments of displacement. In G. Flachbert, & P. Weibel (Eds.), *Disappearing architecture, from real to virtual to quantum* (pp. 18–23). Basel: Birkhauser.

Mumford, E. (2000). *The CIAM discourse on modernism, 1928–1960*. Cambridge, MA: MIT Press.

Mumford, E. (2009). *Defining urban design: CIAM architects and the formation of a discipline, 1937–69*. New Haven, CT: Yale University Press.

Picon, A. (2010). *Digital culture in architecture: An introduction for the design professions*. Basel: Birkhauser.

Picon, A. (2015). *Smart cities a spatialized intelligence*. Chichester: Wiley.

Ratti, C., & Claudel, M. (2016). *The city of tomorrow: Sensors, networks, hackers, and the future of urban life*. New Haven, CT: Yale University Press.

Sassen, S. (2001). *The global city: New York, London, Tokyo*. Princeton, NJ: Princeton University Press.

Sennett, R. (2012). *No-one likes a city that's too smart*. Retrieved from https://www.theguardian.com/commentisfree/2012/dec/04/smart-city-rio-songdo-masdar

Shepard, M. (Ed.). (2011). *The sentient city: Ubiquitous computing, architecture, and the future of urban space*. Cambridge, MA: MIT Press.

Smart Nation Singapore. (2018). Retrieved from https://www.smartnation.sg/

Swyngedouw, E. (2006). Circulations and metabolisms: (Hybrid) natures and (cyborg) cities. *Science as Culture, 15* (2), 105–121.

Thrift, N. (2014). The promise of urban informatics: Some speculations. *Environment and Planning A, 46,* 1263–1266.

Townsend, A. (2013). *Smart cities, big data, civic hackers, and the quest for a new utopia*. New York: W. W. Norton & Company.

Tukiainen, T., Leminen, S., & Westerlund, M. (2015). Cities as collaborative innovation platforms. *Technology Innovation Management Review, 5* (10), 16–23.

Varnelis, K., & Freidberg, A. (2008). *Networked publics*. Cambridge, MA: MIT Press.

Vidler, A. (1990). Case per cyborg: Protesti domestiche da Salvador Dali a Diller e Scofidio [Homes for cyborgs: Domestic prostheses from Salvador Dali to Diller and Scofidio]. *Ottagono, 96,* 36–55.

Waber, B., Magnolfi, J., & Lindsay, G. (2014). Workspaces that move people. *Harvard Business Review*. Retrieved from https://hbr.org/2014/10/workspaces-that-move-people

Wiebenson, D. (1969). *Tony Garnier: The cite industrielle*. New York: George Braziller.

Wiener, N. (1948). *Cybernetics: Or the control and communication in the animal and the machine*. Cambridge, MA: MIT Press.

14

WORK, WELLBEING AND THE CITY

Ian Hesketh and Cary Cooper

Introduction

The nature of our working life is changing dramatically and we can only speculate about what it will be like for generations to come. The recent COVID 19 outbreak has highlighted how future generations may rapidly need to adapt to emergent conditions. Over time, physically challenging work is being gradually, but surely, replaced by mentally challenging work, the so-called knowledge economy. Mental health is defined by the World Health Organization (WHO) as a state of wellbeing in which every individual realises his or her own potential, can cope with the normal stresses of life, can work productively and fruitfully, and is able to make a contribution to his or her community (2014). Furthermore, mental health is determined by a range of socioeconomic, biological and environmental factors, some of which we explore in this chapter.

This chapter considers the changing nature of the workplace, of jobs and of these workforce demographics. In particular, this chapter probes and reports how these will impact upon working in a city, and indeed how this will impact upon our quality of life, our work-life balance and indeed our health and wellbeing. Given that 'millennials' are demanding more flexible working in terms of getting better balance in their lives in an increasing service and knowledge-based economy, there are likely to be more people working partly from home and partly from a central office. Indeed, the recent COVID outbreak has quickened the adaptation of this model of working. In addition, we are likely to have more portfolio workers who will need the support of local working communities. So, how do we re-create cottage-based support communities for freelancers, flexible workers and so on?

As Churchill (1953, as cited in O'Toole, 2007) noted, 'We shape our buildings, and thereafter they shape us'. Churchill was speaking about the rebuilding of the House of Commons in the UK following the bombings during the Second World War. He contested that the size, atmosphere and design should consider the work and atmosphere the chamber created. In essence, he was arguing it should not be made bigger and more modern. The argument stemmed partly out of his desire to set up a confrontational setting (for the British two-party system as it may or may not be when this goes to press!) and to show the Nazis that, post-war, nothing had changed. In effect, this design was to retain the tradition, as is seen sometimes in established long-standing institutions and estates. Ironically, the House of Commons does not have enough seats if all the members of parliament attend, similar to the approach to hot-desking. However, what we argue in this chapter is that cities need breathing spaces where people can commune with nature, taking breaks away from flat screens in their homes and offices. As far as offices are concerned, much more biophilic design, bringing nature into the city offices, will be important for wellbeing, as recent research has indicated. What is analogous is that surrounding the parliament building in London's busy city are a host of walkways, greenspaces, and, of course, the River Thames flows directly by. To this effect, this chapter ponders what we need to consider in the future design of the city to support us in employment and our daily lives.

The Working Population

Our first task is to explain the burgeoning terminology with which we describe the workforce. This will help to create a vivid picture of the future working environment, with up to five generations quite feasibly occupying the same workspace (Figure 14.1).

The importance of generational needs cannot be underestimated. As you will see below, there may be many expectations, and finding compromise may become challenging if there is not a good understanding. Aspects such as technology, environment and appropriate leadership all play critical roles within a

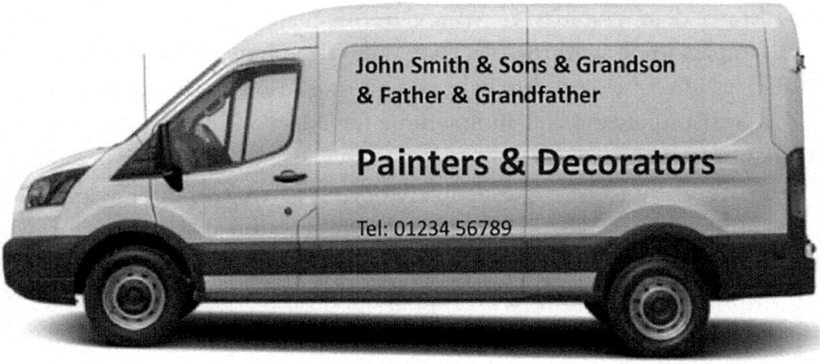
John Smith & Sons & Grandson
& Father & Grandfather
Painters & Decorators
Tel: 01234 56789

FIGURE 14.1 Multi-generational workplace.
Source: Authors.

multi-generational workforce. We will also discuss biophilic design and other advancements as we proceed through this chapter, and once more, you will see how generational understanding is important.

We begin with the so-called *Lost Generation*, who will not feature in the five generations in the workplace. This term refers to those who fought in the First World War and who were born before 1900. While these may not feature in our workplace generation, this marks the beginning of terms for varying generations.

During the Second World War, those born between 1900 and 1924 (though different years are often used) are often referred to as the *GI Generation*. Once more, these may not feature in the new dynamic, but will certainly have had a major influence on our following cohort.

Between 1925 and 1942, people born were referred to as the *Lucky Few*, or *Silent Generation*, in reference to those fighting in the Korean and Vietnam wars. One particular aspect is notable: it is accepted generally that this is pre-feminism and women did not typically work, or if they did, it was as teachers, nurses or in secretarial positions. This cultural aspect may account for some attitudes or even behaviours that were present, especially the cult of masculinity that prevailed through these workers.

From the people who may feature in our five-generation, workforce picture, the first generation is referred to as *Baby Boomers*. This is in reference to the post-war baby boom and referring to those born following the Second World War up until the 1960s. Baby Boomers included hippies and yuppies, an interesting combination: one subset interested in freedom and saving everything, the other with spending, boom and bust and credit cards. Baby Boomers were the first generation to typically have TVs in the home, a car, get divorced (up until this time it was extremely rare) and who saw women taking up positions in the workplace in the same positions as men.

The next cohort is *Generation X*, born mid-1960s to the 1980s. This generation experienced the digital revolution as teens or young adults, and were the first (*en masse*) to live in broken homes, with divorced parents. The term *latchkey kids* referred to them having the keys (worn typically on a chain around their neck) to their homes, which were unoccupied when they returned home from school. This signified working parents and a departure from the earlier depictions as women solely as mothers and housewives. This generation married (and divorced) young, struggled with house prices, ran up debt and were the first to sit watching TV and videos.

Millennials, or *Generation Y*, form the next group, born 1981–1996 (aged 22–37 in 2018). What is interesting about this generation in relation to our previous cohorts is that one in three Millennials still live with their parents. In 1968, 56% of 18–31-year-olds (Baby Boomers) were married and living in their own households, today that is just 23%. Today there are 39% of Millennials who could be described as living in a highly flexible working environment and 32% believe they will be happier than their parents (ONS, 2017). Furthermore, US studies reveal that 35% of the US workforce is now made up of Millennials, overtaking

Baby Boomers in 2016. Also, some 1.2 million Millennial women gave birth for the first time in 2016, raising the total number of US women in this generation who have become mothers to more than 17 million. Gen Y women accounted for 82% of US births in 2016. At the same time, they made up 29% of the adult US population and more than a third of the US workforce (Livingstone, 2018).

The final group, the *iGeneration, Generation Z, Post-millennials* or *Boomlets* are born after 2000. These are the Internet generation, with almost all having a TV or computer in their bedroom, by way of example. According to the Centre for Ageing Better (2017), a girl born today has a 50% chance of living to be 100 years old.

To summarise this overview of the generations in the workforce, there are some breath-taking projections. When we look at the UK population as an example, it estimated that, by 2024, there will be 18 million people aged 60 and over, that is 3.1 million more than in 2014. The number of people aged 85 and over will increase from 1.5 to 2 million, and the retirement age continues on an upward trajectory (Centre for Ageing Better, 2017). Link this with a more knowledge-based economy and less physicality in the workplace and you can clearly see the shifting trends of the working populous. This working population also may have a substantial amount of choice. The Government Office for Science (UK) predicts that 12.5 million people will retire from work between 2012 and 2022, with only seven million available to fill those posts, based on birth rate data, with an additional two million jobs being created (2016).

Workplace Phenomena

In terms of workforce behaviours, we are also seeing the emergence of alternative approaches to managing health. With the advent of zero-hour contracts, flexible, remote, part-time and shared hours, the workforce are responding to ever increasingly complex methods of monitoring performance. This is especially pertinent when the workforce experiences excessive workloads, or when they feel unwell. Mere absence management data does not tell the full story in relation to the workability of employees. We are seeing increasing use of practices such as Presenteeism (Johns, 2010) and Leaveism (Hesketh & Cooper, 2014) to mask over work and sickness.

Presenteeism has a number of interpretations, including so-called *facetime*. Here employees are first in, last out, in order to portray their dedication and commitment. However, studies have concluded that the mere presence of an employee in the workplace may not provide any indication of productivity or performance. In fact, the opposite is very often the case. Further interpretations have viewed Presenteeism as coming to work when one is in fact unwell. There are mixed views on whether this is a good or a bad thing. We conclude the practice is not appropriate or conducive to general health, but we do acknowledge the situation workers may be in when faced with tight contractual arrangements, as we have mentioned earlier, and it may be seen as the lesser of two evils.

In our development of Leaveism, we noted that a further dimension existed in terms of workplace responses to overwork and being unwell. These were when workers found themselves unwell and did not want to report sick. This was very often out of fear of being treated unfairly or being overlooked for development or other advancement. Here, workers preferred to take days off their allocation of annual leave or flexi-time, rather than report sick. A further dimension was noted as employees taking work home with them, or even on holiday. This is work being unable to be completed during normal working hours due to the amount of work they had been given. This workload overload went unchallenged by employees due to the issues we have previously mentioned. Although initially our studies focussed around public sector workers, recent studies have clearly shown the practice extends to public and private sectors alike. A combined study from Chartered Institute of Personnel and Development (CIPD) and Simply Health in the UK asked over 1,000 HR professionals to outline the extent of which Leaveism was practised in a wide variety of occupations. It was reported that 69% practised Leaveism. Not surprisingly, those who noticed Presenteeism, also noticed Leaveism (72%) and considered that technology affected people's ability to switch off out of work hours, taking phone calls and answering emails (CIPD, 2018).

The Organisation for Economic Co-operation and Development (OECD) Employment Outlook (2017) reports that the average UK worker spends 32 hours a week at work. The average German reportedly works just 26 hours, with Mexicans working, on average, a little over 43 hours a week. With a seismic shift to a knowledge-based economy, this time, spent largely in office space, will need carefully thinking through. As we proceed through this chapter, you will hear about the many dimensions one has to consider in the design of work, design of the workplace and the multi-generational needs of the workforce. In terms of office work and city offices, these may need to change significantly in the future in order to attract people into them. The needs of Gen Y and Gen Z being very different from the post-war generations.

The Workplace

The future workplace will most certainly look and feel very different from that of today. The COVID pandemic has undoubtedly accelerated the practice of mass home working, which may lead to lesser physical activity. The growing reliance on technology has now seen us turn to apps to help with monitoring and planning our personal health. For example, most have some sort of step counter attached to them or recording movement via a mobile and wearable device.

Benjamin Franklin once famously stated that, 'An ounce of prevention is worth a pound of cure'. We are also witnessing a burgeoning amount of office ergonomics that offer a plethora of alternates to simply sitting at a desk. Standing desks, although not particularly new, have evolved to include all sorts of exercise regimes that can feel like a full workout, whilst, well, at work.

We have already mentioned that it will be quite feasible and commonplace within the next few years to see up to five generations occupying the same workspace, with improved elderly health, and less physical strain on our bodies. In this 5G workplace, the questions will be how we accommodate the diverse needs; what exactly will those needs be; and how will multiple generations co-exist?

It is obvious to anyone who has worked in a shared space that there are differing views, for example, on the correct working temperature! Will wearable tech provide a way of aggregating, based on individual and collective readings garnered from wearable devices? Similarly, lighting, sounds, humidity and other ergonomic design functions may have to be carefully considered. What will be the new 'reasonable adjustment?' Will the future workplace check food and drink intake for workers, heart rates, blood pressure, blood sugar levels, signs of tiredness, hours of sleep per worker and so on? These are all currently available, but not, as yet, routinely (if at all) monitored by the employer in the interests of productivity or performance. The immediate challenge for employers is to convince the workforce that all these technologies is focussed on their wellbeing, and not to monitor individual performance with a view to having the workforce effectively competing with each other. This competitive working environment is known to be associated with increased stress over time and is not conducive to a sustainable working environment where the workforce can draw meaning and purpose from their work. As with many other metric-driven activities, eventually gaming occurs, which can lead to a toxic working environment, so we urge caution here.

Biophilic Office Design

Most associate biophilia with connections to nature, plants, woods, forests or even a jungle ('bio' means life; 'philic' is to have a fondness, to like, to love or a tendency towards). Of course, we are an integral part of this connected world, too. The concept here is that bringing this nature into the workplace has the effect of bringing meaning and purpose into our working life. So, bringing the outside inside is essentially what we are going to discuss here. Again, technological advances have assisted the quest for nature in the modern office, and what we see now is a move from simply opening a window or two in order to let in some fresh air. Arguably, in our cities the air is not that fresh in any case! Understanding the needs of the modern workforce, with all its peculiarities, and how those needs translate into behaviours, goes some way to us making good judgements on what to include, and exclude, from our modern-day office space.

Furthermore, as well as enabling organisations to make links between their physical spaces and the performance of their people, biophilic office design assists in addressing the cultural differences at work across the world and offers a solution to one of the defining factors of modern life: our ability to cope with urbanisation and the loss of connection with greenspaces. The movement all over the globe of populations from rural to urban environments, and the psychology of work, has conspired to remove the 'outdoors' from our offices. This is in relation to the vista (looking out on other office buildings) and the interior (we will discuss proxemics shortly) design and subsequent layout.

In respect to some of the other theoretical concepts we explore in this chapter, the study of biophilia is a relatively recent phenomenon. The concept is ascribed commonly to Wilson's (1984) comparisons of people's preferences for the feel of nature and the outdoors in terms of their psychological wellbeing, rather than the being in a built-up setting. In the work on human spaces, Browning and Cooper (2015) predicted that 60% of the world's population would live in urban environments by 2030. With this in mind, it is important for organisations to design-in nature to their workspaces, so employees can feel good about their working environment. Of course, the benefit to employers is that they become attractive places to work for employees, and as such experience improvements in all that brings. The advantages are many, including improvements in absence, Presenteeism, Leaveism, productivity, creativity, happiness, enthusiasm, loyalty, trust and engagement. As noted by Bernheimer, 'gazing at a tree can swiftly reduce blood pressure and the circulation of stress hormones' (p. 7, 2017).

One of the more well-known theories of workforce wellbeing can be garnered from Maslow's *hierarchy of needs* (1943). But Maslow, the architect of the hierarchy of needs, also studied office design and workplace aesthetics in the 1950s. His studies, together with subsequent others, concluded that the quality of office design had a positive impact on staff energy levels and morale. Of course, a person's personality impacts on the type of career they may choose, so there may be an attraction to certain settings almost pre-programmed. It is not our intention to draw on aged literature, but Maslow, Yerkes and Dodson and Le Corbusier (1923) all have sound advice for the modern world. Le Corbusier noted that the 'house is a machine for living in', so it would follow that the office may be the machine for working in; and, of course, these may well now be the same place! Yerkes and Dodson (1908) proposed performance directly relates to a person's stimuli, on which, of course, the working environment can have a huge impact. Now, as we have previously mentioned, personality type impacts the workplace, and therefore, environments that are loud and energetic may suit extroverted characters, but not those with introverted traits. Clearly, the needs of the organisation are paramount, but extensive research is suggesting that unless comfortable and conducive working conditions exist, performance and productivity are severely negatively affected. Therefore, it would seem extremely good business sense to design the workplace with these matters at the forefront. In terms of biophilic design, there are several considerations; in the next section, we will look at these design considerations.

Future Design Considerations

Proxemics (Hall, 1966) describes the cultural distinctions between spaces, in this case, personal workspaces, with distinctions between intimate, personal, social and public. This theory can be applied to most working environments.

Hall split workspace into intimacy levels, amount of time in the space and the nature of work being carried out. If we consider entering another working environment other than our own, we immediately become aware of how things operate: the professionalism, the views through windows, the amount of light and the modern or traditional feel. We receive cultural cues and get some idea of what it may be like to work in the place. Hall postulated that this impacted upon work productivity and performance as it influenced how comfortable workers felt in the workplace. For example, we could posit that demands to sit or work too close to others may be seen as intimidation or bullying in the modern workplace if for no other reason than this it becomes worthy of further consideration.

Natural light is often what is lacking when working in urban office environments. However, given the option, most would see this as essential. The famous Hawthorn studies, conducted by researcher Elton Mayo (Bruce & Nyland, 2011), while contested, studied working in various lighting scenarios. Although a well-known study of lighting conditions, it may be unhelpful in the fact that it concluded the largest effect was that of being observed itself. However, the need for outside views, healthy lighting conditions and fresh air are largely accepted as common-sense approaches to good living (and working) standards.

The need for private space, where one can work quietly when needed, is also desirable, but is often missing from modern office space. There is much debate over hot-desking, or non-territorial workspace. Many see it as economically viable and good for social contact, whilst others see it as a bar to productivity, largely due to noise and the lack of privacy (Hedge, 2017).

We have talked already around biophilia and bringing nature into the workplace. This can be done by simply having plenty of plants, pot plants if need be! The addition of bright, happy colours can also help raise the mood.

To emphasise these points, Osmond (1957) identified two systems for allocating workspace, which he termed sociofugal and sociopetal. These concepts may assist in our view of personality types. Sociopetal, according to Osmond's research, which was conducted in a hospital environment, relates to bringing workspaces together. He described this as radial and suggested it promoted social interaction. Polar to this, sociofugal proposes a grid-like system that is designed to give workers their own space, effectively keeping workers apart. This design may be more conducive to people with more introverted characteristics.

Apple and Amazon's future workplace projects in Seattle and California provide a great example of futuristic design in incorporating many of the aspects we have discussed. Amazon's mini-rainforest spheres are based in Seattle and took seven years to design and construct. The spheres hold 40,000 plants from 30 different countries around the world. They were designed as places employees can go to take a break or meet up with others when away from their desks. The spheres also feature living walls, which are vertical gardens with over 25,000 plants woven into 4,000 square feet of mesh. The building structure is made of three, connected spheres constructed from glass and steel, and can accommodate up to 800 people. The biggest sphere is 90 feet high and 130 feet wide, with micro-climates of varying temperature and humidity (Ong, 29 January 2018). As we alluded to earlier, this may help settle debates about comfortable working temperatures. There is also a ventilation system that mimics a windy breeze.

At Apple Park, instead of many buildings spread across a campus, the site features one master, circular structure of 2.8 million square feet called The Ring. The Ring is designed to house 12,000 employees. To get a sense of its scale, The Ring's internal courtyard is wider than St. Peter's Square in Rome and its external wall would surround the Pentagon. The four-story, glass building integrates a long and diverse list of technical achievements.

Summary

In the future, we are going to see workplaces where it will be feasible to commonly have five generations working in the same space. This creates challenges on several fronts in the competitive world of business. Of course, all theory laments the strengths of a diverse workforce; nevertheless, the design and smooth operation of working life can be something wholly different.

Modern commentary, supported by some key foundational readings, champions the notion of bringing nature into the workplace. Natural settings are linked positively to creativity, wellbeing and motivation. This seems to be consistent across generations. So, too, has vibrant colour schemes, greenery, controlled air circulation and natural light, all of which have been linked to increased productivity. Conversely, dull colours, such as grey, have been found to impact negatively on stress levels. This is considered to be down to them relating to the experience of neurophysiological breakdown (Carruthers et al., 2010).

These design aspects pose significant challenges to architects tasked with cramming office space into our already busy city landscapes. The wellbeing of the workforce of the future offers an opportunity to use science and research to inform best practice, improving the working life of people of all ages. The emergence of environmental psychology has assisted our understanding of how both human-made and natural landscapes can combine to create greater wellbeing, identity and improved workplace behaviours.

If the workplace is not conducive to wellbeing, we have described some of the phenomena to look out for. Absence is the obvious class leader, but we have also described some of our earlier research into both Presenteeism and Leaveism, which ought not to be ignored. Wellbeing, work and the city are fascinating facets of modern working life, and with ever-increasing understanding of neuropsychology and the impacts workplaces have on our wellbeing, there seems to be no end of design cues to help us make the workplace better for our ever-diverse working population.

References

Bernheimer, L. (2017). *The shaping of us: How everyday spaces structure our lives, behaviour and wellbeing*. London: Robinson.

Browning, B., & Cooper, C. (2015). *Human spaces: The global impact of biophilic design in the workplace*. Retrieved from: https://greenplantsforgreenbuildings.org/wp content/uploads/2015/08/Human-Spaces-Report-Biophilic-Global_Impact_Biophilic_Design.pdf

Bruce, K., & Nyland, C. (2011). Elton Mayo and the deification of human relations. *Organization Studies*, 32 (3), 383–405.

Carruthers, H. R., Morris, J., Tarrier, N., & Whorwell, P. J. (2010). The Manchester color wheel: Development of a novel way of identifying color choice and its validation in healthy, anxious and depressed individuals. *BMC Medical Research Methodology*, 10, 12.

Centre for Ageing Better. (2017). *People are living longer*. Retrieved from: https://www.ageing-better.org.uk/living-longer

CIPD. (2018). *Health and well-being at work*. Retrieved from: https://www.cipd.co.uk/knowledge/culture/well-being/health-well-being-work

Government Office for Science. (2016). *Future of an ageing population*. Retrieved from: https://www.gov.uk/government/publications/future-of-an-ageing-population

Hall, E. (1966). *The hidden dimension*. Garden City, NY: Doubleday.

Hedge, A. (2016). *Ergonomic workplace design for health, wellness, and productivity*. London: CRC Press.

Hesketh, I. & Cooper, C. L. (2014). Leaveism at work. *Occupational Medicine*, 64 (3), 146–147.

Johns, G. (2010). Presenteeism in the workplace: A review and research agenda. *Journal of Organizational Behaviour*, 31 (4), 519–542.

Le Corbusier. (1923). *Vers une architecture* [Towards a new architecture]. Oxford: Editions Cres. Architectural Press.

Livingstone, G. (2018). *More than a million Millennials are becoming moms each year*. Retrieved from: http://www.pewresearch.org/fact-tank/2018/05/04/more-than-a-million-millennials-are-becoming-moms-each-year/

Maslow, A. H. (1943). A theory of human motivation. *Psychological Review*, 50 (4), 370–396.

OECD. (2017). *OECD Employment outlook 2018*. Retrieved from: http://www.oecd.org/els/oecd-employment-outlook-19991266.htm

Ong, T. (2018, January 29). Amazon's mini rainforest work space spheres are opening in Seattle. Retrieved from: https://www.theverge.com/2018/1/29/16944706/amazon-mini-rainforest-workspace-spheres-seattle

ONS. (2017). *Young adults living with their parents*. Retrieved from: https://www.ons.gov.uk/peoplepopulationandcommunity/birthsdeathsandmarriages/families/datasets/youngadultslivingwiththeirparents

Osmond, H. (1957). Function as the basis of psychiatric ward design. *Mental Hospitals*, 8, 23–29.

O'Toole, R. (2007). *The best-laid plans: How government planning harms your quality of life, your pocketbook, and your future*. Washington, DC: Cato Institute.

WHO. (2014). *Mental health: A state of wellbeing*. Retrieved from: http://www.who.int/features/factfiles/mental_health/en/

Wilson, E. O. (1984). *Biophilia: The human bond with other species*. Cambridge, MA: Harvard University Press.

Yerkes, R. M., & Dodson, J. D. (1908). The relation of strength of stimulus to rapidity of habit-formation. *Journal of Comparative Neurology and Psychology*, 18, 459–482.

15

DESIGNING FUTURE CITIES FOR WELLBEING

A Summary of Implications for Design

Rachel Cooper and Nick Dunn

How Do We Design for Millions of Individuals?

In the introduction to this book, it was illustrated why wellbeing is important and why we need to design cities for wellbeing, that is, to ensure future generations are able to 'do well, feel good, do good and feel well'. The evidence suggests that, in general, we are simply designing our cities to cope with demand, rather than actively and consciously improving wellbeing and quality of life for citizens. A few, leading cities are trying to take a long-term approach yet with wellbeing measured across a wide range of variables and often a factor of underlying systems of governance, tax and so forth, it is not straightforward to identify those which are exemplars and can be easily compared to other cities. This is a challenging process, however, as it requires us not only to understand the multiple perspectives from which to address wellbeing, but also to project our thinking into the far future. The next generation of young people are calling us to task. We know that action must be taken on the way in which we live to save both humanity and the planet. So, when we think of ourselves, we must also think about our neighbours, locally and globally. And we need to consider the wider world in which we live, particularly the legacy of our cities, for that will support and enable the lives of subsequent generations to flourish.

Designing places that are prosperous, sustainable, resilient, liveable and healthy over the long term is a massive challenge, not least since cities are collectives of individuals with different aspirations and values, which may be competing with one another. This raises the first, key challenge, as it is important to understand what we mean by a future city. The diversity of urban environments around the world suggests the current manner in which terminology is applied does not account for such differences, and being able to better understand the granularity of future cities is crucial. This will provide us with the necessary insights to design and develop those aspects that are transferable across contexts whilst being cognisant of those that have specific requirements. Such a process will be successful if it is able to integrate the high-level principles of a city, designed for its people, with local knowledge to articulate the essential perspectives that inform place and its future. Understanding the way in which design can direct, or at least inform, our behaviours is key to unlocking the potential for wellbeing in future cities.

The second, important challenge concerns our ability to explore futures, especially radical ones that may appear very different from existing path dependencies. Most people are not comfortable with imagining alternative futures, yet many do when they are planning new infrastructure that can have significant impacts on the environment and the people that use it or are excluded from it. In such developments as transport or built form, imagination typically does not go much beyond the artefact itself, rarely considering the socio-cultural dimensions and behavioural changes it may bring about, intentionally or otherwise. Before we can fully explore radical alternatives for future cities, we need a better understanding of the multi-dimensional factors that underpin their design so we can identify key principles and practices.

The preceding chapters illustrate many of the intervening variables in the design of a city that have an impact on our wellbeing. In order to develop more holistic and appropriate solutions, the design of places must address the future through multiple lenses. To a certain extent, professional designers are trained to do this. However, when creating places, we are all designers. Many people who have an influence on how a city looks and functions are often brought together by accident, rather than on purpose. They include elected leaders, government officials, local people in business, public, cultural and leisure services and local residents of all ages and social status. It is this collective that must work in partnership to design our cities for future wellbeing. In this final chapter, we draw on a wide range of knowledge set out in the book so far to illustrate the breadth of perspectives on wellbeing in the city and consider the implications for how we should design future cities for wellbeing. We also draw on a research programme through which we attempted to draw this knowledge together, the UK Engineering and Physical Sciences Research Council-funded *Liveable Cities* project, which connected designers with social scientists and physical scientists between 2012 and 2017 to address the multiple aspects of four cities in the UK (Birmingham, Lancaster, London and Southampton) through social, environmental, economic and technological lenses.

First, looking at the various city perspectives, we can identify the criticality of three domains: the physical and technological structures in a city; the services and affordances provided by the place; and the human lens in relation to living in a place throughout the life course.

The Physical and Technological Structures

If we start with the built form, there has been a plethora of knowledge across the centuries on what makes buildings, and specifically buildings in cities, work. Yet the creation of them has been undertaken for the most part in silos. The client, the developer, the architect and the engineer all have particular ways of working and interacting with each other. We have looked at building from a functional point of view, too, whether as an office, a home, a hospital, a school, a theatre or a factory. However, the ways in which we live today, and the digital technology layered onto our lives, means that some of these functions and services need to be rethought – where is it best to deliver care, where should we locate older and younger people, how much do we work at home and where can we make things? It is clear that young children and older people thrive when they are together in some societies, which may suggest principles and practices for intergenerational design in future cities. This would also be beneficial in the long term for many cities, as technological advancements, with their increase in accessibility and adoptability mean that much more healthcare can be delivered in the home or elsewhere in a city rather than via dedicated health centres. Therefore, we need to rethink the purpose of buildings going forward and the need for flexibility of form. We also need to consider how the built environment's form and function affect our health directly. For example, what is light and noise pollution doing to our circadian rhythms, resulting in poor sleep, anxiety, the potential for obesity and for non-communicable diseases? We definitely need to counteract the siloed view that leaves out wider social and psychological aspects of urban life that impact on wellbeing from the design process.

In Chapter 4, Tyler discusses how transport in cities can both connect and separate us. For transport to work well, it needs to be designed and planned *for* people. Thus, we should understand people as individuals, not just numbers and flows. For instance, the transportation of food specifically relates to nutrition, as it supports both doing well and feeling well. However, it also highlights questions of who has access to that food and nutrition. Holistic and effective transport planning must take this into consideration and be cognisant of the larger perspective of city life; integration is key, not only spatially and temporally, but also functionally. Transport enables economic and social connections; as such, it should be viewed as a purveyor of public space, enabling us with the chance to chat and contribute to the human-made environment. Indeed, the changing nature of work places different demands on where and when we want to be according to the need or the desire to be in a different kind of place. Designing transport around walking and providing spaces for encounters (e.g. work hubs, coffee shops, small public spaces and parks, good footways, places to sit and chat) provides a strong core upon which other means of transport can build.

Taking the built environment and transport together, and looking overall at the urban form, we know that the design – purposeful or otherwise – can have an impact on wellbeing. For instance, as Boyko and colleagues explain in Chapter 11, we still need to understand the relationship between social economic circumstances and built form. It is clear that we need more empirical knowledge about the extent to which both density and deprivation impact wellbeing of citizens and the walkability of neighbourhoods. Concentrated efforts are needed to understand the social, environmental and economic value of increasing walkability generally, but especially at different built densities in more deprived neighbourhoods. However, whatever the design that results, the use, management and maintenance of places are critical to their successful adoption, with evidence suggesting that co-designing and co-managing public spaces may be one way to achieve their active use and maintenance.

Considerations of physical infrastructure also often neglect the ecosystems upon which humans depend, the natural and biological systems. We know that 'green and blue' are critical life support systems to humans and the planet. However, there still remains an urgent need to gather better evidence so we can understand all the benefits of these ecosystems and their interrelationships. Furthermore, biodiverse, vegetation-rich, greenspaces are important in the context of public health in urban environments. In Chapter 5, James, Tzoulas and Dennis examine the links between residential proximity and equitable access to natural environments with cardiometabolic disorders and emotional wellbeing. However, we need a wider and deeper evidence base. Moreover, relationships between greenspace and physical activity are empirically inconsistent and may hold only under certain conditions and for certain populations; however, they do consistently predict lower rates of obesity. Therefore, establishing clear associations between ecosystem functions and individual health outcomes are particularly challenging and require further nuance to notions of cascading services. At present, there is very little research in public health that takes recourse to this. In addition, numerous, multi-scalar benefits remain unknown, including large-scale, natural processes such as carbon sequestration, water regulation and pollination. These are very difficult to quantify at local, spatial and temporal scales. There are theoretical gaps that need addressing, and preventative or therapeutic outcomes need clarity so that appropriate architectural and urban design interventions can be implemented with confidence. To do this requires a change in the framing of nature within urban environments.

Finally, the functioning place needs energy, water and waste removal. This is an obvious statement, but one under critical and current concern. Reducing energy consumption and moving to zero-carbon cities are international challenges. Hopes are often pinned on technological solutions: electric cars, sustainable homes, recycling, biofuel and so forth. Yet radical transformation of current infrastructures, technologies and services need to be balanced against people's daily practices and the value placed on behavioural change. For instance, we know that an increased income is related to better health and that better health is related to a decrease in energy consumption as Bahaj and colleagues discuss in Chapter 6. However, a quick, technological change may not work for everyone. In designing for wellbeing, it is critical to examine the opportunity for soft interventions to refine understanding of issues and add design depth (e.g. personalised energy solutions). Liveable, healthy cities need to provide diverse options of mobility and housing that ensure both inclusivity and energy efficiency.

Services and Affordances

Cities exist as an efficient and effective means of exchanging goods and services, sharing knowledge and experiences, that is, they offer a series of affordances. Apart from energy and water, food is a lifeforce within cities. It is not only essential, but also a means of building social ties, through common experience. Furthermore, as Clune and Pollastri demonstrate in Chapter 7, examining food is useful to gain historical insights into issues of production and consumption within cities, and how the design of cities has contributed to illbeing. For instance, there are uneven landscapes in cities, with islands of food abundance and food deserts (i.e. urban areas where fresh food is now very difficult to find, and where fast food is the daily norm), leading to epidemics in obesity, especially among children. Moreover, plastics have been transformative in terms of convenience, but also have fundamentally changed our disposition to the material world by making disposability a new possibility with all the environmental and behavioural issues this raises. Again, here is an opportunity for design orienting scenarios to consider and present a quality to everyday life that enhances liveability and wellbeing rather than viewing humans as merely passive consumers.

Cities that flourish economically mean that there is work in those places. Nowadays, however, the location of that activity has diversified considerably, as has the activity we undertake and when we do it. In Chapter 14, Hesketh and Cooper direct us to the considerable evidence of the effect that work and workplaces have on our health, identifying newer issues to consider, such as the blurring of distinctions between intimate, personal, social and public spaces, and how that applies to both productivity and wellbeing. This is an area that requires much more evidence, as does a better understanding of the role of design in making these boundaries more visible (and less so) where we desire and in ensuring that our health and wellbeing are maximised.

As Pratt in Chapter 12 states, the built environment is the container space for culture, both organisational and physical. Social and cultural diversity are the sources of urban health, and a potential contributor to wellbeing and inclusivity. Yet 'culture' can fall between the cracks of traditional policy silos (i.e. transport, economic development, housing). Indeed, the planning and governance of culture are complex and multi-faceted; it is an ecosystem rather than mono-causal process. We need to develop a more robust understanding of the dynamics of culture, which are both interactive and relational. The wave of 'place-making' strategies that include 'culture' are often well-intended, but deal with the symptoms, not the causes, of inequality and illbeing in cities. In thinking about culture in cities, the role that design should take is to reconceptualise what culture means to the city and to deal with diverse people and viewpoints, rather than introducing top-down diktats.

Finally, the 'lived experience' of the city is key to unlocking how everyday activities, such as our mobilities and our social and work lives, can provide insights for designers. There is – and will be in the design of future cities – a need for more multi-faceted, qualitative analysis of wellbeing in relation to the 'lived experience' of cities so that we can design *with* people, not *at* people. In Chapter 3, Psarikidou explains this by saying that we should be designing 'practices of wellbeing' as activities, like walking and cycling, and 'practices of wellbeing' as destinations that generate positive effects, like meeting friends and bird-watching.

The Human Lens

Talking of lived experiences, this is where we must be concerned with individuals, their specific circumstances and their aspirations. Cities are social spaces, spaces of 'collective effervescence'; much of this occurs on the street but also in 'third spaces', distinct from home or work. Thus, active sidewalks where people socialise outside of both these contexts can nurture a sense of social connectedness and trust between city residents, raising a need for lingering. However, they can also be alienating places where one feels unsafe. The role of weak ties in supporting positive, social connections and the geographic scale of their significance varies from city to city. We require suitable analyses to be conducted to identify those design factors that stimulate interaction and create a lively urban atmosphere. Overall, understanding the nature of interpersonal interaction is key and needs more attention than at present, as it has implications beyond the technological fixes of smart city approaches that dominate much current research and do not easily account for urban ambiances that are the result of complex, social interrelationships. Furthermore, the design of cities should not disregard people's aspirations for affordable, spacious homes with good, indoor air quality and access to greenspace. Ensuring people have secure and sustainable living accommodation is crucial to both mental and physical wellbeing.

Of course, the lived experience depends on one's age, as Hammond, White and Phillipson explain in Chapter 9. Precariousness is a universal insecurity that results from our interdependence, whereas precarity is the unequal distribution of precariousness within different parts of society. The importance of the spatial dimension of precarity and precariousness often can be overlooked in both discourse and programmes seeking to address social inequality. If an age-friendly city is to address the needs of an increasingly older population, interventions need to actively engage with the conditions of precarity, not just the symptoms.

Indeed, in order to know what design can do to improve the wellbeing of cities in the future, we need to understand the reciprocal relationship between the social and physical environment. There is currently an uneven landscape of existing knowledge concerning the negative dimensions of ill-health and illbeing. We need a more holistic appreciation of these issues and increased diversity in the groups with which we research and work. For example, as Ucci identifies in Chapter 8 with regard to housing provision, we need to consider the interconnection of physical hazards, fit to needs, and the security and stability of cities as they relate to older people and children. Another area of evidence emerging from the research is the influence of non-visual effects on the health of older people and children, including light quality, which regulates sleep and alertness. Additional areas for continued research include understanding the health effects of improvements made to housing, particularly improvements in warmth for households facing fuel poverty, the strain of housing instability on teenagers and the impacts of overcrowding in homeless shelters in cities. While technological developments may have positive outcomes for some people's wellbeing, problems still can surface. For example, the ready availability of digital media and technology may result in children being even less likely to play outside; thus, ensuring access to safe, good-quality greenspace and playing areas is one of the most important areas of urban design for the future.

Designing for the life course, for the lived experience, means we must ensure that we have robust evidence upon which to make design decisions. Evidence must include the factors affecting wellbeing today, but also the potential implications for the future. We must find ways of avoiding the creation of siloed knowledge so that we can address the complex systems facing cities in an integrated manner. In Chapter 10, Codinhoto, and colleagues state this means placing more emphasis on considering the economic, environmental, social and cultural contexts of cities and future-proofing interventions as much as possible. More can be done by translating research into interventions and testing them *in situ* with stakeholders who would benefit most from them.

The Essence of a City (Meta-level)

In order to rethink cities, we need another lens through which to gaze, examine and design the future. As we have seen by examining the various, professional and research silos, the city problem coalesces first around people, followed by the place/service/product interface. Looking at these dimensions offers a direction upon which to base the design process and decision-making priorities for all aspects of the city.

People: The Role of Design

At its heart, a city needs people to interact with each other, build connections and ease separations to help create a sense of society, sense of belonging and ways of acting that generate wellbeing. Therefore, the first principle to adopt in designing future cities, and from the brief set out in previous chapters, is to recognise the human dimension of city living. This is central to designing for people. This understanding is dynamic; therefore, there is an ongoing need to keep building and connecting evidence bases, many of which currently are siloed.

We must examine how aspirations – connection to nature, sense of community and safety, and so forth – can be translated into design principles, but we also must recognise the heterogeneity of aspirations that are unique and not necessarily transferable, as Joffe, Smith and Zeeb articulate in Chapter 2.

Designing for people means understanding everyone at all stages of life; therefore, the design perspective must be one of designing for the entire life course: ante-natal through to death. Unfortunately, much of the evidence base is based on research in middle- and high-income countries, as opposed to developing countries, which means conclusions do not necessarily apply. However, what we can do is ensure that developing countries do not make the same mistakes and, therefore, experience the resulting problems of cities in the affluent world.

We also know that design can support culture, which, in turn, provides a means of re-forging and developing identity and community; something we often hear is missing from cities. Conventional, core city functions often become discordant and need to be modified to get them back closer to the intended arrangement; otherwise, transversal dimensions, such as culture and wellbeing, will fail to mesh and unrest will occur.

The way in which design designs, or at least heavily influences, our behaviours are key to unlocking the potential for wellbeing in future cities. We must understand design for behaviour change, the intentional and unintentional consequences of design and their complex interdependencies. This leads us to the issue of designing for the future. Rigorously understanding the interdependencies of people in a complex system; behaviour change; and the impact of technological, social, environmental and economic change, demand a step-change in the way we approach the design of cities.

Place

There is no shortage of guidance on how to design places, and this is the natural habitat for the professional designer. In terms of wellbeing, however, it is important to focus on people and their relationship to place. We know cities are places to enhance social and psychological wellbeing, and this is often engendered by the aesthetic quality of the place, both the buildings and the spaces. We know that the incorporation of greenspaces in urban environments enhances wellbeing, as well as that this must go beyond urban form and needs to be repositioned in policy and practice. Introducing greenspace design into service design as well as into urban design is key; in order to do so, there is a need for a stronger and more diverse evidence base to connect to wider agendas. Furthermore, the scope for interventions aimed at ending homelessness and reducing housing instability is far wider than residential, urban design and planning approaches enabled at present. Using design to redesign housing policy in relation to built form will be an essential part of shaping and supporting wellbeing in future cities.

Services and Products

Designing services and policy are interdependent with the design of the urban environment and infrastructure. However, in the sphere of design, there is a need to raise awareness of urban issues and their impacts on health and wellbeing. For example, research and practice needs to highlight the interdependences between home design, energy consumption, health, improvement in education attainment and independence in old age. Raising awareness of where decisions are made – central or local government, private sector, third sector, residents – can influence how we design products and services to achieve the desired increase in wellbeing. Essential to this process is a better understanding of the impacts of urban life that do not necessarily manifest themselves in the immediate context of the city, but are offshored to areas remote from it, such as the labour and materials needed to provide services and products to people in cities.

Of course, as Laing examines in Chapter 13, there also is an imperative to consider how current trends and innovations, such as AI, IoT, wearable technologies, intelligent products and Smart Cities, might deeply affect our experience of and expectations from the built environment in future. It is plausible that these technologies will allow for greater levels of customisation, adaptability and interactivity with the environment, which might generate not only positive wellbeing outcomes but also unexpected negative ones, as well as a greater risk of inequalities. Core issues of accessibility, ethics, privacy, trust and security will drive the comparative adoption of these new technologies and their application. Understanding who is able to utilise these, and who is excluded and why, will be key to designing ways to support wider inclusion of future cities as a shared and equitable resource for all.

Future Cities by Design

It is critical we understand what we mean by the future city; infrastructure can last for hundreds of years, products and services change rapidly, and behaviour change can take moments or decades, depending on the context and the issue. How do we take this into account? How do we establish the need for a vision of the future city in which millions of individual needs are catered for?

In design terms, it means radically rethinking the boundaries of the design disciplines by considering places as organisms supporting humanity and other species, conceptualising cities as containers for services and the provision of life support throughout our life course. Such rethinking may prove challenging, not least for designers who will need to draw on additional expertise from a diverse range of disciplines and professions, such as the life sciences and public health. Fundamental to this step-change is designing the system for transparency and for the integration of places, products and services. This means including all resident stakeholders in the design process. Radical alternatives will only present themselves through a shift away from path dependencies and careful balancing of urgent needs and contemporary priorities with long-term goals. In order to design future cities there are four principles to consider: where are we now, where we want to be, how will we get there and what are the options.

First, we must establish a baseline of 'what is', including an understanding of what is going on in a place and levels of wellbeing. Greater empirical evidence is needed to challenge assumptions about wellbeing; for example, examining the links between deprivation, built environment and wellbeing, which then can inform discussion and design and can bring about policy change. This will enable the refinement of correlational evidence in terms of the socio-spatial characteristics of the urban environment and how these may impact the wellbeing of residents. Designers and design decision-makers (by which we mean all members of communities, whether professional, elected or resident), therefore, should determine and undertake specific and contextually related enquiry, such as studies of aspirations, energy, mobility and food consumption in relation to wellbeing and public health factors.

Second, we must understand the values, needs and aspirations of people to ensure that any future visions articulate essential perspectives of a city designed for the wellbeing of people (e.g. courteous, active and inclusive, public and aesthetic, healthy, evolving). Our processes for integrating these must enable competing values, needs and aspirations to be expressed and that suitable ways of negotiating towards shared, fundamental principles form the basis of such an agreement. Clearly, the 'who' in such processes is critical to the level of social inclusion, which has a direct correlation to who is able to thrive in our cities.

Third and perhaps most importantly, leadership and governance are critical in bringing together and implementing future visions. The strength of professional designers is that they can look holistically at a situation, diagnose and identify alternatives and opportunities, and then visualise future concepts. However, in order to implement any plans, a process of leadership and articulation needs to be in place whereby alternative voices are addressed, difficult decisions made and trust is established to deliver the preferred outcome. This engagement with the political dynamics of a place is not an easy principle to understand and engage with, yet it is essential for designers and design decision-makers to do. Fundamentally, understanding and applying a system of design decision-making that includes design informers, design decision-shapers, design decision-makers and design decision-takers (Boyko et al., 2010).

Finally, the role of designers in the establishment of future visions is critical. Designing for and with people, and designing throughout the life course, is important; first, though, we must establish the role of design as a 'futuring' practice and designers as facilitators of this practice. Design is a process by which we conceptualise and visualise futures, both near and far, especially through design speculation, design scenarios, world building or narrative creation. The value of these methods has been established in some academic and professional communities. However, there is still a need to bring it into the mainstream, educating designers to design futures in conjunction with all other stakeholders, to enable everyone to speculate and explore scenarios. There are tools to aid us in this process: frameworks that set out quality of place and wellbeing or sustainable development, and tools for addressing complex interdependencies. We have yet to take the leadership mantel. Moving design beyond the individual place, product and service, it is imperative that we now work out the way we can deliver wellbeing in cities for everyone.

Postscript – Covid 19

This chapter was completed before the global crisis around the coronavirus pandemic. Nevertheless, the principles for designing for wellbeing remain the same, it is critical we design with people, that we focus on interdisciplinary approaches towards designing for the future. We will of course bring to design a consideration of how we help to create places that are resilient and that support new ways of living that will result from this pandemic experience, design always focusses on the new challenges and opportunities that arise, Covid 19 is another dimension that will inform design decision for living well in cities over the next century.

Reference

Boyko, C. T., Cooper, R., Davey, C. L., & Wootton, A. B. (2010). Informing an urban design process via a practical example. *Urban Design and Planning, 163* (1), p.17–30.

INDEX

Note: **Bold** page numbers refer to tables; *italic* page numbers refer to figures and page numbers followed by "n" denote endnotes.